# THE

# B

## IG

## OOK

## *of Health Tips*

### by the editors of FC&A

FC&A Publishing
103 Clover Green
Peachtree City, GA 30269

Produced by the staff of FC&A

**Ninth printing September 2000**

ISBN 0-915099-91-8

# Contents

If you don't find what you're looking for here, turn to the Index, which begins on page 379.

**If you don't find what you're looking for here, turn to the Index, which begins on page 379.**

# Publisher's Note

This book is for information only. It does not constitute medical advice and should not be construed as such. We cannot guarantee the safety or effectiveness of any drug, treatment, or advice mentioned. Some of these tips may not be effective for everyone.

A good doctor is the best judge of what medical treatment may be needed for certain conditions and diseases. We recommend in all cases that you contact your personal doctor or health care provider before taking or discontinuing any medication, or before treating yourself in any way.

Is any one of you in trouble? He should pray. Is anyone happy? Let him sing songs of praise. Is any one of you sick? He should call the elders of the church to pray over him and anoint him with oil in the name of the Lord. And the prayer offered in faith will make the sick person well; the Lord will raise him up. If he has sinned, he will be forgiven. Therefore confess your sins to each other and pray for each other so that you may be healed. The prayer of a righteous man is powerful and effective.

James 5:13-16 (NIV)


"But I will restore you to health and heal your wounds," declares the Lord.

Jeremiah 30:17a (NIV)

# Introduction

Did you know that medical knowledge — how much doctors and scientists know about our human bodies — more than doubles every five years? It's hard for doctors to keep up, but it's even more of a challenge for consumers who just want to know the best ways to protect their health and how to get the best medical care available when they need it.

That's why we've put together *The Big Book of Health Tips*. We've organized all the latest health information into 27 chapters chock full of the most up-to-date medical facts. From the latest natural remedy for getting rid of wrinkles to what researchers think may be the cure for AIDS, you'll find it all here, plus much, much more.

After all, your health really is in your hands. Certainly you can't expect your doctor to make your health his number one responsibility. He has hundreds of other people he has to care for as well. That's why you need to keep informed about self-help remedies as well as the latest research and techniques that doctors have easy access to, but everyday folks don't.

To write *The Big Book of Health Tips*, we searched through hundreds and hundreds of the most reputable medical journals in the world to make the best and most recent health information easily accessible to you. Armed with the information you'll find in this book, you'll know when you can safely care for a health problem at home as well as when you should see a doctor. If a doctor's visit is required, you can count on the information you read here to help you discuss your medical condition with your doctor like the informed consumer you want to be.

In addition, the 1,300-plus tips for better health packed into this book give you the keys to a happier, healthier, longer, more fulfilling life right now. Best of all, most of these health tips are easy things you can do at home to keep every part of you strong and vital, from your bones to your brain.

You'll also find out how to deal effectively with the most common health problems people face today, such as high blood pressure, arthritis, hearing difficulties, stuffy sinuses, heart disease, depression, insomnia, headaches, backaches, and allergies. If you've got a problem, you can count on finding a solution in this book.

If you don't have a specific health problem you're trying to solve, just browse through the book at your leisure and choose the best tips for you. Most of the tips are short and concise articles that make reading quick, easy, and fun. You're sure to find something helpful for yourself or a loved one.

Congratulations on your purchase of *The Big Book of Health Tips*. You've just bought the cheapest health insurance you'll ever find — the information you need to help guarantee you better health today, tomorrow, and the rest of your life.

May God bless your good health!

The Editors of FC&A

# Living Longer, Living Better

## 7 secrets to help you live past age 85

Those who have lived to age 85 and beyond are considered master survivors. Although they offer different suggestions as to what helps them live a long life, here are seven of their most mentioned survival secrets.

◆ Talk with friends and/or family every day. People with strong support networks tend to have better emotional health and a better self-image and generally function better mentally and physically than people who don't. They also have increased self-confidence which helps them to deal better with stressful situations.

◆ Face change without fear. This involves accepting illnesses gracefully and philosophically.

◆ Stay involved. This means many different things to different people, from being active in church to staying informed about political issues. People who regularly participate in activities that are meaningful to them, such as helping out family, taking care of a child, volunteering, gardening, and even doing housework and routine house maintenance appear to age more successfully than people who don't regularly participate in such activities.

◆ Recover fairly quickly from difficult situations, such as job loss, disability, or death of children or spouse.

◆ Have a general positive outlook on life. Many of these people rarely felt depressed, dissatisfied with life, lonely, or worried.

◆ Take as much control of life as possible.

◆ Get regular exercise. Not only does this help keep the body healthy, it also helps to hold off mental decline.

*Sources:*
*The Atlanta Journal/Constitution* (April 14, 1996, B1)
*USA Today* (124,2607:10)

## Live longer the Mediterranean way

Ever since the Trojans were burned by the Greeks' "gift" of a gigantic wooden horse to their town of Troy, people have tended to beware of Greeks bearing gifts.

However, this time the Greeks and other people of the Mediterranean have a gift to offer that really stands up under scrutiny. They seemed to have discovered that at least one of the secrets of longer life is as simple as what you eat.

Intrigued by Mediterranean people who lived well beyond age 70 and were rarely bothered by ongoing health problems, researchers began studying the Mediterranean diet in the 1950s. They found the diet to be based on fruits, vegetables, and grains. Olive oil was used rather than hard fats. Fish and chicken were only eaten a couple of times a week. Red meat was limited to a few times a month. Except for cheese and yogurt, Mediterraneans also ate very few dairy products. They ate fruit for dessert. Meals were frequently washed down with a little wine.

Forty years of research later, scientists are still coming to the same conclusions they came to in the early 1950s. If you want to live a long and healthy life, make your meals the Mediterranean way.

*Sources:*
*British Medical Journal* (311,7018:1457)
*The American Journal of Clinical Nutrition* (61,6S)

# Turn back the clock at any age

In the glory days of youth, you could smoke, eat junk food, never exercise, spend your weekends drinking, and still feel pretty good on Monday morning. Times change. Now, in your 50s, 60s, or beyond, you may have accepted your low energy, high blood pressure, or middle-age spread as your just reward for the abuse you've given your body. And, what's worse, you may think you're too old to do anything about it.

Here's good news that could change your mind and your life. Scientists have discovered you can make changes now — whether you're 45 or 105 — to feel better and live longer.

Everyone wants to age successfully. Here are proven ways to help you do just that.

◆ Stop smoking. You can add at least four more years to your life as well as slashing your risk of heart disease by 50 percent in just one year.

◆ Avoid heavy drinking. If you aren't a heavy drinker, you'll likely live about 12 years longer than someone who is. You'll also have a much lower risk of cancer of the esophagus (the tube that connects your throat to your stomach). Plus, you'll reduce your risk of impotence, brain damage, or potentially deadly liver disease, stroke, or aneurysm (tear in an artery). If you must drink, limit your alcohol intake to one drink a day if you're a woman and two drinks a day if you're a man

◆ Lose excess weight. Just carrying around poundage you don't need shaves years off your life. The U.S. Census Bureau has even developed a formula to help you figure out how many years you're likely to lose by carrying extra pounds. They base their formula on a Loss of Life Expectancy (LLE) rating to compute the dangers of various health risks. For every percentage point you are overweight, your LLE amounts to 52 days. So, if you're just 20 percent overweight, you could rob yourself of nearly three years of life. Besides raising your risk of heart disease by 30 percent, being overweight increases your risk of dying from a stroke by 15 percent, and your risk of dying from diabetes by 130 percent.

◆ Exercise regularly. It strengthens your cardiovascular system, lowers your blood pressure, and reduces your risk of diabetes and colon cancer.

Even moderate exercise has been shown to improve blood sugar and cholesterol levels.

Not only is it essential to exercise, it's important to get the right amount. If your doctor gives you the go-ahead, aim for this recent recommendation from the Centers for Disease Control: 30 minutes of moderate to intense physical activity, like walking fast, preferably seven days a week. A recent long-term study reported that people who engage in vigorous activities — like jogging, walking fast, and playing tennis — lived the longest.

Even if you have already been diagnosed with heart disease, don't give up on exercise. Check with your doctor. Many people with heart disease can undertake a safe exercise program that can strengthen the heart's work capacity and improve the quality of life.

While there are a lot of things you can't control in your life, like heredity, you can make changes that will help you age successfully — with independence and the best health possible.

Remember, it's never too late to live a longer, healthier life.

*Sources:*
*American Family Physician* (47,5:1171 and 48,7:1286)
*American Institute for Cancer Research Newsletter* (42:10)
*Archives of Internal Medicine* (154,15:1697)
*British Medical Journal* (299,6715:1547 and 310,6987:1094)
*Circulation* (83:1194)
*Geriatrics* (48,5:61)
*International Journal of Aging & Human Development* (37,4:277)
*Journal of Family Practice* (36,3:271)
*The Journal of the American Medical Association* (273,14:1093; 273,15:1179; and 273,17:1341)
*The Lancet* (342,8881:1201)
*The New England Journal of Medicine* (328,8:574 and 329,2:110)

# Stop aging now

These days growing older means whatever you want it to mean. You can stay strong, fit, and healthy until your life ends, or you can give up and let the aging process take over until you enter The Disability Zone.

If you're determined to be energetic, eager for new adventures, and younger than your years, two professors at Tufts University have developed an anti-aging blueprint just for you.

Designed for people over 50, this program actually reverses the aging process, helping you feel better at 65 than you did at 35.

William Evans, Ph.D., and Irwin H. Rosenberg, M.D., detail this anti-aging plan in their book: *Biomarkers: The 10 Keys to Prolonging Vitality.* The *biomarkers* are the signs of aging that can be controlled, even reversed, through exercise. They include muscle mass, strength, blood pressure, metabolic rate, insulin sensitivity, and bone density.

Bible-history buffs still marvel that Methuselah lived to the ripe old age of 969 years, siring children to the very end. Evans and Rosenberg can't guarantee you that many years, but if you follow their program you will get more life out of your later years than you may have ever thought possible.

Take a look at their anti-aging blueprint, summarized below.

The first step is to stop worrying about how old you are now. The latest scientific evidence shows that older people's bodies respond much better to exercise than younger people's. Starting early is best, but you can catch up.

Next, you need to get used to the idea of strength training. Lifting weights sounds harder than it is. Strong muscles improve your stamina by helping your body use oxygen better. And, muscles store glycogen, our main energy source, so the bigger your muscles, the longer your energy lasts.

Now that you're aware of Evan's and Rosenberg's two most important concepts, you're ready to begin your own anti-aging journey. First, walk a quarter mile as quickly as you can, then check your pulse rate for 30 seconds. That's going to be how you track your improving fitness over the next few months. You'll be able to walk the quarter mile faster and faster, and your pulse rate will get lower and lower.

Except for this test, don't worry about trying to achieve some specific target heart rate, these researchers say. People's heart rates vary a lot. You just want to feel as though you are working fairly hard when you exercise.

If you're really out of shape, do a couple of weeks of plain aerobic exercise before you add any strength training. Walk or bicycle for 30 minutes a day, five days a week.

Then add strength training to your routine at least three days a week — push-ups, bicep curls, chest and shoulder exercises, tricep exercises, knee extensions, partial squats, and stool stepping. Do upper body exercises one day, then lower body the next.

Here's an example of a typical routine:

Warm up by walking around for five to 10 minutes. Stretch for five. Walk or do an aerobic exercise for a minimum of 20 minutes and a maximum of 50 minutes. Include two to three strength training exercises each day. Work up to three sets of eight repetitions. Rest for a few seconds between sets. Cool down for five minutes. This order warms your muscles up slowly and reduces your risk of pulling a muscle or tearing a ligament.

Either buy some hand and ankle weights or make your own. You can use milk cartons filled with sand or water. For leg weights, fill sturdy plastic bags with dirt or lead shot. Weigh your homemade weights on the bathroom scale.

Lift heavy weights. You want to lift 80 percent of the very most you can lift at one time. For example, if the most you can lift is 50 pounds, then do your strength training with 40 pounds. Do eight to 12 repetitions. Young people do it; you can too.

When you get a little sore, don't take aspirin or other over-the-counter painkillers. They may even slow down the good changes exercise is making in your body.

These steps are guaranteed to slow down the ticking of your biological clock. To make sure you stick with your program, sign a written contract with yourself to exercise. Your reward — living longer and living better.

**Source:**
*Biomarkers: The 10 Keys to Prolonging Vitality,* Simon & Schuster, New York, 1991

## Anti-aging exercise tips

◆ Avoid sugar for two hours before intense exercise. This includes candy bars and sugary drinks like Gatorade. Your blood sugar will shoot up, then drop way below normal about an hour after the sugar intake. You may feel dizzy, nauseated, have a headache, and get exhausted quickly.

◆ Don't rob your body of protein. Most Americans get plenty of protein, but some health-conscious athletes stay away from red meat and dairy products. If you regularly avoid meat and dairy products, be sure to eat some tofu or soy protein every day.

◆ Weigh before and after exercise. Drink enough to bring your weight back to the pre-exercise level. Remember, dark urine means you're dehydrated. If you're older, you're particularly at risk of dehydration because you're less likely to notice that you're thirsty than when you were younger. Also, older athletes are particularly at risk for dehydration because kidney function doesn't work as well as it used to.

◆ Don't starve yourself. Recent studies have shown that underweight rats live longer than normal-weight rats. The Tufts researchers say, "Rats aren't people ... Eat a normal, sensible diet."

◆ Take at least one day a week off from exercise. You need a day of complete rest to allow your body time to recover. Your exercise will feel easier after your day off. Many people who exercise every day have learned to live with a constant feeling of fatigue and continual aches and pains.

*Source:*
*Biomarkers: The 10 Keys to Prolonging Vitality,* Simon & Schuster, New York, 1991

## Fitness not affected by break in routine

No matter how well you plan, life happens. And it seems like whatever surprise or new responsibility arises, your exercise program is always the extra that gets cut to make room for those unexpected interruptions.

However, don't let little interferences (even if they last several weeks) discourage you from your exercise program. A recent study shows that very little of your previous exercise efforts will be lost.

A group of men and women over age 60 participated in a 16-week program of strength training or treadmill exercise. Then, for 10 weeks, they did not exercise at all. Researchers found that the exercisers retained any increases in muscle strength for at least five weeks. Even after 10 weeks, the decrease in lung and heart capacity was very small. Once they began exercising again, they returned very quickly to their previous fitness levels.

You may find it heartening to hear that even if you have to put aside your training shoes for a while, it's easy to get right back on track.

*Source:*
*Journal of American Geriatrics Society* (43,3:209)

## Cholesterol: should you worry after age 70?

You may have heard that once you hit age 70 you don't have to concern yourself with cholesterol levels any more. Don't count on it. The most recent study still shows that abnormal cholesterol levels increase risks of heart disease.

Researchers found that total cholesterol level is a good predictor of heart disease for older women, although not for older men. For some unknown reason, cholesterol behaves differently in men and women.

Total cholesterol levels rise in both sexes throughout middle age. About the time of menopause, though, the total cholesterol level in women continues to rise while men of the same age experience a decline.

But gentlemen, these findings are certainly not a green light for you to indulge in high-fat and cholesterol-laden foods. Once you reach age 70, your level of HDL cholesterol, the good cholesterol, is the most reliable predictor of your chances of dying of heart disease.

The higher your HDL, the lower your risk for heart disease. The lower your HDL, the greater the chance that you may experience a heart attack or stroke. After the study was over, the researchers realized that men in their 70s with low HDL were nearly five times as likely to die of heart disease as men with normal HDL.

To be on the safe side, both men and women should have their cholesterol checked and their HDL measured. If you discover your HDL level is lower than it should be, talk with your doctor about lifestyle changes which may help to bring it up, such as increasing the amount of exercise you do and eating low-fat foods. You can also raise your HDL by abstaining from alcohol and quitting smoking.

*Sources:*
*The Brown University Long-Term Quality Care Letter* (7,19:9)
*The Journal of the American Medical Association* (274,7:539,575)

## High iron levels and heart disease

You've no doubt heard that very high iron levels may increase your risk of heart disease. Well if you're over age 71, a new study shows just the opposite.

According to a study conducted at the National Institute of Aging in Bethesda, Md., of almost 4,000 people aged 71 or older, low iron levels appear to increase the risk of heart disease. In fact, men with the highest blood levels of iron (104 or more milligrams of iron per deciliter of blood) had less than half the risk of heart disease as men who had the lowest blood levels of iron. Women with the highest blood levels of iron (95 or more milligrams of iron per deciliter of blood) had one-third the heart disease risk of women with very low iron levels.

With all the conflicting information that's floating around these days, what's a wise person to do? Your best bet is to work with your doctor to be sure your iron levels stay within a healthy range. Other than that, don't worry.

*Source:*
Geriatrics (51,2:35)

## Popular painkillers jeopardize heart health

The most prescribed drugs in the U.S., nonsteroidal anti-inflammatory drugs

(NSAIDs) such as Motrin, Relafen, and Lodine, are a no-no for people age 65 or older who want to avoid having to take medication for high blood pressure.

That's the conclusion of a recent study of more than 19,000 people age 65 or over, half of whom took prescription NSAIDs and half of whom did not. Many of the people who had slightly higher blood pressures than normal, but who wouldn't normally have to take blood pressure drugs, ended up taking blood pressure lowering medications if they also took NSAIDs.

The researchers found that the higher the NSAID dose, the greater the risk of high blood pressure. If you've recently been diagnosed with high blood pressure that your doctor says should be treated with drugs, be sure you tell him exactly what drugs, both prescription and over-the-counter, you take regularly. Any type of NSAID you're currently taking could be the cause of your high blood pressure. Treatment may be as simple as switching to a drug which isn't an NSAID.

If your doctor suggests NSAIDs to relieve arthritis or another type of pain, make sure he's exhausted all other avenues of treatment. In the case of osteoarthritis (a painful condition commonly relieved by NSAIDs), weight loss, gentle exercise, and acetaminophen (such as Tylenol) should all be tried before turning to NSAIDs for relief. These alternatives are often very effective in treating osteoarthritis.

If using NSAIDs is your only option, work with your doctor to try to use the lowest dose for the shortest period of time possible. Have your blood pressure checked regularly while you're using NSAIDs.

*Sources:*
*Geriatrics* (50,1:57)
*The Journal of the American Medical Association* (272,10:781)

# 16 steps to fight the fear of falling

Falling, or fear of falling, is one of the most common problems that plagues people as they age.

While growing older has its benefits, better balance is not one of them. If you often find yourself struggling to stay upright, try these suggestions:

◆ First, see your doctor to make sure you don't have underlying medical conditions, such as heart or eye problems, which could be contributing to your wobbly woes. Proper treatment may solve your balance problems.

◆ Be sure to ask your doctor if any medicines you're taking could cause dizziness or otherwise raise your risk of falls.

◆ Get your doctor's approval and then enroll in an exercise program that fits your level of fitness. Many community centers offer a wide variety of choices. A regular exercise program will build and maintain your strength and flexibility so you can keep your balance better.

◆ Finally, fallproof your house. Here are some suggestions to help you do that:
 ▶ Make sure all rugs are skidproof. Nonskid tape or pads placed on the bottom of a slippery rug will do the trick.

- ▶ Remove clutter from all walk areas.
- ▶ Install night lights from the bedroom to the bathroom.
- ▶ Cover bathroom tiles with nonskid strips or indoor/outdoor carpet to prevent slipping on wet floors. Carpet offers the added benefit of providing cushioning in case of a fall.
- ▶ Be sure all rooms are well lit and have light switches at each entrance. Stairways or step-ups should also have plenty of light.
- ▶ Avoid glare from exposed light bulbs by using frosted bulbs or covering all lights with some type of shade.
- ▶ Use only nonskid floor wax.
- ▶ Tape down any loose extension cords or carpet edges.
- ▶ Place plenty of stable furnishings along commonly used pathways for support.
- ▶ Put a nonskid mat in the bottom of your bathtub.
- ▶ Use a long-handled reaching device to help you get difficult-to-reach objects. This is less risky than standing and stretching on a slippery stool.
- ▶ Install round handrails along stairs and grab bars in the bathtub.

*Source:*
*Geriatrics* (51,2:43)

## How to defend against a hip fracture

Besides the pain and hardship a hip fracture can cause, it often also restricts how well you get around. Only half of the people who undergo surgery for a hip fracture can walk normally afterward. The other half require a cane, walker, or another person's assistance.

Both men and women have a greater risk of hip fracture after age 65, although women's risk is almost double that of men's. In fact, one out of every six white women over age 65 breaks a hip. (Generally, very few black women break their hips.)

Although more hip fracture studies have been done on women than men, many of the safety suggestions researchers make are the same for both men and women. So, if hip fracture is one hazard you'd just as soon avoid, here's how to keep your hips happy and safe:

- ◆ If you take any long-acting benzodiazepines (such as Valium), talk with your doctor about stopping the drug completely or switching to a safer alternative. Anticonvulsant drugs used to control seizures may also cause problems.
- ◆ Walk for exercise. Women who walk regularly have a 30 percent lower risk of hip fracture than women who don't. Walking longer distances (more than just a few blocks) helps lower your risk of hip fracture even more. And, men, what's good for the goose is good for the gander, so slip on those sneakers and get started.
- ◆ Stop smoking. Current smokers have double the risk of a hip fracture than

women who've never smoked or stopped smoking. Several studies indicate smoking also increases men's risk.

◆ Cut back on caffeine. Drinking more than two cups of coffee a day increases women's risk of hip fracture. No word yet on how caffeine affects men's risk.

◆ Count on calcium. Both men and women over age 65 need 1,500 milligrams of calcium every day.

◆ Maintain a normal weight for your height. Women who've lost a lot of weight since age 25 seem to have a higher hip fracture risk. A healthy weight is also important for men.

◆ Have any vision problems, such as cataracts, glaucoma, or diabetic retinopathy (a disorder of the retina caused by diabetes), treated by your eye doctor.

◆ Get a hip guard if you have an especially high risk for hip fracture. People with osteoporosis ("brittle bones") or balance problems often benefit from this device. Sold in drugstores or medical supply catalogs, you wear this padded protector in the same way you'd wear a girdle.

If you fall, the hip guard helps cushion your hips against the impact. Studies show that people who wear hip guards reduce their risk of fracture by half.

In addition to the above tips, men should also avoid drinking large amounts of alcohol (more than two drinks per day). Research is still being done on how alcohol affects women's bone density.

*Sources:*
*American Journal of Public Health* (84,11:1843)
*Geriatrics* (51,2:43)
*Journal of Bone and Mineral Research* (6,8:865)
*The New England Journal of Medicine* (332,12:767)

## Ancient exercise improves balance

When it comes to improving balance, *tai chi* is tops.

Several recent studies have suggested that balance training seems more helpful to people with a high risk of falling than flexibility training, endurance training, or strength training.

Tai chi is an ideal form of balance training with its emphasis on slow, stable, controlled, continual movements. Because of the concentration required to perform tai chi movements correctly, it also provides a mini-mental workout.

Formally known as t'ai chi ch'uan, tai chi (pronounced tie gee) is an ancient Chinese martial art that has gradually evolved more into a form of relaxation and balance exercise than an active type of self defense. It's the most widely practiced form of exercise in the world. Over 200 million people in the Republic of China alone regularly perform tai chi.

Tai chi emphasizes continual flowing movements, designed to develop good breathing. Some people even go so far as to describe tai chi as a form of moving meditation — in movement, you find inner stillness. Whatever the philosophy behind tai chi, it definitely can beat your balance blues.

There are six styles of tai chi. Yang is the most common form taught in the

U.S. Although there are tai chi videos and books available, you'll probably get the most benefit attending classes taught by a qualified instructor. To find a tai chi teacher in your area, ask around or check the Yellow Pages for a martial arts school specializing in Chinese techniques.

Try to sit in on at least one class before you sign up. This will give you some idea of how well the instructor communicates with the students as well as what the tai chi class emphasizes. Some emphasize fitness, others relaxation or self-defense.

Although tai chi can take years to master, your balance should start to benefit from the exercises within a few weeks. An added bonus — two recent studies indicate that regularly performed tai chi works the heart as much as other moderate types of aerobic exercise.

*Sources:*
*American Fitness* (10,5:46)
*Physical Therapy* (73,4:254)
*The New England Journal of Medicine* (273,17:1341)
*Women's Sports and Fitness* (17,1:45)

# Special instructions for good bones

If you want to keep your teeth and bones healthy and strong, do the D thing — the vitamin D thing, that is. You need vitamin D to regulate the balance of calcium and phosphate salts in your body and to help your body absorb calcium, all of which keep your teeth and bones healthy.

As you get older, you need to carefully monitor the amount of vitamin D you get because you're more likely to suffer from osteoporosis, bone fractures, weakness, and pain if you're vitamin D deficient.

To protect yourself from these preventable problems, be sure you get sufficient sunlight exposure, especially during the winter months. Vitamin D deficiency is most common during the winter season. You should expose your hands, face, and arms to the sun two to three times a week for at least 15 minutes. If possible, keep clothing from covering your hands, face, or arms. Any type of material will interfere with your body's ability to turn ultraviolet B rays from the sun into vitamin D.

Don't use sunscreen during these first 15 minutes. This will also prevent your body from absorbing the ultraviolet B rays it needs to produce vitamin D. However, if you plan to be outside longer than 15 minutes, it's still important to apply sunscreen with a sun protection factor (SPF) of 15 or more.

If for some reason you can't get outside regularly, don't count on getting all the sunlight you need just standing by a window. Both glass and plastic windowpanes absorb the ultraviolet B rays your body needs to produce vitamin D.

If you can't regularly enjoy outside sunshine, especially during the winter months, you should take a multivitamin that contains 400 International Units (IU) of vitamin D. Although that's twice the Recommended Daily Allowance (RDA), studies indicate you need at least that much vitamin D if you don't get regular sunlight exposure. Don't go beyond the 400 IU per day, however. Too much vitamin D can be toxic.

Although fortified milk (has vitamin D added during processing) is often promoted as a good source of vitamin D, you can't depend on it to meet all your needs. One cup of fortified milk should contain about 100 IU of vitamin D. However, many of the milk samples tested in the U.S. are underfortified with vitamin D. Vitamin D deficiency is even more of a problem for skim milk lovers because between 14 and 21 percent of the skim milk samples tested had no detectable levels of vitamin D.

Whatever you do and however you do it, just be sure to get enough vitamin D every day. It really does do a body good.

*Sources:*
*The American Journal of Clinical Nutrition* (61,3S:638S)
*The Journal of the American Medical Association* (274,21:1683)

## Put the shine back in your golden years

Your golden years are supposed to be just that — golden. You've worked hard all your life, and your post-retirement days are supposed to be time for you to do all those things you enjoy. You're supposed to be happy.

But sometimes life doesn't go the way it's supposed to. Many people find those golden years tarnished by depression.

Everyone feels down sometimes, but about 3 percent of the elderly in America are clinically depressed, which is quite different from sadness. It's more than the low moods you experience when you lose a loved one or argue with a friend. It's a disorder that can affect the way you think and feel.

In fact, what appear to be symptoms of high blood pressure, diabetes, heart disease, arthritis, or stomach, back, or lung disorders may actually be symptoms of depression. To make sure that you aren't misdiagnosed and perhaps even prescribed medicines you don't need, make sure any symptoms you have are not actually signaling depression.

Take this test to see if depression might be a problem for you.

- ◆ Do you cry more often than you did a year ago?
- ◆ Have you lost interest in things you used to enjoy?
- ◆ Do you constantly feel sad?
- ◆ Do you feel hopeless about the future?
- ◆ Are you losing your appetite?
- ◆ Do you feel that you are not useful or needed?
- ◆ Are you restless?
- ◆ Do you have trouble sleeping through the night?
- ◆ Are you irritable?
- ◆ Are you losing weight without trying?
- ◆ Is your mind less clear than it used to be?
- ◆ Have you lost a lot of motivation?
- ◆ Is morning the worst part of your day?
- ◆ Do you spend a lot of time thinking about the past?
- ◆ Do you have more physical problems, like headaches, upset stomach, constipation, and rapid heartbeat than you did a year ago?

◆ Do you think life is not worth living?

◆ Do you think other people would be better off if you were dead?

If you answered yes to seven or more of these questions, or if you answered yes to any of the first three, you may be depressed. If you are depressed, you should take steps to help yourself because depression can get worse, leaving you withdrawn and potentially suicidal.

Even though your depression may make you think your situation is hopeless, there are many things you can do to get back into the swing of enjoying life.

What you eat can have a powerful effect on how you feel. Maybe your diet isn't well-balanced and you're missing out on some key nutrients.

Foods rich in carbohydrates, like sugar, are natural antidepressants. Sugar will lift your mood, but other carbohydrates like dried beans, pasta, vegetables, cereal, bread, and crackers are healthier alternatives because of their vitamin and fiber content.

Folic acid, which is found in beans, peas, and green leafy vegetables, is another natural anti-depressant. Seafood and Brazil nuts can also be mood-lifters because of their high levels of the mineral selenium. In addition, garlic and chili peppers have been reported to have good effects on depression.

While a little caffeine can help relieve depression in some people, more than a couple of cups of coffee a day may make the problem worse.

Sometimes prescription drugs can cause depression, especially in the elderly. Some blood pressure medications and corticosteroids have been linked to depression. If you think your depression might be related to drugs you are taking, talk to your doctor. He may be able to change your medication or the dosage.

Some other steps you might consider to fight depression include:

◆ Accept responsibility. You should recognize that many factors which affect your depression are under your control. Low self-esteem, loneliness, and a lack of intimacy with God are three factors which can cause depression or make it worse. Make yourself feel valuable by volunteering. You'll raise your self-esteem and meet new friends. If you've lost contact with God, return to church where you will find spiritual comfort and friends. Remember that you have a choice in how you handle life's problems and traumas.

◆ Pray for guidance. Many people find that a daily prayer or meditation on scripture can help them keep a positive attitude. Pray for peace, joy, self-control, and forgiveness.

◆ Monitor your thinking. When you start to think critically about yourself or think angry, resentful, painful, or gloomy thoughts, you are reinforcing your depression. When these thoughts occur, immediately start a new activity or call a friend — anything to get your thoughts moving in a different direction.

◆ Ask for professional help. Sometimes people with depression need more than just a change in diet or the ability to control their negative thoughts.

Psychiatrists, psychologists, and Christian counselors are available to help you. Talking through your problems with a professional may be one of the best ways to beat depression.

Depression is a serious problem, but you don't have to suffer. Take charge of your situation, find help, and get back those golden years you so richly deserve.

***Sources:***
*Encyclopedia of Natural Medicine,* Prima Publishing, Rocklin, Calif., 1991
*Food —Your Miracle Medicine,* HarperCollins Publishers, New York, 1993
*Geriatrics* (50,1:S4)
*"If You're Over 65 and Feeling Depressed... Treatment Brings New Hope,"* National Institute of Mental Health, 5600 Fishers Lane, Room 15C0-05, Rockville, Md. 20857, 1990
*The Complete Life Encyclopedia,* Thomas Nelson Publishers, Nashville, Tenn., 1995

# Stay mentally active to keep your mind sharp

Your billion-celled brain is the most complex known object in the universe. And just like a car or any other piece of complicated mechanical machinery, you have to use it regularly if you expect to keep it running well.

Studies carried out in the 1960s demonstrated that rats raised in cages with lots of toys and companions had better functioning brains than rats raised in boring environments. More recent experiments confirm that an interesting environment is important for brain development at any stage in life.

So, if you want to keep your brain running smoothly and working well, you need to provide it with an environment that's stimulating, interesting, and challenging. If you need suggestions, here are several fun ones to consider:

◆ Go back to school. There is a wide variety of educational opportunities available for older adults. Many colleges and universities require only a minimal fee to let you sit in on regular college classes. If you want credit, many colleges offer reduced rates to older adults.

If you're not near a local college or university, consider taking classes by mail. The American Association of Retired Persons (AARP) offers a booklet called *Learning Opportunities for Older Persons*, which describes various correspondence continuing education programs. The AARP also offers its own courses through its Institute of Lifetime Learning. You can request the booklet or get more information on the Institute of Lifetime Learning by writing to the American Association of Retired Persons, 1909 K Street, NW, Washington, D.C. 20049.

◆ Engage in some Elderhosteling. This is a worldwide travel/educational program that brings older people together for a week at a time to take an in-depth look at a variety of subjects, such as art, nature, history, literature, and medicine. Total cost includes meals, accommodations, and educational materials.

The only requirement to participate is that you be older than age 60. You can't beat Elderhosteling if you want to expand your knowledge but don't want to fool with homework, tests, or grades. For more information, write to Elderhostel, 80

Boyleston Street, Suite 400, Boston, Mass. 02116

◆ Learn a new language. Many older people find this an especially enjoyable way to keep their brains active and agile. Researchers suggest that this may be because the left side of the brain, which is responsible for language learning, appears to decline less quickly than the right side of the brain.

Many older people who've mastered a foreign language say that all it takes is a fascination with words, curiosity about different cultures, and an organized approach to learning the new material. However, if you have a hearing problem, you may find language learning more frustrating than fun.

Other good options for keeping your brain happy and healthy include volunteering, traveling, pursuing hobbies, or even taking up a second or third career.

By keeping your brain active, you can actually stimulate the growth of new neurons. This means that as you age you won't be bothered by any apparent loss of mental skills. In addition to giving your brain big challenges, give your brain regular mini-workouts, such as balancing your checkbook without a calculator or doodling creatively while you're talking on the phone.

Just remember that as in all activities, moderation is the key. Not thinking will atrophy your brain, but thinking too much can also kill brain cells. So, to rephrase a popular cliché, use it, but don't abuse it. An overworked brain cell can reabsorb some of the same chemicals it excretes as waste, which can poison the cell and may cause it to die. Your best bet is to use common sense. Don't wear yourself out or get overstressed.

Finally, you must move your body if you want to maximize your brain power. This means getting involved in a regular exercise program. Be sure to get your doctor's approval before you begin.

Regular exercise helps keep plenty of blood and oxygen pumping to your brain, which it needs to function efficiently. In addition, regular exercise will help protect you from depression, which can cause memory problems.

If you regularly work out, both mentally and physically, and you still seem to be experiencing major mental loss, see your doctor. You may have suffered some sort of injury or have a serious illness that is interfering with your memory.

For more memory/mind skill tips, see the ***Boost Your Brain Power*** chapter.

***Sources:***
Canadian Maturity (16,1:25)
Look Ten Years Younger, Live Ten Years Longer , Prentice Hall, Englewood Cliffs, N.J., 1995
Successful Aging: A Sourcebook for Older People and Their Families, Ballantine Books, New York, 1987
The Economist (338,7954:85)
The National Geographic (187,6:2)

## Mental skills that get stronger with age

If you keep yourself healthy and physically fit, your ability to reason, remember, and solve problems can be superior to what it was when you were younger. You'll also find that you become a better communicator as you age, as well as a better judge of art. Other skills that continue to develop well into your mature years are making speeches, writing, and the fine art of philosophy.

*Source:*
Look Ten Years Younger, Live Ten Years Longer, Prentice Hall, Englewood Cliffs, N.J., 1995

# A prescription for confusion

If you're feeling mentally fuzzy, check your medicine cabinet. You may be taking a drug that commonly causes confusion in older folks.

Check the chart below for a list of drugs that can cause confusion. Keep in mind that even if a drug you're taking is listed below, it may not necessarily cause you any problems. The opposite also may be true. If you suspect a drug you're taking may be causing you to feel confused and it's not listed on the chart, you should still discuss your suspicions with your doctor. All drugs affect people differently.

If a drug is causing you problems, ask your doctor about trying a smaller dose or a different drug. However, NEVER stop taking any prescription drug without your doctor's permission. That could be a deadly mistake.

### Anticholinergics
*Used to help block impulses from the nervous system which aren't under voluntary control.*

| Drug | Common brand names |
|------|--------------------|
| Atropine | None available. Included in a variety of drug combinations. |
| Benztropine | Cogentin |
| Scopolamine | Transderm Scop |

### Antiparkinsonians
*Used to control the symptoms of Parkinson's disease.*

| Drug | Common brand names |
|------|--------------------|
| Amantadine | None available. Sold only as generic. |
| Benzotropine | Cogentin |
| Bromocriptine | Parlodel |
| Diphenhydramine | Benadryl |
| Levodopa | Dopar, Larodopa |
| Pergolide | Permax |
| Selegiline | Eldepryl |
| Trihexyphenidyl | Artane |

### Anticonvulsants

| Drug | Common brand names |
|------|--------------------|

*Used to prevent or treat convulsions.*

| Drug | Common brand names |
|------|--------------------|
| Acetazolamide | Diamox |
| Clonazepam | Klonopin |
| Clorazepate | Tranxene |
| Diazepam | Valium, Valrelease |
| Phenytoin | Dilantin |

## Antiemetics
*Used to control nausea or motion sickness.*

| Drug | Common brand names |
|------|-------------------|
| Chlorpromazine | Thorazine |
| Diphenhydramine | Benadryl |
| Prochlorperazine | Compazine |
| Promethazine | Phenergan, Prometh Syrup Plain, Prometh VC Plain |
| Scopolamine | Transderm Scop |

## Antihistamines
*Used to relieve allergy symptoms.*

| Drug | Common brand names |
|------|-------------------|
| Brompheniramine with phenylpropanolamine and codeine | Dimetane-DC, Poly-Histine CS |
| Clemastine | Tavist |
| Cyproheptadine | Periactin |
| Diphenhydramine | Benadryl |
| Orphenadrine | Norflex |
| Orphenadrine with aspirin and caffeine | Norgesic, Norgesic Forte |
| Promethazine | Phenergan, Prometh Syrup Plain, Prometh VC Plain |
| Tripelennamine | PBZ, PBZ-SR |

## Antipsychotics
*Used to control the symptoms of severe mental illness.*

| Drug | Common brand names |
|------|-------------------|
| Haloperidol | Haldol |
| Thioridazine hydrochloride | Mellaril |
| Thiothixene | Navane |

## Beta blockers
*Used to treat high blood pressure, chest pain, and irregular heart rhythms.*

| Drug | Common brand names |
|------|-------------------|
| Acebutolol | Sectral |
| Atenolol | Tenormin |
| Betaxolol | Betoptic, Betoptic S, Kerlone |
| Labetalol | Normodyne, Trandate |
| Metoprolol | Lopressor, Toprol-XL |
| Nadolol | None available. Sold only as generic. |
| Penbutolol | Levatol |
| Pindolol | Visken |
| Propranolol | Inderal, Inderal LA |
| Timolol | Blocadren, Timoptic, Timoptic-XF |

## Benzodiazepines
*Used to treat anxiety, sleeping problems, seizures, and muscle tension.*

| Drug | Common brand names |
|------|-------------------|
| Alprazolam | Xanax |

**Benzodiazepines** *(continued)*
*Used to treat anxiety, sleeping problems, seizures, and muscle tension.*

| Drug | Common brand names |
|---|---|
| Chlordiazepoxide | Librium, Libritabs |
| Clonazepam | Klonopin |
| Clorazepate | Tranxene-SD, Tranxene-SD Half Strength, Tranxene T-TAB, Gen-XENE |
| Diazepam | Valium, Valrelease |
| Flurazepam | Dalmane |
| Quazepam | Doral |
| Triazolam | Halcion |

## H2 blockers
*Used to treat stomach and intestinal problems.*

| Drug | Common brand names |
|---|---|
| Cimetidine | Tagamet |
| Famotidine | Pepcid |
| Nizatidine | Axid Pulvules |
| Ranitidine | Zantac |

## Narcotics
*Used to relieve pain.*

| Drug | Common brand names |
|---|---|
| Codeine | Included in a variety of drug combinations. |
| Meperidine | Demerol |
| Methadone | Dolophine |
| Morphine | Astramorph/PF, Duramorph, MS Contin, MSIR, Roxanol, Oramorph SR, MS/L, MS/S, OMS, RMS |
| Oxycodone | Roxicodone |
| Propoxyphene | Darvon, PP-CAP |

## NSAIDs
*Used to relieve pain, fever, or swelling.*

| Drug | Common brand names |
|---|---|
| Diclofenac | Cataflam, Voltaren |
| Diflunisal | Dolobid |
| Etodolac | Lodine |
| Fenoprofen calcium | Nalfon |
| Flurbiprofen | Ansaid |
| Ibuprofen | IBU, IBU-TAB, Motrin |
| Indomethacin | Indocin, Indocin SR |
| Ketoprofen | Orudis, Oruvail |
| Ketorolac tromethamine | Acular, Toradol |
| Meclofenamate sodium | None available. Sold only as generic. |
| Nabumetone | Relafen |
| Naproxen | Naprosyn |
| Naproxen sodium | Anaprox, Anaprox DS, Aflaxen |
| Piroxicam | Feldene |
| Sulindac | Clinoril |
| Tolmetin | Tolectin |

**Steroids**
*Used to treat a variety of symptoms.*

| Drug | Common brand names |
|------|--------------------|
| Beclomethasone dipropionate | Beclovent, Beconase, Beconase AQ, Vancenase, Vanceril |
| Betamethasone dipropionate | Alphatrex, Diprolene, Diprolene AF |
| Flunisolide | AeroBid, Nasalide |
| Methylprednisolone | Depo-Medrol, Medrol, Solu-Medrol |
| Prednisone | Deltasone, Liquid Pred, Prednicen-M, Sterapred, Sterapred DS |
| Triamcinolone acetonide | Aristocort A, Azmacort, Nasacort, Tac-3 |

**Tricyclic antidepressants**
*Used to treat depression.*

| Drug | Common brand names |
|------|--------------------|
| Amitriptyline | Elavil, Endep |
| Amoxapine | Asendin |
| Desipramine | Norpramin |
| Doxepin | Sinequan, Zonalon |
| Imipramine | Tofranil |
| Nortriptyline | Pamelor |
| Protriptyline | Vivactil |

*Sources:*
*801 Prescription Drugs: Good Effects, Side Effects, and Natural Healing Alternatives,* FC&A Publishing, Peachtree City, Ga., 1996
*Geriatrics* (50,2:41)
*Physicians' Desk Reference,* Medical Economics Company, Montvale, N.J., 1996
*The Essential Guide to Prescription Drugs,* HarperPerennial, New York, 1994

# When over-the-counter drugs turn deadly

Moderation is the magic word when it comes to magnesium. That's because too much can make you very sick, causing nausea, vomiting, or even paralysis and death.

If you regularly consume large amounts of over-the-counter antacids, laxatives, or pain relievers that contain magnesium, you may be poisoning yourself. One woman who had been taking two bottles of antacids containing magnesium a day for several months learned that lesson the hard way. She ended up paralyzed, in a hospital on life support, before routine blood work uncovered her massive magnesium overload. And she was one of the lucky ones. According to a study from the Food and Drug Administration, 14 people have died and several others have been hospitalized or disabled from magnesium poisoning since 1968.

Older people are particularly prone to magnesium poisoning because they often have indigestion and constipation and frequently turn to over-the-counter remedies for relief. In addition, many people think that if a little works well, a lot works better so they take far more than recommended. Problems also arise because older people's kidneys don't work as well as they used to, and they don't remove excess magnesium from the body as well as they should.

If you have a stomach or intestinal disorder and take several drugs, especially narcotics or anticholinergics (drugs used to help block impulses from the central nervous system which aren't under voluntary control, including some antidepressants, antihistamines, antiparkinsonism drugs, and muscle relaxers), you have an especially high risk of experiencing serious side effects from a magnesium overdose.

To protect yourself, carefully read all labels on any over-the-counter medicines you take. If possible, substitute a product that contains magnesium for another product that doesn't. Never take a higher dosage than the manufacturer recommends. In addition, don't take antacids and laxatives at the same time. And be sure to let your doctor know about any over-the-counter medicines you use regularly.

**Source:**
*Medical Tribune for the Internist and Cardiologist* (36,18:17)

# How to avoid the hazards of misprescribed medications

A recent study revealed that too many nursing homes are prescribing too many medications to older people. If you have a parent or relative in a nursing home, here's how you can help protect your loved one from deadly interactions or side effects caused by overprescribing.

◆ Ask about laxative use. Laxatives are the most prescribed drugs in long-term care nursing homes. However, long-term use of laxatives will just make constipation worse. Try to make sure your relative gets a high-fiber diet, plenty of water, and regular exercise, if possible. These natural treatments are safer and more effective solutions for constipation than drugs.

◆ Find out what the nursing home typically gives residents for pain. Although nonsteroidal anti-inflammatory drugs (NSAIDs), including aspirin, are often prescribed, low doses of acetaminophen are the best choice for mild to moderate pain. NSAIDs can cause ulcers and kidney damage. Request that your relative be given acetaminophen whenever possible.

◆ Suggest that your relative be given more personal attention and support for problems caused by senility, such as babbling, aimless wandering, or agitation, instead of being prescribed sedatives. These drugs significantly increase older people's risks of falling and hip fractures. Besides being less dangerous, personal attention and support are often more effective than the drugs.

◆ Request that caregivers try behavioral therapy for sleeping problems before they turn to sleeping pills. Some effective behavior changes include regular exercise, not letting a person who's having trouble sleeping have coffee after 1 p.m., and not allowing daytime naps. Also, an older person should not necessarily be made to go to bed by 9 p.m. Often, older adults need as little as six hours of sleep per night, which means that if they go to bed at 9, they're likely to be wide awake at 3 a.m.

◆ Inquire about antidepressant drug therapy if you suspect your loved one may be struggling with depression. Older people often respond remarkably well to this type of treatment and have a much improved quality of life. Usually, the best antidepressants are those from the secondary amine family, such as desipramine or nortriptyline, because these drugs have fewer side effects.

*Source:*
*Medical Tribune for the Internist and Cardiologist* (36,16:19)

## Gift from the sea speeds healing

In most everyone's home, there lives at least one sharp corner on a table or countertop that has an uncanny ability to reach out and snag you every time you go by, leaving a scrape, a bruise, or a cut in the same spot. These furniture battle scars are hard to heal, especially for older people.

Aging skin has more trouble healing because the top layer of skin can easily pull away from lower layers. Older skin tears more easily because it isn't anchored as securely. Bruising can be a lot worse too because blood vessels lie closer to the surface of the skin. Once aging skin is injured, it takes longer to heal because cell growth is slower.

For these and other reasons, researchers have been working for decades to develop more effective bandages for aging skin. In recent years they've come up with a totally new kind of bandage that can actually speed healing and cut down on scarring, particularly in bed sores, burns, and surgical wounds. Much better than the old cotton gauze, it's made from a chemical called calcium alginate which is found in seaweed. This special gift from the sea stimulates the natural healing process and helps fight off infection like no adhesive bandage ever could.

The amazing seaweed bandage is one of a number of new hydrocolloid bandages. These high-tech bandages can be used for all kinds of surface wounds as well as deep wounds. The plastic outer layer of the bandage holds fluids in close to the wound so that your body's natural enzymes and white blood cells can speed healing. Because it's moist, it can be removed easily and doesn't stick to the wound. Instead of several times a day, hydrocolloid bandages only need to be changed about once a week on some kinds of wounds. These innovative bandages are especially useful in nursing homes where residents often get hard-to-heal bed sores and diabetic ulcers.

Gauze bandages have been used for centuries, but not without problems. As late as the 1970s, nurses were still taught to use gauze to keep wounds dry. But recent studies show that when the natural fluid that oozes from the wound is kept close to the wound, the wound heals faster. The old tried-and-true gauze bandage actually delays the natural healing process because it soaks up that natural fluid and takes it away from the wound's surface. Gauze bandages also cause other problems:

◆ They have to be changed several times a day.

◆ They require additional material, such as scissors, tape, and gloves.

◆ They don't protect the wound from bacteria in the environment.

◆ They can stick to wounds and reopen them each time the gauze is removed, causing unnecessary pain and delaying healing.

Hydrocolloid bandages are available through home medical care suppliers. The cost is usually higher than a typical gauze bandage. But when you consider the time and money saved in faster healing, less scarring, and significantly less pain, it may be worth the extra cost.

As for the tricky furniture corners, try taping a layer of foam padding on the offending obstacle. Or you might stick a bright orange hazard sticker on them — anything to get your attention and guide you away from an unwanted encounter.

*Sources:*
American Journal of Surgery (167,1:21S)
British Journal of Surgery (77,5:568)
Drug Topics (138,22:40)
Harvard Health Letter (20,10:6)
Nursing Homes (43,1:27)
Science News (145,13:206)

## Weight loss not always wise

Over 65 and still trying to shed those few unwanted pounds? Maybe you shouldn't, suggest two recent studies.

In a study of 247 men over age 65, researchers found that those men who intentionally lost 4 percent or more of their body weight doubled their risk of dying within two years compared with men who simply maintained their current weight.

Researchers speculated that the higher death rate was due to older people's bodies not being able to cope with the stresses of weight loss as well as younger people's bodies.

Another study indicates that after age 70 being slightly heavier than you should be may lengthen your life span, report researchers at the National Institutes of Health Obesity Research Center at St. Luke's-Roosevelt Hospital in New York.

Women with the lowest death rates had a body mass index (BMI) of 30.2. Men with the lowest death rates had a BMI of 28.4. For women, the healthiest BMIs (in terms of life span) ranged from 28 to 32, and from 26 to 30 for men. Body mass index is a formula comparing height and weight that doctors use to determine risk of heart disease, diabetes, and high blood pressure.

To figure your own BMI, first calculate your height in inches. For example, if you're 5 feet 8 inches tall, this number would be 68. Now square your height in inches. In this example, 68 squared would be 4,624 (68x68).

Next, divide your weight (in pounds) by your squared height. Let's say you weigh 185 pounds. You would divide 185 by 4,624, which equals .0400. Now multiply this number by 705 to find the BMI, which in this case would be 28.2.

The moral of these studies is that a fairly wide range of weights can be healthy for older people. While you shouldn't try to gain weight if your BMI is in the low range, you may not need to lose weight either. Let your doctor be the judge. Unless he suggests slimming down for health reasons, consider maintaining your current weight.

*Sources:*
*Healthy Weight Journal* (Jan./Feb., 1996)
*Journal of the American Geriatrics Society* (43,4:329)

## Dealing with dry mouth

As you get older, dry mouth is often a problem that makes eating difficult and unpleasant. It can actually cause you enough discomfort that you severely limit the types of foods you eat, avoiding all chewy, crunchy, dry, or sticky foods such as beef, carrots, bread, and peanut butter.

If you avoid enough foods long enough, you'll deplete your body of much needed nutrients. Don't deprive yourself by settling for dry mouth. Here are some suggestions to help you stimulate some saliva:

◆ Monitor your medicines. Many different drugs can cause your mouth to feel dry, including ipratropium, triamcinolone, amitriptyline, triazolam, and oxybutynin. Ask your doctor if any other medicines you're taking could cause your dry mouth. See if he can suggest an alternative drug that doesn't dry out your mouth.

◆ Drink more water. This will help keep your mouth moist.

◆ Zap dry mouth with xylitol, a sugar substitute that stimulates saliva. Check your local stores for sugar-free chewing gum containing xylitol.

◆ Try a saliva substitute. A variety of these products are available without a prescription at your local drug store. Although all saliva substitutes are sugar-free, you can buy ones that contain fluoride if you have a history of cavities.

*Sources:*
*Medical Tribune for the Internist and Cardiologist* (36,10:19)
*Pharmacy Times* (61,3:55)

## Reclaim your lost appetite

If your doctor says a loss of appetite is normal with aging, don't believe him. In fact, you should see another doctor. A number of underlying causes can lead to lack of appetite including heart or lung disease, cancer, senility, alcohol addiction, depression, and even certain medicines.

If you don't get these problems treated and your appetite loss under control, you're likely to suffer from increasingly serious problems including muscle loss, general weakness, tiredness, depression, and even a reduced ability to fight off disease or recover from surgery or sickness.

In addition to consulting a doctor, try these tips to turn on your taste buds again:

**Eat with a companion whenever possible.** If you don't have a live-in partner, participate in church and community gatherings and meet family or friends for a meal as often as possible. You may be surprised to find how much just getting out and socializing can arouse your appetite.

**Be sure you rest enough.** If you're tired in the evenings, you're less likely to want to prepare the meal that can make up as much as one-third of your daily calories. If you need to, take a nap or two during the day so you'll feel like fixing your supper at night. Some people prefer to fix and freeze meals ahead of time.

**Get your doctor's approval, then get physical.** Regular exercise, such as walking, will improve your sense of well-being and may stimulate your appetite.

**Make the most of your favorite meal.** You may want to add additional foods to this meal to make up for other meals at which you typically eat very little. If you always look forward to breakfast, consider adding another food or two that you really like but don't normally eat in the mornings. For example, if you normally only eat toast and cereal for breakfast, try adding some cheese to your toast and fruit to your cereal.

**Fill your favorite foods with extra calories if you need to maintain or gain weight.** This way, even if you can't eat all the foods you know you should, you'll at least get energy from the extra calories you pack into your favorite foods. An easy way to get extra calories is to add nonfat dry milk or breakfast powders to cereals, casseroles, and soups.

You may also want to try stimulating your appetite before a meal with a high-calorie nutritional supplement, such as a liquid meal drink or even yogurt. A recent study of 16 older men found that the older men ate a heartier lunch than they normally did if they ate some high-calorie yogurt beforehand.

**Save drinks for the last part of the meal.** If you drink too much too soon, you may not eat as much food as you should because you feel so full from drinking. If you need to take medicine with your meal, wait until you've finished eating, if possible.

**Avoid gassy foods and drinks.** Stay away from foods you know cause you to feel bloated. These foods vary from person to person, but some common culprits for many people are beans, broccoli, cabbage, carbonated drinks, and coffee.

**Control constipation.** If you're constipated, be sure to drink at least eight to 10 glasses of water a day and avoid caffeine. Ask your doctor if you're taking any drugs that could be causing constipation. He may be able to switch you to a less constipating alternative.

**Deal with diarrhea.** Eat a low-fiber diet and avoid milk until your diarrhea has run its course.

**Avoid high-fiber foods when you're having a problem with appetite loss.** They'll make you feel fuller than you really are, possibly reducing your intake of other foods.

**Make your mouth work for you.** If you don't like to eat because your mouth tends to be dry, moisten your foods with gravy, include soup with your meals, and drink plenty of liquids (but not caffeine). If poorly fitting dentures are a problem, have them adjusted or replaced.

If you have trouble chewing, consider cooking meats in a pressure cooker or for a longer period of time than normal to make them extra tender. If you still have trouble chewing, replace whole meats with ground meats or get your protein in the form of eggs or cheese.

**Knock out nausea.** Suck on hard candies, eat very dry bread, or sip some flat soda to help relieve nausea. Don't eat too much at one time, but be sure to eat on a regular schedule. Small, frequent meals are your best bet. Getting overly hungry can increase your feeling of nausea.

Don't eat your favorite foods when feeling nauseated. If you do, you run the risk of never liking those foods again.

*Sources:*
*American Journal of Clinical Nutrition* (62,5:923)
*Geriatrics* (49,3:54)

## Fever is serious symptom for people over age 65

If you're over 65 and develop a fever of 100 degrees Fahrenheit or higher, see a doctor immediately, especially if you have diabetes or a lung disorder, suggests a recent study conducted at the Johns Hopkins Bayview Medical Center in Baltimore, Md.

You're likely to have a serious illness which may require hospitalization, such as pneumonia, a urinary tract infection, or sepsis (a bacterial infection which can lead to blood poisoning, a life-threatening condition).

Researchers reached these conclusions after observing 470 people over age 65 who went to a Baltimore emergency room with a fever over 100 degrees. Nearly half the people diagnosed with a serious illness had no other symptoms besides a fever. The higher your fever, the higher your risk of being seriously ill.

A fever is one of the ways your body fights infection. However, older people's immune systems are often slow to begin the battle. When an older person does have a fever (a sure sign the body is fighting off infection), doctors know that something serious is going on.

If you feel a little fuzzy-headed or hotter than usual, take your temperature. If it's 100 degrees or higher, don't worry about whether you should feed a fever or starve it. Just see your doctor immediately.

*Source:*
*Medical Tribune for the Internist and Cardiologist* (36,14:1)

## Defend yourself from dehydration

Dehydration, or a shortage of water in your body, can be deadly at any age.

However, as you grow older, it's even more important to protect yourself from dehydration. That's because you're less likely to recognize signs of thirst, which is your body's natural defense mechanism against dehydration. As many as half of all older people who suffer from dehydration and don't get treatment end up dying from it.

To protect yourself, be sure you drink enough liquids every day to keep your urine a clear or very pale color. Drink even if you don't feel thirsty. Be especially careful to drink enough liquids to keep your urine clear if you're suffering from any disorders likely to trigger dehydration, such as vomiting, diarrhea, diabetes, or kidney problems.

Some symptoms of dehydration include extreme thirst; dry lips, tongue, and skin; faster breathing or heartbeat than normal; dizziness; and confusion. If you've lost a lot of salt in addition to being dehydrated (which may happen if you've vomited, had diarrhea, or been sweating heavily), you may also feel extremely weak, be very pale, and suffer cramps and headaches.

If you develop any of these symptoms, see a doctor immediately. Since dehydration can be such a serious problem, especially in older people, it's best to have this condition treated by a doctor.

*Sources:*
*Medical Tribune for the Internist and Cardiologist* (36,23:18)
*The American Medical Association Encyclopedia of Medicine*, Random House, New York, 1989

# Easy pill popping

Mary Poppins always said a spoonful of sugar made medicine go down in the most delightful way. Nurse Emma Maendel of Elka Park, N.Y. finds that to be sound advice, only she suggests a spoonful of applesauce instead of sugar.

Just place the pill you need to take into a spoonful of applesauce and swallow. It will go down easily, and if you have to take pills before bedtime, you won't have to worry about drinking too much water right before bed. You can actually swallow as many as four to five pills at once in a spoonful of applesauce.

*Source:*
*Emergency Medicine* (27,2:114)

# What to do about a never ending nose

Toucan Sam says, "Follow your nose. It always knows."

Actually, "it always grows" would be a more accurate description of what most people's noses really do. Most people will find, if they care to keep measurements, that noses and ears grow larger with age.

In fact, in a recent British study, doctors measured the ears of 206 people, aged 30 to 93 years, and found that ears generally grow about 3/4 of an inch over a period of 80 years or so. That's such a small amount each year you usually won't notice any difference — until the morning you look in the mirror and find yourself sporting a pair of elephant ears.

While there's not a lot you can do about ever-growing ears (except hide them under your hair), you can prevent, and even reverse, a Pinocchio nose.

As you age, gravity gradually lengthens your nose. In addition, your mouth and cheek muscles weaken and start to sag, which creates hollow areas around your nostrils and can give your nose a rather unpleasant pointy look. Some people's noses just get wider instead of pointier. However, with a little practice you can put gravity in its place and have your nose looking shorter and more pert in as little as six days.

The secret to success is *Facercise*. Created by Carole Maggio, Facercise focuses on a set of exercises designed to tone the 57 muscles of the face, which helps people's faces look firmer and younger. You'll see results quickly because facial muscles are small and respond rapidly to the exercises.

**Nose Shortening Exercise**

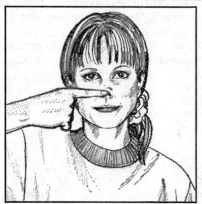 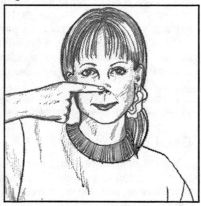

**Figure 1**                    **Figure 2**

Here's how to give yourself a natural nose job. Using your forefinger, push the tip of your nose up toward your eyebrows (Figure 1). Now, flex your nose downward by stretching your upper lip down over your top teeth (Figure 2). Hold for one second, then release. You may experience a slight tingling sensation around your nose. This is normal and is simply a result of increased blood circulation.

Repeat the exercise 35 times, twice a day for six to eight weeks. If you're already fairly happy with your nose and just want to prevent it from growing longer, then do the exercise only once a day. Once you've reached a point where you're satisfied with your nose, you can do the exercise every other day or as your nose needs it.

*Sources:*
*British Medical Journal* (311,7021:1668)
*Facercise*, Perigee, New York, 1995

## Straw sipping made simple

As you get older, you may find that you have more and more difficulty drinking through a straw. Dr. Louis C. Barricelli of Brooklyn suggests that you'll find sipping through a straw easier if you snip the straw in half.

*Source:*
*Emergency Medicine* (28,10:47)

# Your Emotional Health

## Stress-stopping solutions

In today's hurry-scurry world, it's easy to succumb to stress, low spirits, and lack of energy.

Working constantly without a break contributes to those feelings. While your conscience may con you into thinking that's how you should work, that's really not the case. You'll work better and more efficiently if you treat yourself to a stress-buster break every few hours or so during the day.

Dr. Marcia Yudkin, editor of *The Creative Glow* newsletter, recommends trying one of the following five minute stress busters the next time you feel pressure building or your spirits sagging:

- Exercise. Take a quick walk around the block, up and down the stairs, or lift hand weights for a few minutes.
- Read a magazine article or a chapter from a favorite book.
- Go outside. Look at the flowers, the sky, or just watch the cars go by.
- Call a friend for a quick chat.
- Listen to a favorite song. Sing your favorite song.
- Fix something.
- Watch fish in an aquarium.
- Work a crossword puzzle.
- Treat yourself to a favorite food you don't eat very often.
- Close your eyes and visualize a pleasant experience. It can be anything that makes you feel good, such as a fond memory, a favorite place or person, or even a fantasy.
- Pet a purring cat.
- Trade shoulder massages with a friend.

Not all these stress busters will work for everyone. "What is a stress buster for one person could actually add stress to somebody else," says Dr. Yudkin. The key to successfully controlling stress and energizing yourself is to find out what works for you.

One of the keys to identifying your best source of stress relief is to know which of your five senses — taste, touch, sight, smell, or sound — tends to relax you the most.

If you're having trouble deciding, jot down your answers to the following questions:

1) What are your favorite things to do?
2) What is your dream vacation?
3) What types of activities appeal to you?

4) What are your bad habits?

5) What are others' most common complaints about you?

Whichever of your senses is represented most in your list of answers is probably the sense most likely to relieve your stress.

On the other hand, if sensory experiences don't seem to relieve your stress, you may be the type of person who best works off excess stress through exercise. This is often the case for very fidgety people. Walking or squeezing a stress ball would probably be helpful for you.

*Source:*
Dr. Marcia Yudkin, *The Creative Glow* newsletter, P.O. Box 1310, Boston, Mass. 02117

## A stitch in time stops stress

No doubt you've heard that a stitch in time saves nine. Did you also know it can save you from stress?

You may be thinking that taking care of a small problem before it turns into a big one, or sewing up a little hole with one stitch before you must sew nine stitches to repair a big rip, would certainly save you a lot of stress. That's true, but it isn't the only way stitching can stop stress.

According to a recent study commissioned by the American Home Sewing & Craft Association (AHSCA), women who sew have lower heart rates, lower blood pressures, and lower perspiration rates (all signs of lower stress levels) than women who relax by playing cards, painting, reading the paper, or playing a hand-held video game.

Researchers at the New York University Medical Center who conducted the study found that experienced sewers' heart rates dropped an average of 11 beats per minute. Inexperienced sewers' heart rates dropped an average of seven beats a minute. Women who performed the other activities had their heart rates increase by four to eight beats a minute.

AHSCA's executive vice-president, Len Ennis, says some women even report that sewing is "better than therapy." The results of the study seem to suggest that sewing relaxes women while allowing them to enjoy their creativity.

Ogden Nash titled one of his poetry collections *A Stitch Too Late Is My Fate.* Don't let his fate be yours. Remember that a stitch in time stops stress.

*Sources:*
*Arthritis Today* (10,1:15)
*The Journal of the American Medical Association* (274,4:291)

## Lessons for a healthier heart

"Hard work never hurt anybody." Bet you've heard that old adage at least once in your life.

A few years ago, studies linking job strain and heart attack threatened to make that homily history. Eager to shift responsibility for their poor health from their shoulders, people eagerly embraced researchers' theory and began blaming their heart attacks on job strain.

Guess what? Heart attack victims are going to have to come up with a new excuse. According to a study from the Stanford University School of Medicine in California, job strain is no longer a justifiable excuse for having a heart attack.

A four-year study of 1,500 people who had *coronary angiography* (a test to determine if the coronary arteries are narrowed or blocked) to determine their heart health revealed that people with high levels of job strain had no higher risk of heart disease or heart attack than people who reported low levels of job strain.

In this study, researchers defined job strain as working in an environment with many mental demands but few opportunities to make independent decisions. Generally, laborers had the highest levels of job strain, managers and professionals the lowest. People working in technical and sales jobs, farming, fishing, forestry, precision crafts, and service jobs experienced moderate levels of job strain.

In fact, this study suggests that people with a history of heart disease may actually benefit from working, even in a stressful job. The benefits that work offers include social support from friends and colleagues and feelings of productivity. These benefits seem to balance out job strain caused by stressful work.

Still, some researchers aren't convinced. Because stress is difficult to measure and because more studies show a link between job stain and heart disease than don't, those researchers remain skeptical.

However, one thing researchers do agree on is how anger affects your health. The bottom line is simple. If you don't control your anger, it will kill you, probably sooner than later. Only one outburst of anger doubles your risk of heart attack.

Some research has shown that regularly using aspirin can reduce the risk an anger outburst can cause. However, regular use of aspirin can lead to intestinal bleeding. You should never use aspirin to self-treat yourself unless your doctor recommends it. Your best bet is to control your anger in natural ways.

A good place to start learning natural, healthy methods for controlling anger is Redford and Virginia Williams' book *Anger Kills*. They offer an overview of how hostility and anger harms your health, then take you step-by-step through 17 strategies for controlling anger. Change is not always an easy process, but in this case it's worth the effort. A less angry, hostile lifestyle is not only healthier, it's happier, too.

*Sources:*
American Heart Association Press Release (NR95–4326)
*Medical Tribune for the Internist and Cardiologist* (36,16:4)

# Simple, cheap, drug-free way to defeat depression

If you're tired of spending money on drugs to treat your depression, suffering from unwanted side effects, and seeing no real improvement in your condition, consider problem-solving therapy.

This natural treatment offers hope to millions of people who deal daily with depression. Studies show that problem-solving therapy relieves depression as effectively as antidepressants.

This therapy is based on the idea that everyday problems of living sometimes become completely overwhelming and lead to emotional difficulties. Learning to deal effectively with these problems can help relieve your symptoms of depression.

This cost-effective treatment works wonders, and it doesn't involve any drugs or long-term treatment. In as little as six sessions, a therapist trained in problem-solving therapy can help you identify your problems, brainstorm solutions, set goals, and show you how to map out a plan to reach those goals. He'll also help you evaluate your progress. Expect to see improvement in about three months.

For more information on effective problem solving see *How to solve a problem in 6 easy steps* below.

*Source:*
British Medical Journal (310,6977:441)

# How to solve a problem in 6 easy steps

Too many people go round the mulberry bush of worry and frustration when confronted with a problem. One common reason for this is that people are searching for the "perfect" solution. The truth is, perfect solutions don't exist. One solution may be better suited to your particular situation than another, but no solution will ever be completely perfect. Just knowing you don't have to make a perfect decision should take a load off your mind. So will this six-step system for solving a problem.

**Step 1)** Identify the problem. You may have more than one problem that needs solving, but you should work through each problem separately.

**Step 2)** Make a list of all possible solutions, no matter how ridiculous or outrageous they seem.

**Step 3)** Choose the solution that seems best. If two solutions are very close and you can't decide, toss a coin. You can try one and if it doesn't work, try the other one.

**Step 4)** Take action.

**Step 5)** Re-evaluate. Ask yourself: How are things going? Is the problem solved? If the problem is not solved, what additional action should I take to solve the problem?

**Step 6)** Repeat steps four and five until the problem is resolved.

Work through this process on paper. Sometimes you will come up with a really great solution but forget about it when the time comes to make your decision. This is because the brain tends to discard original ideas and opt for old tried and true favorites or what seems more likely to work.

There. Now don't you feel better already?

*Source:*
Confessions of a Healer: The Truth from an Unconventional Family Doctor, MacMurray & Beck, Aspen, Colo., 1994

## The down side of dieting

If you've ever tried dieting, no doubt you know that it certainly isn't one of life's most uplifting experiences.

While dieting is supposed to make your weight go down, it's also likely to have a depressing effect on your mental state, according to a recent study.

Researchers surveyed 2,000 adults by phone. Participants were asked to rate themselves for symptoms of depression. They were also asked how many times they had gone on a diet in the past year.

Dieting was linked to depression whether dieters were extremely overweight or only needed to lose a few pounds. Overweight people were more likely to be depressed than normal weight people.

The solution? Eat healthy and exercise regularly, then depression triggered by dieting will be one less worry you'll have to deal with.

*Source:*
*Healthy Weight Journal* (July/August 1995)

## Exercise eases depression

Don't those aerobic exercise instructors ever get depressed? Whatever channel you flip to or wherever you turn in the video store, you're surrounded by them. Sometimes those goofy grins are enough to send you into the depths of despair.

Actually, people who exercise regularly are less likely to experience depression than most people. Several studies have found that exercise is an effective way to prevent depression. It also helps treat depression once it starts.

So, as the old saying goes, if you can't beat 'em, join 'em. You'll probably feel better. Who knows? You may even end up with a goofy grin yourself.

Depression robs a person of natural enthusiasm and energy. If you're depressed, you may also experience:

- A down attitude or "the blues."
- A lack of motivation.
- Tiredness because of changes in sleep habits.
- Weight gain or loss.
- Appetite changes.
- Concentration problems.

If the depression doesn't disappear on its own after a few weeks, traditional treatment includes drugs or counseling or both. However, many doctors now prescribe exercise along with other treatments.

Several studies have compared the effects of counseling with the effects of exercise on depressed people. These studies revealed that exercise resulted in as much improvement as counseling. Exercise plus counseling led to an even greater improvement than exercise alone.

Antidepressant drugs are the most common and the most effective single treatment for depression. However, when people on antidepressants also participate in an exercise program, they make greater improvements than on drugs alone.

Exercise may also help prevent depression. People with higher levels of fitness are less likely to suffer from depression and anxiety. Regular exercise probably helps protect you from developing depressive symptoms.

There are several ways in which exercise fights depression:

◆ Distraction. Depression causes you to feel overwhelmed by your problems. Exercise provides a positive focus for your attention.

◆ Control. When you're down, you often feel out of control. Exercise gives you an opportunity to regain control of your body and master a new skill.

◆ Social interaction. Exercise can offer more social opportunities. Aerobic classes, tennis lessons, etc. put you in new situations. You get to meet new people and make new friends.

◆ Chemical changes. Exercise causes your brain to secrete more of certain chemicals, such as dopamine, serotonin, or norepinephrine. These chemicals can help reduce symptoms of depression.

Studies show that low-intensity exercise reduces depression just as effectively as more vigorous activity. So, choose an exercise program you can stick with. If the exercise is too difficult, you may become discouraged. An ideal exercise program should be easy and enjoyable. Try a variety of activities to keep it interesting.

Doctors usually recommend aerobic exercise since it also strengthens the heart and lungs. Thirty to 40 minutes of aerobic exercise, such as brisk walking or jogging, three to five times a week is best. Don't forget to warm up and cool down for five to 10 minutes every time you exercise.

If you want to beat depression through exercise, plan on starting slowly and building up gradually. Work closely with your doctor to find the best mix of drugs, counseling, and exercise.

There's one possible downside to this approach, however. Excessive exercise can actually lead to depression. Take care not to overdo it. Because vigorous exercise can alter your brain chemicals, some people can become addicted to it just like drugs. If you begin to devote so much time to exercise that other areas of your life suffer, you need to exercise some common sense and cut back.

**Source:**
*The Physician and Sportsmedicine* (23,9:44)

# Well-nourished way to happiness

Sometimes getting in a good mood seems more impossible than finding the fabled pot of gold at the end of the rainbow.

Actually, a good mood may not be as much of a mission impossible as you might think. A recent study suggests that the way to happiness could be as simple as a well-rounded diet.

In a study of 100 middle managers in British factories, with an average age of 39, researchers found that people who took a vitamin/mineral supplement plus ginseng felt better than those people who didn't take the supplement.

Those folks taking the supplement reported feeling less stressed and more pepped. People with poor eating habits who took the supplement felt even better. Not only did they have an improved mood, they felt calmer, less confused, and less angry.

The only problem is that at this point researchers aren't sure which part of the supplement was responsible for the improved mood — the extra vitamins and minerals or the ginseng.

However, researchers do know that even slightly low levels of certain nutrients, such as the B vitamins, can lead to anxiety, confusion, and depression.

It looks like the road to happiness may be paved with good food instead of gold. If you eat less than 2,500 calories a day or you regularly eat fast food on the run, you may not be getting all the nutrients you need. If that's the case, consider a supplement. Good nutrition may be your ticket to a good mood.

*Sources:*
Food and Mood: The Complete Guide to Eating Well and Feeling Your Best, Henry Holt and Company, New York, 1995
Psychology and Health (10,2:97)

## Best way to banish a bad mood fast

Want to banish your bad mood fast? Then, distract yourself instead of dwelling on your problems.

According to a study of 79 men conducted at the State University of New York at Stony Brook, this tactic is your best bet for improving a bad mood.

Although you may have always heard that seeking a sympathetic ear to listen to your troubles works wonders for soothing a ruffled soul, the Stony Brook study didn't provide support for that theory. In fact, spouting off just seemed to make a bad mood worse.

Instead, accept the fact that the problem or annoyance occurred. Then, focus on relaxing and distracting yourself. Good ways to distract yourself include listening to music and exercising. For men, at least, acceptance, relaxation, and distraction work a lot better at improving a bad mood than vocally venting frustrations. That method appears to just add fuel to the flame.

Although the distraction technique works well at banishing a bad mood fast, you shouldn't always depend on it. Sometimes, you should talk out your problems, especially if they concern someone close to you. In that case, little molehills can quickly mushroom into looming mountains.

However, for minor gripes which really won't matter tomorrow anyway, remember the good mood rule: distract, don't dwell.

*Source:*
Health Psychology (14,4:341)

## Good news about your Monday morning pick me upper

What can improve your mood, thrust your thinking powers into high gear, and increase your sense of happiness and calmness at the same time?

If you guessed caffeine, congratulations, you're correct.

Although caffeine has been the center of much controversy, people continue to rely on it to help them charge out of the house in the mornings and to improve concentration during a crunch

Still, critics of caffeine suggest that any apparent performance-enhancing benefits really just relieve withdrawal symptoms that occur after going several hours without caffeine.

However, new research crumbles that theory. In a study of 18 men, ages 18 to 30, results showed that caffeine's ability to reduce tension while improving clearheadedness, happiness, and calmness occurred independently of relieving withdrawal symptoms.

The researchers also found that caffeine often improved performance on attention tests and recall as well as the ability to process information and solve problems.

Although it's been declared as addictive as cocaine, this study suggests that caffeine certainly helps many people keep a clear head. And even though it may be addictive, caffeine, unlike cocaine, is fairly harmless. If you indulge in too much, the worst side effects you can expect will be the jitters, a headache, a stomachache, or a sleepless night.

Of course, caffeine affects each person differently. While a cup of coffee may be just what your friend needs to get his day off to a soaring start, it may give you a serious case of the shakes.

If you seem extra sensitive to caffeine, you may want to have less or avoid caffeine altogether. You may want to consider finding another way of boosting your brain power since caffeine can trigger anxiety attacks in people with extremely sensitive nervous systems.

On the positive side, however, a cup or two of coffee or tea can help you get maximum mileage out of your mental efforts. For the best brain boost, have your cup of coffee or tea when you first get up. Then, if you feel draggy, have another cup in late afternoon.

Just remember not to overdo your caffeine intake late in the day or you may suffer a restless night of sleep.

*Sources:*
*Psychopharmacology* (119,1:66)
*The Food Pharmacy*, Bantam Books, New York, 1988

# The crying cure

Crying comes so naturally you sometimes wish it didn't — because a flood of tears in an emotionally charged or painful moment can leave you wishing for a chair to crawl under.

Most people are programmed from childhood not to cry because tears often make others feel helpless and uncomfortable.

At certain times, however, whether you'll cry or not is completely out of your control. Most people can't cry on command and find it almost as difficult to turn tears off.

Maybe because tears offer healing therapy during tough times is the very reason they're so hard to control. In fact, studies show that people who cry have fewer stress-related diseases, such as ulcers and colitis, than people who don't. In addition, crying can relieve symptoms of asthma and hives, as well as lowering blood pressure, heart rate, and body temperature.

How do tears heal? Researchers have two theories. One is that tears help rid the body of chemicals caused by stress and grief. The other theory is that tears prompt you to seek support from family and friends when you're facing a tough situation. In general, tears help people cope by reducing stress, relieving negative feelings, and recharging their spirits.

So, as uncomfortable as it may feel, it's not always healthy to hold back tears. You also shouldn't encourage other people not to cry. Repressed tears can lead to repressed emotions, which can affect your ability to think clearly.

By attempting to hide your emotions from others, you may end up not knowing how you really feel. This limits your ability to empathize and be compassionate to others.

However, you can't increase your compassion or improve your general health by peeling onions to make yourself cry. Scientists have known for some time that tears caused by peeling onions have a different chemical content than tears triggered by stress or grief.

Also, a tendency to cry every time you receive criticism isn't particularly healthy. That response indicates you may have some deep hurt or loss of self-esteem that you need to deal with. If you aren't able to cope with the problem on your own, consider consulting a therapist.

Generally, however, crying has great curative powers. Although researchers aren't absolutely sure how this natural therapy works, they do know that tears triggered by stress or grief have the power to heal. So, even if it hurts, a good cry can help.

**Sources:**
*Arthritis Today* (5,5:44)
*Mothering* (62:52)

# The healing power of plants

Not only do plants provide the basic resources people need to survive, such as food, clothes, shelter, and oxygen, many of today's most powerful medicines are derived from plants. However, that's not the only way plants heal. Recent research indicates that merely being in the presence of plants is a powerful healing tool.

Dr. Paula Diane Relf, a professor of horticulture at Virginia Polytechnic Institute and State University, has collected a variety of research documenting plants' natural healing powers.

A study from the University of Delaware noted that people who had undergone gallbladder surgery recovered quicker and were able to leave the hospital sooner when they had a view of the landscape from their hospital windows compared to people who only had a view of a brick wall. The people with the landscape view also required fewer, less potent drugs to control pain.

Another study conducted at the Sloan Kettering Institute in New York City revealed that women recovering from breast cancer surgery were better able to focus, concentrate, and relieve depression if they took 20 to 30 minute walks in a garden at least three times a week for three months.

Researchers think that plants may also be useful in reducing office anxiety and stress. They are currently testing this theory.

Although research on the healing power of plants is not complete, one thing is sure. Indulging yourself in the pleasures plants offer is a healthy habit you can feel good about enjoying.

*Source:*
*"Horticulture for Human Health and Happiness,"* by Dr. Paula Diane Relf, Extension Specialist, Horticulture, Virginia Tech, PDRELF@VTVM1.CC.VT.EDU, August 1994

## Conquer chronic foot and leg ulcers with mind control

Leg and foot ulcers are common complaints of people with poor circulation. Among those affected include older folks, people with varicose veins, and people with diabetes.

Unfortunately, there is no easy or completely effective cure for this common problem. However, researchers think they may have discovered a natural way to speed up the healing process of ulcers.

In a recent study of 32 people with foot ulcers, researchers found that people who used *biofeedback relaxation* in addition to standard medical treatment had 10 times greater healing of their leg ulcers than the people who didn't practice biofeedback.

Biofeedback is a relaxation technique that uses special sensors attached to your body to help you learn to control body functions, such as blood pressure, muscle tension, and heart rate, that you normally control unconsciously.

In this study, participants were taught to increase blood flow to their feet using progressive relaxation and special breathing rhythms. They performed the exercises daily following the instructions of a specially prepared cassette tape. The improvement in the healing rates of their ulcers was impressive.

If chronic leg and foot ulcers are a constant challenge you cope with, ask your doctor about biofeedback. Make sure any biofeedback practitioner you consult is certified by the Biofeedback Certification Institute of America. For more information on biofeedback, you can reach this organization by calling 1–303–420–2902.

*Sources:*
*American Family Physician* (50,5:1067)
*Alternative Medicine: The Definitive Guide,* Future Medicine Publishing, Puyallup, Wash., 1993

## Scared to death: fact or fiction?

Scared to death may be more than just a commonly used cliché. Recent Harvard research reveals that in some people this old expression takes on a frightening new meaning.

For years, researchers have suspected that during times of crisis, such as wars or natural disasters, death rates from heart failure rise dramatically. Studies of the 1981 earthquake in Greece, the 1989 earthquake in Australia, and the Iraqi-Israeli conflict in 1991 confirmed researchers' theories.

During times of terror, anxiety is at least a natural, if not always healthy, response. But what about the anxieties that accompany everyday living? Do they take their toll?

They do, according to Dr. Ichiro Kawachi, assistant professor at the Harvard School of Public Health. He has found that if you're prone to everyday anxiety, you're more likely to die of heart failure.

Kawachi based his findings on 32 years of data collected by the Veterans Administration. In addition to standard tests, 2,280 Boston-area men were asked five questions to determine their anxiety levels.

Men who scored two or higher on the test were 4 1/2 times more likely to die of sudden heart failure than men who did not have high anxiety levels.

Kawachi speculates that anxiety triggers electrical "storms" in the heart, which cause an irregular heartbeat that can be fatal.

So far, the researchers have only studied men. Kawachi and his team are in the process of looking at how anxiety affects women. He says that he suspects they will observe a similar effect in women.

Are you at risk? To find out, take the same test the researchers used in their study. Answer yes or no to each question.

1. Do strange people or places make you afraid?
2. Are you considered a nervous person?
3. Are you constantly keyed up and jittery?
4. Do you often become scared for no good reason?
5. Do you often break out in a cold sweat?

If you answered yes to two or more questions, research suggests that you probably have an increased risk of sudden heart failure.

Now for the good news. That's not a risk you have to live with. By regularly practicing relaxation techniques, you can reduce your anxiety levels. Try these six suggestions:

◆ Take time for a walk or a talk. Physical exercise helps relieve tension, and talking with a trusted friend or family member is a time-tested way to work out problems. Doing both together just doubles the benefits.

◆ Concentrate on deep breathing that forces your stomach muscles in and out. Often, feeling stressed or anxious causes you to breathe shallowly from your chest, which only increases fatigue and anxiety.

◆ Focus on now. Concentrate all your energies and attention on whatever you're doing or whomever you're with at the present moment. This type of focusing helps you replace worries with more pleasurable, productive feelings.

◆ Take a mini vacation. Close your eyes and transport yourself to a favorite place. Try to mentally recreate all the sights, smells, sounds, and pleasurable sensations you associate with your favorite spot.

◆ Put your feelings on paper. This technique will often help you discover any hidden conflicts that may be bothering you. Throw the paper away afterward if that makes you more comfortable.

◆ Wash your worries away. Sitting by a fountain or stream; taking a swim, shower, or bath; or simply washing your hands and face work wonders for relieving anxiety.

If none of these methods works for you, talk with your doctor. He may be able to suggest a qualified therapist or recommend other alternatives.

However you do it, just make sure you stop your stress before it stops you — permanently.

*Sources:*
*Circulation* (90,5:2225)
*44 Easy Ways to Relieve Stress,* Arborvitae Publications, P.O. Box 2431, Ann Arbor, Mich. 48106–2431, 1994
*The Journal of the American Medical Association* (273,15:1208)

# Virtually fearless: How to conquer your fears face to face

If a fear of heights is keeping you from enjoying experiences others take for granted, consider conquering your fears the virtual way — through *virtual reality.*

Virtual reality is a computer-generated environment that lets you experience the sensations of being in another place although you never actually leave the spot you're in. Specially wired gloves, helmet, and body gear allow the computer to send your body the same signals you'd receive if you were really in a different location. This gear also allows you to react intuitively in your new virtual environment.

If you have a frustrating fear of heights, situations simulated through virtual reality can allow you to experience heights you might never dare attempt in real life for fear that dizziness, weak knees, or sweaty palms might somehow turn your fear of falling into reality.

The first controlled study of virtual reality therapy for treating fear of heights looks promising. A research team led by Dr. Larry F. Hodges, associate professor in the College of Computing at the Georgia Institute of Technology, and Dr. Barbara O. Rothbaum, assistant professor in the Department of Psychiatry at Emory University's School of Medicine, analyzed 17 students who displayed classic symptoms of *acrophobia* (fear of heights).

Ten of the students received virtual reality treatment to help them overcome their fear of heights. The other students received no treatment.

Each week for two months the students who received treatment were exposed to a variety of situations likely to produce anxiety in people with a fear of heights, including balconies, bridges, and an open glass elevator. Eventually, all

10 students were able to function in each virtual environment.

Seven of the 10 treated students were so encouraged by their improved ability to handle heights that they were able to deal with real life height situations they voluntarily exposed themselves to between virtual reality treatments.

Currently, virtual reality therapy is still in the testing stages so it's not widely available. Only the few people who've participated in the studies have actually been able to receive virtual reality therapy.

Also, no study has yet compared the effectiveness of virtual reality therapy with *traditional exposure treatment* therapists generally provide. In traditional exposure treatment, therapists actually accompany the person to the feared place and, during a series of visits, coach him through the fear. However, researchers suspect that even if virtual reality therapy turns out to be no more effective than traditional therapy, it will save significant amounts of time and money.

Dr. Hodges and his team hope to have a virtual reality system ready to market in the spring of 1997. This system will be used to treat people with a fear of flying. He says, "Then our goal is to keep adding systems, such as fear of heights, fear of driving, etc."

*Sources:*
*American Journal of Psychiatry* (152,4:626)
Dr. Larry Hodges, Associate Professor, College of Computing, Georgia Institute of Technology, Atlanta, Ga.
*Research Horizons* (13,1)

## Is there a hoarder in your house?

Hoarders can be hard to understand, not to mention hard to live with. Not only can you not touch their stuff, you often don't have any place to put your possessions because their things are spilling out of every closet and cubby available.

The habit of hoarding, which begins in childhood and tends to run in families, can be especially annoying to nonhoarders. If you're not a saver of stuff, it can be difficult to accept a hoarder's need to hold on to everything, especially things that are never used. It can also be difficult to comprehend why hoarders are so protective of their stuff, getting upset when their things are moved, and becoming extremely agitated if their things are thrown away.

Actually, hoarders and nonhoarders are likely to save the same type of stuff. The only difference is the quantity of stuff that hoarders save. Hoarders also make sure they have extras of things they use a lot, like shampoo and soap. In addition, they tend to carry a well-stocked supply of "just-in-case" items, such as pens, aspirin, and tissues. They want to be sure they have the proper possession when an occasion arises.

How do super savers develop the hoarding habit? Researchers have noticed that many hoarders have problems with perfection and difficulties making decisions. Because they're afraid of making an imperfect decision, they put off deciding whether to throw an item away or not. It's almost as if the hoarding develops as a byproduct of not being able to make a decision.

In general, hoarders also have a great sense of responsibility. They feel a need to be prepared for any possible future situation. Therefore, they collect all sorts of stuff. Then, because they are such responsible people, they feel compelled to take good care of what they've collected. In addition, hoarders often view their possessions as part of themselves, becoming emotionally attached to and even deriving comfort from their things. That helps explain why hoarders become so upset when someone touches or throws away their stuff.

Is there any hope that a hoarder can ever cut loose and be clutter-free? Yes, a chronic saver who wants to change can change. Often the motivation for change comes in the form of an irritated partner. Forced to face losing or alienating their partner further, many hoarders have been able to change their habits.

A great self-help resource for hoarders who hope to kick the saving habit is the book *Stop Obsessing: How to Overcome Your Obsessions and Compulsions* by Edna B. Foa, Ph.D., and Reid Wilson, Ph.D. Some people also find it beneficial to consult with a qualified mental health professional.

*Sources:*
*Behavior Research and Therapy* (33,8:897)
*Stop Obsessing: How to Overcome Your Obsessions and Compulsions,* Bantam Books, New York, 1991

# Secrets of
# Sound Sleep

## Put insomnia to bed

"I couldn't sleep at all last night." Sound familiar? It's not just a line from a popular old song, it's a phrase spoken by millions of tired people every day. About a third of all adults experience significant insomnia sometime in their lives.

Occasional insomnia happens to almost everyone. It can be caused by stress, a change in work hours, trying to sleep in a strange place, or a change in time zones (jet lag). A sleepless night every now and then probably won't hurt you, but if your insomnia continues, it could cause problems. Lack of sleep can cause you to feel fatigued, sad, lonely, and tense. Your ability to perform everyday tasks may be impaired, and your thoughts may be foggy.

Insomnia is usually a passing phase which crops up during times of stress and then goes away. However, sometimes this temporary insomnia can turn into long-term insomnia which is much harder to get rid of.

Sometimes when you experience a bout of insomnia that should be temporary, you may come to associate the idea of going to bed with a restless, sleepless night. This can lead to stubborn chronic insomnia. The trick is to treat insomnia before it becomes a chronic problem, so don't ignore insomnia and expect it to go away on its own.

Don't hesitate to see your doctor. Insomnia can be a symptom of depression, heart disease, or anxiety disorders. Any condition that causes pain may make sleep more difficult. Once you're sure that there's not a medical reason for your sleepless nights, you can try to help yourself put insomnia to rest.

**Stick to a schedule.** Try to go to bed at the same time every night, get up at the same time every morning, and avoid taking frequent naps. Your body has an internal sleep clock that works best on a regular schedule. Stick to your schedule, even on weekends. If you stay up late, you should still get up at the usual time, rather than sleeping in.

**Control your sleep environment.** Like Goldilocks, if your bed is too hard, too soft, or too lumpy, you won't be able to sleep well. Make sure your bed and your bedclothes are comfortable and the room isn't too hot or too cold. Keeping the light and noise level down also helps.

**Use your bed for only two activities.** Sleep and sex should be the only things you do in bed. Don't eat, drink, or watch television in bed, and leave your paperwork and laptop computer at your desk.

**Unwind slowly.** You've been dashing about all day long, and you need some time to unwind. Try to do some quiet activities, like reading, before you go to bed. This will help calm you and put you in a better frame of mind for sleep.

**Don't stay in bed if you're not sleepy.** If you don't fall asleep within a half hour, get out of bed. Do some type of quiet activity and go back to bed when you feel sleepy. Do this as many times a night as you need.

**Exercise regularly.** Daily exercise will help you sleep, but avoid exercising just before bedtime.

**Relax.** As you lie in bed, try to relax all your muscles. Start at your feet and work your way up.

*Sources:*
*American Family Physician* (51,1:191)
*Medical Tribune for the Internist and Cardiologist* (36,10:2)
*The Shuteye News* (1,1:3)

## Exercise improves snooze

A daily jog or brisk walk can help you sleep, according to a study of people ages 50 to 76 with sleep problems. The people engaged in aerobic exercise four times a week. After four months on the exercise program, the people were able to sleep an average of one hour longer than before and fell asleep 10 minutes faster.

However, another study found that exercise can sometimes interfere with your slumber. If you exercise too long or too hard late in the day, you may find it more difficult to fall asleep, especially if you're not physically fit. If you exercise in the afternoon, try to keep it at a mild to moderate intensity and make your session short. Morning exercise shouldn't interfere with your slumber at all, even if it is vigorous.

People who are physically fit tend to sleep better than those who aren't, so keep moving. Just be careful how and when you do it.

*Sources:*
*American Family Physician* (51,1:203)
*Health News* (2:4,7)

## 'Scent'sational sleep aid

The sweet scent of lavender oil could solve your insomnia problem. British researchers discovered that when elderly people with insomnia were treated to the aroma of lavender in their sleep, they rested easier and had more normal sleep patterns. This finding could provide a "scent-sational" alternative to the tranquilizers and hypnotic drugs that are usually prescribed for insomnia.

*Source:*
*Alternative and Complementary Therapies* (2,1:56)

## Turn out the lights on sleep problems

We all have an internal clock that tells us when we need to sleep and when we need to wake up. If you frequently dash in late for work because you overslept, you may need to reset your internal clock. One of the things that can throw off your internal clock is the amount of light you get.

Our ancestors slept at night, when it was dark, and worked during the day, when it was light. Makes sense, right? However, we now have artificial light and can stay up and work (or play) into the wee hours. Unfortunately, when you want to sleep, you may not be able to doze off, or you may wake up in the middle of the night. One of the reasons for this could be exposure to artificial light.

Researchers have long known that very bright light can affect your sleep/wake cycle. However, a recent Harvard study found that even low indoor light can cause changes in your internal clock. The brighter the light, the greater the effect. Exposure to light during the evening can shift your sleep cycle forward, causing your body to think it's earlier than it really is. This could make it more difficult to drag yourself out of bed in the morning.

If you're having trouble sleeping, maybe you should dim the lights and get romantic. It could help you get to work on time and make your boss and your spouse happier.

*Sources:*
*Health News* (2,5:3)
*Journal Watch* (16,6:51)

# Smoking steals shut-eye

If you're a night-owl smoker who can't seem to get enough shut-eye, perhaps you should chuck the cigarettes. Researchers in Kentucky found that smokers were more likely to have trouble sleeping at night and trouble staying awake during the day. Smokers were also more likely to have minor traffic accidents.

The nicotine in cigarettes could be the sleep thief because it acts as a stimulant. However, smokers were also more likely to engage in other slumber-robbing activities, like drinking lots of coffee. Smoking also increases your risk of snoring, which could interfere with restful sleep, and smokers reported having more unusual dreams and nightmares than nonsmokers.

If you decide to kick the habit for the sake of your shut-eye, be aware that, at first, withdrawal from nicotine will cause you to get even less sleep. However, if you persevere, soon you should see a great improvement in your snooze time.

*Sources:*
*Archives of Internal Medicine* (155,7:734)
*Medical Tribune for the Internist and Cardiologist* (36,9:4)

# Common drugs that cause insomnia

If you're walking around like a zombie with bags under your eyes, you probably have insomnia. You've tried everything from warm milk to sleeping pills, and nothing seems to help. A peek in your cupboard or medicine cabinet could provide the solution.

Most people know that caffeine can keep them awake, but many people think that drinking a glass of wine before bed relaxes them and helps them sleep. The opposite is actually true. Alcohol may make you sleepy at first, but it can cause you to wake up later in the night. Some other common drugs that can cause insomnia include:

- Amphetamines
- Appetite suppressants
- Blood pressure medicine
- Corticosteroids

- ◆ Decongestants
- ◆ Diuretics
- ◆ Nicotine
- ◆ Oral contraceptives

Follow your doctor's directions when taking prescription medicine. If you have insomnia, let him know. A change in medicine could help you rest easy.

*Source:*
*Medical Tribune for the Internist and Cardiologist* (36,10:2)

## Melatonin: miracle or myth?

If you're lying awake and counting more sheep as you get older, a simple supplement may help.

Melatonin, a chemical produced by the pineal gland in your brain, may hold the key to swifter, sweeter slumber. Melatonin levels are highest at night and lowest during the day. This leads researchers to believe that melatonin helps regulate your sleep cycle.

Melatonin tends to decrease as you age. In an Israeli study, elderly people who had trouble sleeping were found to have melatonin levels much lower than younger people. They also had less melatonin than people their own age who had no sleep problems. Melatonin supplements helped these people sleep better.

Melatonin can also help people suffering from jet lag and workers who change shifts frequently. When you change your sleep patterns, like when you travel to another time zone or change your working hours, your body sometimes protests the change by refusing to sleep at all. Taking melatonin just a few hours before you go to bed may trigger the sleep response that your body usually generates naturally.

A dose of as little as 0.3 mg of melatonin can improve sleep. However, many stores sell melatonin in much higher doses. Since no one knows what side effects higher doses may cause, be careful not to overdo it. If you have insomnia, you may need to take melatonin for a couple of months before you notice a significant improvement.

Melatonin has been hailed as the latest medical miracle. It has been claimed that melatonin can cure or help with diabetes, heart disease, cancer, Alzheimer's disease, and even AIDS. Researchers continue to explore melatonin's possible effect on these disorders. However, the only use for melatonin that has significant evidence to support it is for treatment of sleep disorders.

*Sources:*
*British Medical Journal* (309,6948:167)
*The Lancet* (345,8962:1408; 346,8974:541; and 347,8995:184)
*Medical Tribune for the Internist and Cardiologist* (37,4:1)

## 7 steps to snore-free sleeping

Laugh and the world laughs with you. Snore and you sleep alone. Snoring occurs when inhaled air passes through the narrow airway where your mouth meets your throat. The air rattles the soft tissue there, creating a harsh noise.

It affects more men than women, and the likelihood of snoring increases with age. In their early 30s, 20 percent of men and 5 percent of women snore, but by their 60s, 60 percent of men and 40 percent of women are "sawing logs" in their sleep. This is probably caused by loss of muscle tone in the throat as people age.

One of the most obvious effects of snoring is loss of sleep. The snorer's bed partner may lose sleep, but the snorer himself is not getting a good night's sleep, though he may not realize it. Snorers often experience extreme daytime drowsiness. This can cause problems at work, as well as dangerous sleepiness behind the wheel.

Fight the effects of snoring with these hints:

◆ Sleep on your side. To help keep yourself on your side during the night, you can sew a tennis ball into the back of your pajamas, or simply stuff a couple of tennis balls into a sock, and pin it to the back of your pajamas.

◆ Avoid thick pillows that cause your neck to bend forward. This pinches the airways, making snoring worse. However, if you can elevate your entire upper body with pillows, that may help. (If you can sleep sitting halfway up!)

◆ Stop smoking. Smoking can cause the tissues of the throat to swell, and nicotine can disturb sleep patterns.

◆ Avoid alcohol, sleeping pills, and tranquilizers at bedtime. These relax the muscles of your throat, making snoring more likely.

◆ Use a decongestant spray before bedtime, especially if you suffer from allergies. These help to open nasal passages so you don't breathe through your mouth.

◆ Use a humidifier in your bedroom. Low humidity can dry out mucous membranes, increasing irritation and adding to your snoring problem.

◆ Lose weight. Extra weight, especially in the neck area, can put pressure on your throat, collapsing already narrow air passages.

Although most snoring causes no harm, it may still annoy others and embarrass you. Try some of these suggestions. If you won't do it for yourself, do it for your loved ones. Otherwise you may find yourself sleeping alone.

*Sources:*
*American Review of Respiratory Diseases* (144,5:1130)
*British Medical Journal* (300,6739:1557)
*Chest* (99,6:1378 and 107,5:1283)
*The Home Remedies Handbook,* Publications International, Lincolnwood, Ill., 1993
*The Wellness Encyclopedia,* Houghton Mifflin, Boston, 1991

# When snoring can kill

Sometimes snoring can cause more problems than just a poor night's sleep. Even if your snoring doesn't drive your bed partner to smother you with a pillow, you may still be in danger.

Snoring may be an indication that you suffer from sleep apnea. This disorder interrupts normal breathing patterns, causing you to stop breathing for short periods of time during the night. When these interruptions take place, the lack of oxygen in your blood causes you to snort, gasp for air, then settle back down to sleep. These gaps in breathing usually last only about 10 seconds, but they can occur up to 400 times a night.

You may not be aware that you have sleep apnea, because it usually doesn't cause you to wake up. The person you sleep with may notice it, or you may be drowsy, irritable, and tired during the day. You may also have morning headaches, forgetfulness, mood changes, and a decreased interest in sex.

People with sleep apnea have a higher risk of heart attack, stroke, and high blood pressure. They also have seven times more automobile accidents than the general population. Therefore, sleep apnea is a potentially fatal condition.

Though drugs have been ineffective in treating sleep apnea, some medical devices may help. Continuous positive airway pressure, the most common treatment, uses air pressure to keep breathing passageways open during the night. However, because it involves wearing a face mask all night, many people discontinue using it.

Dental devices that help hold airways open by pulling the jaw forward may also be an option. If your condition is severe enough, and if other remedies don't help, surgery is another option. The operation widens the airway in your throat and tightens loose tissue.

Don't ignore a snore. It may be trying to tell you something. If you think you have sleep apnea, follow the above tips for snorers, and see your doctor.

*Sources:*
*American Family Physician* (52,3:871)
*The New England Journal of Medicine* (334,2:99)

# Dreams may be a warning sign of illness

"Dreams can come true, it can happen to you, if you're young at heart." Remember this old song? Well, some medical researchers think that dreams can sometimes tell you when you're sick at heart.

Many ancient scholars believed that dreams could predict or cause illness. Aristotle, for example, believed that dreams were the products of information received by the brain during sleep from inside and outside the body. Sigmund Freud, who wrote a famous book about dreams, also believed that illness could affect a person's dreams.

Modern scientists began to investigate the relationship between dreams and a person's health when it was discovered that dreams occurred during REM (rapid eye movement) sleep. During REM sleep, changes occur in a person's temperature, heart rate, and blood pressure which are similar to the changes experienced during stress. This discovery led scientists to think that dreams could indeed be a reflection of a person's health.

Studies find that dreams may be an indication of illness even when you are unaware that you are ill. For example, dreams of death and dying seem to be common among people with a serious illness, particularly heart disease. Men who are seriously ill tend to dream of death, while women dream about separation. Dreams of lost wealth or possessions often occur among people with brain disease. People with narcolepsy (a sleep disorder which causes people to suddenly and unexpectedly fall asleep) frequently have vivid and bizarre dreams, probably because their REM sleep pattern is disturbed.

Drugs may also affect your dreams. People with Parkinson's disease may have vivid and unusual dreams caused by levodopa, a drug used to treat Parkinson's.

Antidepressants, sedatives, and alcohol can all affect your dreams, causing them to be disturbing or disappear altogether.

Having one disturbing dream should not be cause for alarm. We all have them from time to time. However, if you have recurring disturbing dreams, perhaps your subconscious is trying to tell you it's time for a checkup.

*Source:*
*British Medical Journal* (306,6883:993)

# A happy ending for nightmares

Do monsters, goblins, or disasters disturb your sleep every night, keeping you from the peaceful rest that you need? Ending the nightmares may be as easy as making up a new ending.

In a recent study, people who suffered from chronic nightmares were told to make up a happy ending to their nightmares. They wrote the endings down, and then rehearsed them in their minds all day. Most people found that their nightmares decreased, and their sleep improved. Think up a happy ending and end your nightmares. Sweet dreams.

*Source:*
*Medical Abstracts Newsletter* (16,1:8)

# Safety tips for sleepwalkers

Have you ever seen someone take a stroll in their sleep? While it might seem amusing, a sleepwalker could take a tumble down a flight of stairs or otherwise seriously harm himself.

Sleepwalking is a parasomnia, an abnormal occurrence during the deepest part of your sleep cycle. It tends to run in families, and you are 10 times more likely to sleepwalk if you have a close relative who also sleepwalks. Episodes of sleepwalking may last from a few minutes to an hour.

Sleepwalkers should take the following steps to make sure their sleep environment is safe:

◆ Put bars on upstairs windows.
◆ Install locks on all outside doors.
◆ Keep the area clear of dangerous objects like knives.
◆ Put gates at the head and foot of stairs.
◆ When travelling, request a room on the ground floor of hotels.
◆ Avoid alcohol, especially just before bedtime.
◆ Try to keep regular hours, and take afternoon naps.

*Sources:*
*British Medical Journal* (306,6882:921)
*The Good Night Guide,* Better Sleep Council, Washington, D.C., 1993

# Defend yourself from time change danger

Do you grumble every spring when daylight savings time causes you to lose an hour of sleep? You may have even more reason to grumble if you're not careful. According to a recent Canadian study, automobile accidents increase by 8 percent on the Monday following the spring time change. In the fall, when people get an extra hour of sleep after the time change, accidents decrease by about the same amount.

When the spring time change occurs, if you want to avoid a crunched fender (or worse), be sure to keep your eyes open because the other driver may not.

*Source:*
*Medical Abstracts* (16:5,4)

## Tooth wear and tear: Get out of the grind

Did you know that your teeth can exert an average biting force of 162 pounds per square inch (psi), and the record for biting force during teeth-grinding is 975 psi? It's easy to see why bruxism, or teeth-grinding during sleep, can result in serious dental damage.

Bruxism occurs more often during periods of stress, and people who have high-stress jobs are more likely to grind their teeth in their sleep. Since bruxism usually occurs during sleep, many people are unaware they have the condition. Often, the person's bed partner notices the grinding noise. Signs of bruxism include:

◆ Abnormal wear on teeth
◆ Sensitive teeth
◆ Sore jaw muscles
◆ Headaches
◆ Decreased jaw-opening ability

Most people will experience bruxism at some time in their lives. Usually it is stress-related and goes away on its own. However, people with ongoing bruxism can damage their teeth severely. Try these suggestions to end bruxism and save your smile.

**Relaxation exercises.** Certain relaxation techniques sometimes work well in treating bruxism. One involves relaxing the jaw with your lips closed and your teeth not touching. Repeat this 50 times a day. As soon as you're comfortable with this exercise, practice visualizing sleeping with your jaw in this position.

**Change your sleep position.** Sleep on your back with pillows under your knees and neck. This allows the lower jaw to relax.

**Clench your teeth.** This treatment is called massed negative practice. You clench your teeth firmly for five seconds, then relax for five. Repeat this five times in a row, six times a day. In one study, this method helped over 75 percent of the participants in just 21 days.

**Have someone wake you.** If you're lucky enough to have a cooperative spouse, ask him to wake you every time he hears you begin to grind your teeth. This can at least reduce your bruxism.

If these self-help techniques don't work, or if you have already experienced damage from bruxism, see your dentist. He may prescribe a rubber mouth guard to protect your teeth.

*Sources:*
*American Family Physician* (49,7:1617)
*The Good Night Guide,* Better Sleep Council, Washington, D.C. 1993

# Boost Your Brain Power

## The 9 best ways to beat brain drain

**Be on time for breakfast.** If you skip breakfast, you're basically asking your body to run on the fumes of food you consumed the day before. People who eat breakfast are able to think clearer, faster, and more creatively than people who don't.

**Eat a little a lot.** To think and feel better, divide the three traditional big meals into six small ones. Research shows that people who divide their daily calories into a series of evenly spaced mini-meals and snacks throughout the day have more even moods, and fewer problems with tiredness, depression, insomnia, illness, and unwanted weight gain. Light meals also leave you feeling more alert than heavy meals, which make most people sleepy.

**Pack some protein for lunch.** Protein fuels your brain better for after-lunch work than carbohydrates, which tend to make you sleepy this time of day. Some good lunch choices: a turkey sandwich on whole wheat bread (hold the mayo) or extra-lean meatballs with a little spaghetti. Don't forget to include one or two fresh fruits and vegetables as well.

**Avoid alcohol.** It kills the brain cells you need to think. See the article *Don't drink if you want to think* later in this chapter.

**Nix nicotine.** Tobacco smoke constricts blood vessels, which reduces the amount of blood and oxygen flowing through your body, including your brain. The less oxygen your brain cells get, the less able they are to function effectively.

**Stop the stress.** Uncontrolled stress saps your ability to pay attention, remember, and concentrate. Exercise is a great solution for stress.

**Stay slim.** Study after study shows being slim lengthens life span and improves mental functioning. Eat enough daily calories to get all the vitamins and minerals you need, but don't overeat.

Make sure your daily calories include three servings of fruit, four servings of vegetables, seven servings of breads/grains, and one serving of legumes (dried beans or peas). If you eat less than 2,500 calories a day, you should take a daily multivitamin.

**"B" smart with vitamins.** A low intake of the B vitamins niacin, folic acid, B1, B2, B6, and B12 can interfere with maximum mental functioning. If you don't eat 2,500 calories a day and include the recommended servings from each food group, make sure your multivitamin contains the recommended daily allowance (RDA) for all these vitamins.

You can check the back of your multivitamin bottle to see how your supplement measures up. If your multivitamin leaves the B vitamins out or provides an amount lower than the RDA, consider taking a vitamin B complex, a supplement which contains a combination of all essential B vitamins.

**Get up and get moving**. If you just sit around, your brain will get as sluggish as your body. If you want your brain to run like a well-tuned hot rod, you've got to rev its engines with exercise. You'll remember better, concentrate better, and think better. Recent research indicates that physical activities which also involve thinking and coordination, such as dancing, can even boost IQ.

*Sources:*
*Food and Mood: The Complete Guide to Eating Well and Feeling Your Best*, Henry Holt and Company, New York, 1995
*The Economist* (338,7954:85)

## Low blood pressure boosts brain power

You can have a mind as strong as a steel trap for as long as you live. However, expect senility and memory loss to set in if high-pressure blood is damaging your brain.

A sharp mind depends on a steady supply of healthy blood. If you have high blood pressure, your brain doesn't get that steady blood supply. Your arteries are either weak and flimsy or they have a thick, callous-like buildup that prevents good blood flow.

A 25-year study of 3,700 men in Honolulu showed that men who had high blood pressure in middle age had a decreased ability to think and reason in later life.

So, if you want to increase your powers of memory and concentration as you grow older, keep your blood pressure under control. You'll need to have your pressure checked regularly and follow your doctor's orders, including taking any medication he recommends.

With weight loss, a healthy diet, and exercise, you can lower your blood pressure. You'll not only baby your brain, but you'll also reduce your risk of heart attack, stroke, and kidney damage.

*Sources:*
*The Atlanta Journal/Constitution* (Jan. 4, 1996, B6)
*The Journal of the American Medical Association* (274,23:1846)

## Beat brain disorders with a dose of B12

If you or someone you know is suffering from depression, memory loss, confusion, or senility, the solution could be as simple as taking some extra vitamin B12 (also called cobalamin).

Because B12 is essential for proper functioning of the nervous system, it's not surprising that even a borderline deficiency of this vitamin can lead to mental problems. A recent study revealed that low levels of B12 can lead to permanent brain damage. However, if the deficiency is caught and treated soon enough (usually within a year), brain damage can be prevented. If you are deficient and you don't receive treatment promptly, you have an eight in 10 chance of developing a nervous system disorder as you grow older.

People prone to a deficiency of B12 include older people, vegetarians, alcoholics, people with digestive difficulties, or people who have recently suffered severe stress or undergone surgery. Every person age 65 or older should have B12 levels tested because 5 to 15 percent of people in this age group suffer from a deficiency of this mind-nurturing nutrient. In older people, even low-normal levels can cause complications.

If you're age 65 or older or you suspect a lack of B12 is causing mental problems in yourself or a loved one, ask your family doctor about testing B12 levels. If the test shows a definite deficiency or even just levels in the low-normal range, consider supplements. Once you have healthy levels of B12 in your body, you'll not only think better, you'll feel better, too.

If your B12 deficiency is caused by a digestive problem, you may need to take shots to enable your body to absorb and benefit from the vitamin B12. If not, you may only need to take a daily supplement or increase the number of foods you eat that are rich in B12, such as beef, chicken, dairy products, eggs, fish, kidney, liver, and pork.

*Sources:*
*Archives of Family Medicine* (4,4:304)
*Complete Guide to Vitamins, Minerals and Supplements,* Fisher Books, Tucson, Ariz., 1988
*Scientific American Medical Bulletin* (18,8:4)

# Don't drink if you want to think

You know not to drink and drive, but did you know you shouldn't drink if you want to think?

A recent study shows that regular drinking, even in moderate amounts, kills brain cells.

You're born with about 100 billion brain cells, also called neurons. Between birth and your early 20s, your brain mass triples due to new connections you create between neurons each time you learn something. Once you've passed your early 20s, you lose 100,000 neurons every day for the rest of your life.

If you regularly drink alcohol, you're likely losing more than that. A heavy drinker (one who regularly drinks more than two alcoholic beverages a day) may lose up to 60,000 more neurons a day in addition to the normal loss of 100,000.

Alcohol generally kills cells in your brain's left hemisphere, the area responsible for language and logic. Men who are alcoholics also have reduced blood flow to the front of the brain, the area responsible for thinking creatively, making memories, and solving problems.

According to Ernest Noble at the UCLA School of Medicine, even two to three drinks a day four days a week will worsen brain function. The effect seems to be especially pronounced in people over age 40. In addition to causing a badly functioning brain, this amount of regular alcohol intake will make you age faster. Alcohol also makes your brain more susceptible to damage.

One recent study suggested that drinking three or more beers or glasses of wine a day may cause permanent brain damage that affects motor skills, such as driving.

If you want your brain to be at its best, you really shouldn't consume more than 1 ounce of pure alcohol a day, which is equal to two regular beers or two small glasses of wine. Women shouldn't drink more than one beer or one glass of wine per day because they seem to be more sensitive to the effects of alcohol than men.

If you drink heavily every day for 30 to 40 years, your brain will weigh 105 grams less than the brains of people who were only light drinkers or those who didn't drink at all. The less brain you have, the less able you are to think.

A body without a working brain is just a bunch of parts. Before you down that next drink, think about it — while you're still able.

*Sources:*
*British Medical Journal* (308,6945:1663)
*If You Drink Alcoholic Beverages, Do So in Moderation,* United States Department of Agriculture, Home and Garden Bulletin No. 253-8, 1993
*The Owner's Manual for the Brain: Everyday Applications for Mind-Brain Research,* Leornian Press, Austin, Texas, 1994

# Maximize your memory

Have you ever started to talk about an upcoming event and forgotten the date? Ever hesitated while trying to remember someone's name? If you have (and it's rare to find the person who hasn't), you know just how embarrassing momentary memory lapses can be.

To save yourself from future embarrassment in such situations, here are some tips to help you maximize your memory power:

◆ Substitute the stuff you need to remember for the lyrics of a favorite song. This is a fun and simple way of remembering all sorts of stuff.

◆ Make memories last by using wacky associations. One way to do this is by associating information with different body parts. If you have a list to remember, link items on your list with various body parts. For example, if you need cantaloupe, chicken, and bread, you might mentally picture your head as a cantaloupe, a chicken clucking on your chest, and see yourself wearing loaves of bread for shoes. The crazier the associations you make, the easier they will be to remember.

In addition to creating crazy images, it also helps to logically organize the material you need to remember. For example, if you have a grocery list that includes produce and meat items, you're more likely to remember them all if you group similar items, such as fruits and vegetables, together.

◆ Take advantage of the acronym. If you've got a list of items you have to remember, take the first letter of each item to make up a new nonsense word — your acronym. For some reason, this is often easier than trying to recall each item individually. The fairly famous acronym ROY G. BIV has been used to help countless students remember the colors of the rainbow in their correct order: Red, Orange, Yellow, Green, Blue, Indigo, and Violet.

◆ Do things as you think of them. If you do what you need to do as you think of it, you won't forget to do it later.

◆ Group important numbers you need to remember into twos and threes. This makes remembering them easier.

◆ Make use of notes. Besides helping you not forget, using notes frees up your brain to focus on whatever you're doing at the moment instead of trying not to forget what you're supposed to do sometime in the future.

◆ Practice having a positive attitude. The more negative, self-critical, unhappy thoughts you think, the less well your brain will work. If you persist in thinking you're going to lose your memory just because you're getting older, the more likely it is to happen. Think good thoughts about yourself and your memory and realize that it's natural to be forgetful now and then.

◆ Pump up your memory power by playing games. This is a fun way to improve memory skills. Some good games to try include bridge, Concentration, Memory, Solitaire, Trivial Pursuit, and Twenty Questions.

◆ Get enough rest. Anyone who's tired, whether he's 7 or 70, won't remember as well as someone who's well-rested.

◆ Eat a well-balanced diet. Just like your car, your brain needs fuel to function efficiently. In a typical day, your brain uses up one-fifth of the calories you eat.

*Sources:*
Look Ten Years Younger, Live Ten Years Longer, Prentice Hall, Englewood Cliffs, N.J., 1995
Successful Aging: A Sourcebook for Older People and Their Families, Ballantine Books, New York, 1987
The Compass in Your Nose and Other Astonishing Facts about Humans, Jeremy P. Tarcher, Los Angeles, 1989

# Get your memory up to speed with sugar

Despite all those naysayers who always said sugar was a no-no, you just knew there was something good about sugar besides its sweet taste, didn't you?

The latest study says you may be right. Researchers at the University of Virginia in Charlottesville say a spoonful of sugar not only makes medicine taste better, it also improves learning and memory. Sugar seems to be an especially sweet solution to memory problems for older people because their brains are often hit extra hard when blood-sugar levels drop.

Researchers tested their theory on a group of generally healthy 60- to 80-year olds. Each participant was tested early in the morning before breakfast. Before the test began, they were given a glass of lemonade to drink, which was sweetened either with sugar or the artificial sweetener saccharin.

Then they were asked to read a short story. A few minutes later, each participant was requested to retell the story in his own words. The participants who had lemonade with sugar did much better than the participants who had lemonade sweetened with saccharin.

The positive effects of the sugar lasted even into the next day after blood sugar had leveled off. People who received sugar-sweetened lemonade had better recall of the story they'd read the day before than people who had the saccharin-sweetened lemonade.

Several earlier studies indicate that sugar can even enhance the memory and learning capabilities of people with Alzheimer's or Down syndrome.

Since a little sugar works so well at improving memory and learning, does that mean more sugar will work even better? Not necessarily. The key to success seems to be stable blood sugar levels, so huge amounts of sugar won't help. Plus, too much sugar can lead to unwanted cavities or weight gain.

However, the study does seem to suggest that researchers need to look into how eating many small, healthy meals throughout the day, instead of three fairly large meals, affects brain functioning. By keeping blood sugar levels steady, many small meals may boost brain power better than three square meals.

In the meantime, researchers hope to learn enough about how sugar affects brain functioning to be able to develop specific drugs to provide some form of relief for memory and learning problems, whether they're caused by aging, Alzheimer's, or Down syndrome.

*Source:*
*The American Journal of Clinical Nutrition* (61,4S:987S)

## Getting a grip on forgetfulness

No one likes to feel forgetful, so it would be really nice if the brain came with a lifetime guarantee. Then you could trade in the old model for a new one when things like remembering became a troublesome task.

As nice as that would be, it just isn't possible at this point, so here are two easy tips to make remembering simpler:

- ◆ Hang a bulletin board someplace where you'll see it everyday. Post important reminders on it.
- ◆ Keep a large calendar handy and note important dates and appointments. Some people prefer a small calendar so they can carry it with them at all times.

And don't find so much fault with yourself if you're a little forgetful now and then. It happens to everybody.

*Source:*
*Geriatric Nursing* (16,2:55)

## Make-believe memories?

Ever been surprised to discover that a memory you thought was crystal clear in your mind was the same as a picture in a family scrapbook or that the way you remembered some incident was completely different from how someone else remembered the same event?

Jenya Weaver of Atlanta was stunned to see a photograph from her childhood she thought only existed in her mind. Fairly often in her adulthood, she would find herself mulling over a memory of herself as a child attempting to climb into the family bathtub. Only after she saw the photograph did she realize that what she considered an actual memory was really a memory of the photograph she must have seen as a child.

How could she tell the difference? When she recalled her memory, she realized she always saw a back view of herself getting into the bath, the same exact angle at which the photo was taken. If the experience had truly been a memory, she realized she would have remembered looking into the water in the bathtub, not seeing herself from behind.

Based on reports of similar experiences, more and more researchers are beginning to realize just how unreliable memories may be. It might be more accurate to refer to a sea of memories instead of describing memories as set in stone.

For years, there has been a theory that the mind can't tell the difference between a memory of an actual event and a memory of a vividly imagined incident. New research appears to support this theory.

A recent conference held at Harvard Medical School indicated that the way memories are stored in the brain almost guarantees that some memories will be false. Whole memories are literally stored in pieces in different parts of the brain.

The visual parts of the memory are stored in the brain area called the visual cortex; the sound sections of the memory are stored in the auditory cortex; sensations are stored in the sensory cortex; and smells are stored in the olfactory cortex (the smell center of the brain). When you want to recall a memory, something called the limbic system is responsible for pulling all these parts together again correctly.

Because so many connections are involved in the storage of one memory and your brain can hold many, many memories (generating too many connections to count), Harvard researchers seem to think that it's inevitable you will occasionally have memories of things that never really happened.

Part of the problem is that the mind forgets the origin of the memory faster than any other part of the recollection. Unfortunately, it's the origin of the memory that's most important in determining its relationship to actual events.

According to Harvard psychologist Daniel Schacter, it is possible to remember a dream, a fear, or someone else's story of something that happened to them as a real memory of your own.

Sometimes, even a simple suggestion can generate a memory that seems real. According to one study, one out of four people are likely to take some suggestion and turn it into a memory they believe is their own. This study was conducted in a low-stress situation. If greater stress levels had been present, researchers believe that the false memory rate would have been even higher.

Basically a suggestion that leads to a false memory occurs in four steps:

1. The suggestion leaves traces of its presence in your brain and unconscious mind.
2. The ever-busy brain links the suggestion with a real memory you may have stored which could be similar to the suggestion.
3. The origin of the new memory, which was the original suggestion, gets lost in the shuffle.
4. Suddenly, you have a new false memory. Later, when describing this memory to others, it's very common to add extra details that weren't there before.

For your peace of mind, and before you go off making wild accusations at somebody over a disturbing memory you've recently recalled, just remember that many things which arise out of the unconscious mind may actually be symbolic. In fact, researchers believe that much of what comes from the unconscious in the form of dreams or sometimes disturbing memories is actually just referring to some other situation in your life your subconscious is trying to solve.

*Source:*
*Subconsciously Speaking* (10,1:1)

# Easier learning

"You can't teach an old dog new tricks" is a saying that's been around forever, but it's just not true. In fact, the authors of *Forever Mind: Eight Ways to Unleash the Power of Your Mature Mind* say you can learn things better now than you did when you were younger.

However, it may take you a little longer to learn new things than it used to. Still, it seems that once you do learn something you're just as likely to remember it as a 25 year old. You've just got to figure out your personal learning style.

You've had a personal learning style since you were a child, but over the years you've probably gotten better at that one style of learning and worse at other styles. Now, it's more important than ever to figure out how your mind likes to learn.

◆ Visual learners. You learn best by reading, looking at drawings or graphs, and taking notes. You probably find objects you've lost by visualizing where you last put them. After listening to a lecture or speech, it takes colorful description to remember what you've learned. *Easiest learning techniques:* Reading, drawing, and making outlines or diagrams.

◆ Verbal learners. You talk to yourself when you learn something new. You may mutter out loud: "First, you slide this bolt in place. ..." You used to love to talk in class, and you like to read to people out loud. *Easiest learning techniques:* Workshops with a lot of participation required, discussion with others. Putting what you've learned into your own words is a great learning tool for you.

◆ Auditory learners. Listening is how you learn best. College lectures were easy for you. You probably like music. *Easiest learning techniques:* Listening to tapes or lectures. You're lucky; you can learn while you drive. Take full advantage of tapes you can check out at your local library.

◆ Kinesthetic learners. You learn best by doing. You like to take things apart and put them back together again. *Easiest learning techniques:* Role-playing, hands-on projects. You learn well by teaching others. Demonstrating how something works is right up your alley.

In addition to identifying your own personal learning style, knowing how your learning needs may change as you grow older can also make learning easier.

Generally, adults learn best when information is presented at a slower pace than when they were younger. Realize that it's OK and even normal if it takes you two or three repetitions to completely master the material.

Many older adults hinder their learning by being anxious about their performance because they've heard it said so many times that you can't teach an old dog new tricks. Now that you know that old saying is nothing more than mere myth, relax and enjoy yourself. You'll find learning much easier and more enjoyable.

Get back in the groove. Like any skill, learning gets better with practice. The more time you spend learning, the better you'll be at it. If you think someone younger than you is a quicker learner, it's probably just because he's had more recent practice.

*Sources:*
*Forever Mind: Eight Ways to Unleash the Power of Your Mature Mind,* William Morrow and Co., New York, 1996
*Successful Aging: A Sourcebook for Older People and Their Families,* Ballantine Books, New York, 1987

## The truth about subliminal self-help tapes

P.T. Barnum knew what he was talking about when he said, "There's a sucker born every minute." And every unscrupulous seller since P.T. Barnum has attempted to make every buyer a sucker by preying on buyers' deep-seated desires and fears.

In this era of the information age where knowledge is power, everyone wants to be smarter, know more, and have healthier habits to live longer and take advantage of all this awesome information.

That's why subliminal self-help tapes are such a booming business. "Learn while you sleep," "Stop smoking the easy way," shout announcers and advertisements. With so much to do these days and so little free time, learning new stuff and breaking bad habits while you sleep seems like the perfect solution.

It isn't. It's only a good solution for parting you from your money without giving you anything in return, except perhaps a poor night's sleep. You have to be consciously aware for learning to take place. In addition, many of these tapes don't actually have any of the subliminal images or messages that advertisers claim will revolutionize your life.

Save your money, your sleep, and any other time you might be tempted to waste listening to subliminal self-help tapes. The only people these tapes help are the people who sell them.

*Source:*
*The Owner's Manual for the Brain: Everyday Applications from Mind-Brain Research,* Leornian Press, Austin, Texas, 1994

## ADD and the art of success

Creative, inspirational, intuitive, visionary ...

If you've been diagnosed with Attention Deficit Disorder (ADD), it's likely that you haven't had your condition described this way. You're more likely to hear disorganized, inattentive, and impulsive.

But did you know that the ability to be creative, inspirational, intuitive, and visionary are just a few of the characteristics that people with ADD share with some of the most successful people the world has ever seen? In fact, some people are successful because they've learned how to use ADD to their advantage.

Most people with ADD have incredible imaginations. Unlike many other people, you have the ability to see great possibilities in small opportunities. Here are some tips to help you harness your unique brain organization and achieve the success you've always dreamed of.

- Recognize that many of the difficulties people with ADD experience, everything from frequent mood swings to being easily distracted, is caused by a genetic glitch in the brain. ADD has nothing to do with a weakness of character or will or lack of maturity. You simply have to learn to create an environment for yourself that makes the most of your brain setup.
- Have hope. This may be very difficult after enduring years of embarrassment trying to cope with ADD. Because of the number of failures people with ADD often experience, they also frequently have very little self-confidence. However, you must have hope to travel down the road to success. Hope will also help rebuild your self-confidence.
- Educate yourself and others. Understanding ADD is the most powerful treatment you can get. Share your knowledge with family and friends so they can provide the kind of support you need. Reading books, joining or creating a support group, and talking with professionals are some of the best ways to learn about ADD.
- Find a coach (a good friend, a colleague, or a therapist) to encourage you and help you stay organized. Sometimes spouses serve as coaches, but this can be a risky venture. The coach you choose should have a sense of humor and be willing to give you feedback and a friendly push when you need it.
- Structure your world to keep yourself on track. Use lists, reminders, notes, rituals, and files to keep yourself organized. Since people with ADD are often visually oriented, make use of colors to attract and keep your attention. For example, use different colored file folders for filing and different colored marking pens to help you remember important schedules or text.
- Liven up your living and working spaces. Many ADD'ers find it easier and more productive to work in a visually stimulating environment.
- Figure out how and when you work best and take advantage of that time. People with ADD often work best in situations other people might find disruptive, such as a noisy room or while listening to music. Just do whatever works for you. Also, recognize that it's OK if you need to be doing several things at once, such as talking and typing or walking and reading. Doing several things at the same time is the only way some ADD'ers can get anything done at all.
- Set priorities and make deadlines. If you're having a day when this seems impossible, get someone to help you. By setting priorities and disciplining yourself to stick with them, you can beat procrastination, one of the biggest problems many adults with ADD face.
- Break big tasks down into a series of smaller ones. Be sure to set deadlines for the completion of each small task. This process makes big jobs much more manageable.
- Realize and accept that not every commitment and project will be completed. Give yourself a break now and then.
- Exercise every day. This is one of the best natural treatments for ADD. It soothes and calms the body by allowing you to work off aggression and excess energy in a healthy way.

♦ Schedule some "let-loose" time each week. Do something you really like to do, such as listening to loud music or dancing the night away in a downtown disco, that helps you release extra energy.

♦ Give yourself time to relax and recharge. You really need this time, so don't feel guilty about taking it. Do something calming and restful, such as reading or napping.

*Source:*
"50 Tips on the Treatment of Adult Attention Deficit Disorder," by Edward M. Hallowell M.D. and John J. Ratey, M.D.

## A little pill more powerful than Alzheimer's?

Can popping a popular painkiller really put the brakes on Alzheimer's? The possibility looks promising, say researchers.

According to a 15-year study of 1,828 older people conducted at Johns Hopkins University, ibuprofen, the painkiller used in drugs like Advil, Motrin, and Nuprin, may reduce the risk of developing Alzheimer's by 60 percent.

This study supports earlier studies which suggested that nonsteroidal anti-inflammatory drugs (NSAIDs) like ibuprofen (the most commonly used NSAID) may be able to help the brain fight off Alzheimer's.

Although earlier studies suggested that aspirin might offer protection against Alzheimer's, this study found aspirin to offer only weak protection, if any. Acetaminophen, the pain reliever used in Tylenol, appeared to provide no protection at all.

Before you rush to the drugstore to stock up on ibuprofen or other NSAIDs, remember that these studies are still in the early stages. Researchers are hopeful, but they aren't ready to make any definite recommendations.

Considering the severe side effects that regular use of NSAIDs can cause, including stomach and intestinal bleeding, you should hold off on that trip to the drugstore until researchers feel more confident about making recommendations.

You probably won't have to wait long for definite answers. Some scientists speculate that a definite yes or no on NSAIDs preventing Alzheimer's will be available within the next five years.

*Sources:*
*Science News* (145,8:116)
*The Atlanta Journal/Constitution* (March 29, 1996, A1)
*The Journal of the American Medical Association* (275,18:1389)

## Estrogen replacement therapy may reduce risk of Alzheimer's

Many women are already well aware of the various benefits of estrogen replacement therapy, from relieving the discomforts of menopause to helping prevent more serious problems, such as heart disease and osteoporosis.

The latest research seems to suggest yet another benefit of estrogen replacement therapy — a reduced risk of Alzheimer's disease.

In a study of 514 menopausal women conducted at Johns Hopkins University, researchers found that the women who received estrogen replacement therapy had less than half the risk of developing Alzheimer's as women who had not taken estrogen.

Previous studies had suggested that there might be a link between estrogen replacement therapy and a reduced risk of Alzheimer's. However, this study, the most recent and the largest done so far, offers the strongest evidence yet that estrogen may have a protective effect against Alzheimer's.

Because the research is still in the early stages, estrogen replacement therapy is not currently offered as a treatment for Alzheimer's. However, more studies are underway, and researchers hope to soon discover why and how estrogen seems to offer protection against this devastating disease.

*Source:*
*The Journal of the American Medical Association* (275,18:1389)

# Unproven Alzheimer remedies can be more harmful than helpful

The slow search for an Alzheimer's cure tempts many Alzheimer caregivers to turn to alternative therapies.

In a recent study, over half of the 101 caregivers interviewed revealed that they had given the Alzheimer's victim in their care at least one alternative remedy, hoping to see some improvement in memory or behavior. The most common treatments tried included vitamins, health foods, herbal medicines, smart pills, and home remedies. The majority of caregivers reported seeing no signs of improvement.

Besides the often high costs of these alternative therapies, there is also the risk of harmful side effects. For example, certain herbal preparations can be toxic as can megadoses of some vitamins. In addition, they may interact adversely with another drug a person with Alzheimer's may already be taking.

If you care for a person with Alzheimer's, be sure to let his doctor know if you plan to try any alternative treatments. That way, he can keep an eye out for possible interactions or side effects or warn you if he feels the alternative treatment may be more harmful than helpful.

*Source:*
*The Journal of the American Geriatric Society* (43,7:747)

## Art therapy for Alzheimer's

Probably the most devastating aspect of Alzheimer's is the continued loss of memory. Things, people, and places that used to be important slowly slip from the Alzheimer victim's grasp.

While no cure for this destructive disease is yet available, Genesis Health Ventures has developed an art therapy program designed to help people with Alzheimer's rediscover and hold on to parts of their past.

Based in Kennett, Pa., Genesis Health Ventures use art therapy and other techniques to help people with Alzheimer's cope with the physical, emotional, and psychological challenges of this disease. The company now offers programs in Connecticut, Florida, Maryland, and New Jersey.

In the art portion of the program, professional artists work one-on-one with Alzheimer victims, teaching them to express themselves through a variety of art forms, including painting, photography, quilting, sculpting, playing music, dancing, and playacting.

Usually, each Alzheimer artist's work reflects some aspect of the past he considered important. Because the hands sometimes remember what the mind has forgotten, this therapy gives victims of Alzheimer's a chance to recapture pleasures they enjoyed in the past.

One man, a former auto mechanic, took great pride and pleasure in sculpting clay into parts of an automobile engine, and then explaining to others how the various parts fit together. Before the therapy began, no one knew what his former profession had been.

Not only does this therapy give people with Alzheimer's an avenue for expressing themselves, they also get a sense of pride from the work they've done. Sometimes the finished works are displayed in local art galleries.

While many of the Alzheimer victims don't completely understand the purpose of the art exhibits, they take pleasure in knowing that others want to see their works, and briefly take a peek into a past that is almost forgotten.

*Source:*
Hospitals and Health Networks (69,14:55)

## Living well with Parkinson's

As devastating as a diagnosis of Parkinson's may seem, you don't have to let this disease control your life. A prognosis of Parkinson's is not a death sentence or a trial of torture. A healthy combination of diet, exercise, and other self-help measures can enable you to continue living a happy and productive life.

**Keep a diet diary.** Note which, if any, foods seem to worsen your condition. For example, some people with Parkinson's say spicy foods can set off violent, uncontrollable body movements. Other people, who have no problem with spicy foods, find that meats or other foods full of protein make them feel stiffer and move slower. If certain foods seem to affect you more than others, let your doctor know.

Work closely with your doctor or a dietitian to develop a food plan that helps your body make maximum use of any medication you're taking. For example: Some people respond better to medication if they eat protein only in the evening. Others respond better by eating a little protein in combination with carbohydrates at regular intervals throughout the day.

**Take any medicine for Parkinson's** 30 to 45 minutes before you eat, if possible, to prevent any protein in the meal from reducing the medicine's effectiveness.

**Exercise.** Regular exercise can keep muscles stiffened by Parkinson's mobile and strong. A big benefit of regular exercise is being able to move around easier.

A good exercise program may include a regular walk, simple stretching and strengthening exercises, and range of motion exercises, which moves joints through as many movements as possible to keep them flexible. Talk to your doctor or physical therapist about developing an exercise program to meet your particular needs.

Don't force yourself to exercise when you're having a particularly bad or "off" day. Exercise during these periods can be painful as well as dangerous.

**Laugh for the health of it.** Many people with Parkinson's, or Parkinsonians as they call themselves, find laughter a good way of coping. If you, too, can laugh at the sometimes preposterous positions Parkinson's puts you in, you'll find other people laughing with you instead of at you.

**Learn all you can about your condition.** Keep up with the latest research on Parkinson's. Have hope in research and future treatments because you never know when a new treatment will turn up that can help you deal with or even defeat this disease.

**Join a support group.** To find a support group in your area, call your local American Parkinson Disease Association Information and Referral Center. If there is no local office near you, call the APDA office in New York at 1–800–223–2732.

**Develop a strong working relationship with your doctor** as this disorder may require that you take several medicines at the same time. You should also let your doctor know if you're self-treating your condition with any alternative therapies, such as megadoses of vitamins. Sometimes these therapies may interfere with your regular medication or even make your condition worse.

**Use self-help aids,** such as jar openers, doorknob turners, and special silverware, to make daily living easier and less frustrating. For a complete guide to the different types of self-help aids available as well as a list of suppliers, call The American Parkinson Disease Association at 1-800-223-2732 and request the booklet "Be Independent! A Guide for People with Parkinson's Disease." If you prefer, you can write to them at 60 Bay Street, Suite 401, Staten Island, N.Y. 10301.

They have a number of other helpful pamphlets available as well, including:
*34 Helpful Hints to Ease the Daily Life of Parkinson's Disease Victims*
*Good Nutrition in Parkinson's Disease*
*Coping with Parkinson's Disease*
*Parkinson's Disease Handbook: A Guide for Patients and Their Families*
*Be Active! A Suggested Exercise Program for People with Parkinson's Disease*

**Sources:**
Coping with Parkinson's Disease, American Parkinson Disease Association, 60 Bay Street, Suite 401, Staten Island, N.Y. 10301
Parkinson's Disease Handbook: A Guide for Patients and Their Families, American Parkinson's Disease Association, 60 Bay Street, Staten Island, N.Y. 10301
Postgraduate Medicine (99,1:52)

# Recovery from Addictions

## The great debate about alcohol

From a nutrition point of view, alcohol is a big fat zero. It supplies plenty of calories, but no nutrients. However, alcohol is getting some good press these days, since current evidence points to moderate drinking as a factor that lowers the risk of coronary heart disease in some people.

What exactly is moderate drinking? According to the government-issued Dietary Guidelines for Americans, moderation means "no more than one drink per day for women and no more than two drinks per day for men."

So, what is one drink? Here are the equivalents:

◆ 12 ounces of regular beer (150 calories)
◆ 5 ounces of wine (100 calories)
◆ 1.5 ounces of 80-proof distilled spirits (100 calories)

On the flip side, levels of alcohol intake higher than moderate raise your risk of high blood pressure, stroke, heart disease, certain cancers, accidents, suicide, violence, birth defects, and death. Malnutrition is a risk because heavy drinkers tend to substitute alcohol for food. Too much alcohol can also damage the brain and heart and cause cirrhosis of the liver and inflammation of the pancreas.

There are certain people who should not drink alcohol under any circumstances. Here's the list:

◆ Children and adolescents.
◆ Women who are pregnant or trying to conceive. Fetal alcohol syndrome and other birth defects have been attributed to heavy drinking by the mother during pregnancy. A safe level of alcohol intake during pregnancy has not been established.
◆ People who plan to drive a vehicle or to take part in activities that require attention or skill. You can retain alcohol in your blood for two to three hours after a single drink.
◆ People taking any type of medicine. Alcohol can alter the effects of medications and make them toxic, and medicine can increase the harmful effects of alcohol.
◆ People who cannot restrict their drinking to moderate levels. Recovering alcoholics and those with alcoholism in their families should be especially careful.

If you do decide to drink alcoholic beverages, be sure that you understand the risks. Drink only in moderation, and only with meals. Never let your alcohol consumption put other people at risk.

*Source:*
*Nutrition and Your Health: Dietary Guidelines for Americans,* United States Department of Agriculture, United States Department of Health and Human Services, Washington, D.C., 1995

# How to tell if alcoholism is a problem

More than three million Americans over the age of 60 are alcoholics or have some kind of drinking problem. Unfortunately, most of them slip through the medical system without ever being diagnosed. Now the American Medical Association is recognizing the problem and has published guidelines to help doctors tell if an elderly person has a problem with alcohol.

Changes occur to your body as you age, so the amount of alcohol that didn't seem to bother you in younger years may be far too much now. An older person can slip into alcoholism without even knowing it.

Alcoholism in the elderly can be mistaken for dementia. A person may develop symptoms that go untreated because they are assumed to be a part of mental dysfunction or "normal" aging.

Doctors are being encouraged today to look closely for symptoms of alcoholism. If you drink alcohol, ask yourself the following questions to help determine if you have an alcohol problem.

♦ Do I ever feel bad or guilty about my drinking?
♦ Do I feel that I could cut down on my drinking?
♦ Do I feel annoyed when people criticize my drinking?
♦ Do I need a drink first thing in the morning to steady my nerves or get rid of a hangover?

If the answer to any of these questions is yes, seek your doctor's advice to determine whether you are an alcoholic. Alcoholism is a disease, and treating it can improve your quality of life.

*Source:*
*Medical Tribune for the Internist and Cardiologist* (36,19:2)

# Alcohol raises breast cancer risk

The controversy continues over the risks versus the benefits of alcohol consumption. If you are a woman who has consumed a drink a day over the course of a lifetime, a new study shows that you may have a 39 percent higher risk of breast cancer. The risk goes up to 69 percent if you consume two drinks a day, and to 230 percent for three drinks a day. Doctors are not sure of the reason, but alcohol may raise levels of the natural steroid *estradiol*, which is similar to the hormone *estrogen*. High levels of estrogen may put you at higher risk of breast cancer.

In this study, the alcohol in wine did not seem to be as harmful as that in beer and hard liquor. However, other studies have found no difference in the risk among alcoholic beverages.

Interestingly, women who gave up alcohol completely by around age 30 did not have a higher risk of breast cancer.

*Sources:*
*Medical Tribune for the Internist and Cardiologist* (36,13:25)
*Taber's Cyclopedic Medical Dictionary,* F.A. Davis Company, Philadelphia, 1989

## Alcohol-related injuries

Every year in the United States, an estimated 48,000 people die of alcohol-related injuries. If you consume even a moderate amount of alcohol, you are at higher risk of injury, according to a new study. Of course, your risk of injury increases with the number of drinks you consume.

The study investigated 350 people who went to emergency rooms for medical aid. Those who had consumed alcohol in the previous six hours more than doubled their risk of injury. Those who consumed four or more drinks six hours before injury were five times more likely to get hurt than those who consumed three or less.

Half of the people who drank alcohol prior to their injuries said they believed that alcohol played a role in their getting hurt.

*Sources:*
*Archives of Family Medicine* (1995,4:505)
*Medical Tribune for the Internist and Cardiologist* (36,13:3)

## New hope for alcoholics

Until recently, there had not been a new drug approved to treat alcoholism in the last 47 years. Now *Revia,* a drug previously approved for treating narcotic addiction, has been studied and approved for treating alcoholism. Revia works by counteracting the receptors in your brain that cause feelings of pleasure from drug or alcohol use.

In two studies sponsored by the National Institute of Alcohol Abuse and Alcoholism, Revia increased abstinence and reduced alcohol craving. In one of the studies, only 23 percent of the alcohol-dependent people who took Revia went back to drinking, compared to 54 percent who were given a placebo (a harmless, unmedicated pill). In the second study, alcohol-dependent people were about twice as successful in giving up their drinking when they took Revia.

Revia is not habit-forming and is not a drug that can be abused. However, your best chance of success is in using it along with a larger treatment plan for alcohol dependency, such as Alcoholics Anonymous.

If you have a problem with alcohol that has not responded to other treatments, check with your doctor to see if taking Revia might be helpful to you.

*Sources:*
*FDA Consumer* (29,3:2)
*Taber's Cyclopedic Medical Dictionary,* F.A. Davis Company, Philadelphia, 1989

## New link between smoking and pancreatic cancer

You already know about the link between smoking and lung cancer. The warning is even on packages of cigarettes. But do you know that smoking is also linked to other types of cancer?

The fifth most common fatal cancer in the United States today is pancreatic cancer. Because people who get it usually die so quickly, it has been difficult to pin down some of the suspected causes. Twenty-nine previous studies have linked smoking to pancreatic cancer, but they were usually based on interviews with surviving relatives of the cancer patients.

Now a new study, based on direct interviews, shows a definite link between smoking and cancer of the pancreas. In fact, smokers were found to have a risk of pancreatic cancer up to 70 percent higher than people who don't smoke. The longer you smoke, the higher your risk.

For people who had stopped smoking more than 10 years before the study, there was a significant decrease in risk. The authors of this study believe that 6,750 lives lost to pancreatic cancer would be saved in the United States each year if everyone stopped smoking.

*Source:*
*Nutrition Research Newsletter* (14,1:10)

## Improve your odds against breast cancer

For women, there are additional risks in smoking. A woman who has smoked for 30 years has a 60 percent higher risk of developing breast cancer than a woman who has not smoked. For a woman who has smoked for 20 years, the risk is 30 percent higher. Another serious concern for smokers is that they may develop breast cancer as much as eight years earlier than nonsmokers.

Breast cancer is occurring more frequently, even in young women. Smoking is a risk factor for cancer that you can definitely control and even eliminate. You can help beat cancer by not smoking.

*Source:*
*Medical Tribune for the Internist and Cardiologist* (36,25:17)

## Smoking may lead to diabetes

A new, long-term study of more than 41,000 men has shown a link between smoking and adult-onset diabetes. This kind of diabetes, called noninsulin-dependent diabetes mellitus, or NIDDM, is usually controlled by diet and weight management.

Doctors are not exactly sure how smoking is a factor in causing diabetes. They think it may damage the pancreas, where insulin is manufactured in your body. Previous studies have shown that smokers' bodies must work harder to produce enough insulin to lower glucose levels. It may be that, over time, the pancreas simply burns out. When your pancreas can no longer produce the amount of insulin your body needs, diabetes can be the result.

If you smoke, your risk of developing diabetes is much greater. If you smoke as many as 25 cigarettes a day, your risk is almost doubled.

*Source:*
*Medical Tribune for the Internist and Cardiologist* (36,7:18)

## Passive smoke puts heart health at risk

You would never knowingly expose your loved ones to poison, electrical shock, or any type of physical injury. But when you smoke around them, you are increasing their risk of developing lung cancer and heart disease. If you don't smoke, but someone in your family does, he's putting you at risk.

The link between passive smoking and lung cancer is already established. Now a new Australian study of young adults shows the connection between exposure to secondhand smoke and heart disease.

According to researchers, exposure to someone else's cigarette smoke contributes to heart disease by damaging the lining of your blood vessels. The vessels can't expand normally, and blood flow is slowed down. Even as little as one hour of exposure a day for three or more years can damage your blood vessels.

The authors of the study believe that up to 20,000 deaths of middle-aged and elderly nonsmokers a year are due to heart disease from secondhand smoke. There is a danger to healthy young people, as well. Exposure and damage to blood vessels can start when people are young.

If you're routinely exposed to passive smoke, the healthiest thing to do is remove yourself from the situation. Your body may be able to heal the damage, but the longer it goes on, the less the damage can be reversed.

If you're routinely exposing someone else to the health risks of your bad habit, quit smoking. Don't expose your loved ones to a dangerous situation that *you* can prevent.

*Source:*
*Medical Tribune for the Internist and Cardiologist* (37,3:3)

## Bypass smoking to help your heart

If you watch television, listen to the radio, or read magazines or newspapers, you know that smoking increases your risk of heart disease. According to a recent study, 34 percent of people who had coronary bypass surgery either continued to smoke or started again within five years.

People who had bypass surgery and kept smoking more than doubled their risk of suffering a heart attack and of needing more surgery within a year. People who had bypass surgery and were smoking five years later more than doubled their risk of heart attack, and tripled their risk of needing another bypass surgery. They also doubled their risk of developing angina (chest pain).

Chemicals from cigarette smoke cause arteries to harden and constrict. The damage to old and even new replacement blood vessels continues if you don't stop smoking.

Cigarettes may be the reason you needed the bypass surgery in the first place. Do yourself and your heart a big favor and throw your cigarettes out. You can start fresh with new, healthier habits and a healthier heart.

**Source:**
*Medical Tribune for the Internist and Cardiologist* (37,3:18)

# Dying to stay thin

Are you a smoker who's just dying to stay thin? You could literally be dying from your diet strategy, if you use smoking to control your weight.

For some people, using cigarettes is like taking an appetite suppressant. Nicotine changes your body's metabolism so that you burn calories faster, but the price of this kind of weight control is too high.

The average weight gain for a person who stops smoking is only five to 10 pounds. Smoking to avoid weight gain puts your heart, your lungs, and your whole life at risk.

If you're a smoker who wants to quit, but you're worried about weight gain, here are some strategies you can use to regain your health and maintain a desirable weight:

◆ Set a date to quit smoking, and write it on your calendar.

◆ Begin to eat a healthier diet before your "quit date."

◆ Start exercising regularly. It will make you feel better, help you control your weight, and give you the same tension relief that cigarettes do.

◆ Don't try to quit smoking and lose weight at the same time. That's too much deprivation at once. After you are a secure nonsmoker, you can begin to lose any weight you may have gained when you quit.

◆ Realize that quitting smoking is much more important to your health than the small amount of weight you might gain when you quit. If your dieting triggers cigarette cravings, remind yourself of this fact.

◆ Consider using a nicotine replacement product, such as gum or a patch, to help you quit. The gum seems to be better at preventing weight gain.

If you do gain weight when you quit smoking, don't blame yourself. Just realize that you are in control once again, instead of the cigarettes, and give yourself enough time to correct the problem.

**Source:**
*The Wall Street Journal* (March 4, 1996, B1)

# Stop low back pain: Say no to nicotine

If you are a smoker, you are more likely to suffer low back pain from an on-the-job injury. Researchers in North Carolina surveyed people with low back injuries to see what factors made their risk of injury higher.

They didn't find a relationship between low back pain and repetitive job tasks, leisure activities, specific jobs, or income. They did find that 50 percent of the smokers, but only 20 percent of the nonsmokers, had low back pain as a result of injuries on the job.

Researchers aren't sure what accounts for the higher percentage of injuries among smokers. But it could be due to nicotine's effect of decreasing blood flow to the discs in the spine.

Smokers with back pain were affected by the number of cigarettes they smoked. People who smoked more than a pack a day were more influenced by the pain to restrict their activities.

Some studies in the past have suggested that chronic smoker's cough may also be a factor in low back pain. This seems to be more of a problem if you are overweight.

No one wants to carry the burden of constant, nagging, low back pain. If you want to give your back a real "break," stop smoking.

*Source:*
*Arthritis Today* (9,5:16)

# 8 reasons to stop smoking right now

There's no doubt of the long-term ill effects of smoking. Each year, more than 350,000 people die from smoking-related illnesses in the United States. People who smoke have much higher risks of heart disease, lung and other types of cancer, stroke, diabetes, and many other health problems. So, the long-term advantages of quitting smoking are obvious, but are there any short-term payoffs for throwing away your pack of smokes? Definitely.

Here are some positive aspects of becoming a nonsmoker:

◆ You won't feel like an outcast. These days, smokers are often forced into awkward, embarrassing situations in order to indulge their habit. Some people will think better of you if you don't smoke.

◆ Your sense of taste and smell will return. Food will taste better, and you can really enjoy the aromas of delicate spring blossoms and crackling autumn fires.

◆ You'll smell better. You won't see people wrinkling their noses from the stale, smoky smell when you walk in the room.

◆ Your chronic smoker's cough will begin to get better, and may even disappear.

◆ You'll probably get fewer colds and other respiratory problems.

◆ You'll save money. If you smoke one pack a day, you're spending about $500 a year on cigarettes.

◆ You'll improve your cardiovascular fitness, endurance, and athletic performance.

◆ You'll simply feel better.

*Source:*
*Dr. Dean Ornish's Program for Reversing Heart Disease,* Random House, New York, 1990

## Snuff out smokeless tobacco

It can be as addictive as cigarette smoking, and terrible for your health. In the short term, smokeless tobacco can cause bad breath, stained and worn teeth, receding gums, and mouth sores. In the long run, it may cause cancer of the mouth.

The nicotine smokeless tobacco contains can also raise your blood pressure and cholesterol levels, and your risk of heart attack. So why would anyone want to keep using it?

Smokeless tobacco puts more nicotine into your bloodstream than cigarettes, and some people say it's even harder to quit than smoking. But you can quit.

Many of the previous tips for quitting smoking also apply to quitting smokeless tobacco. Here are some specific tips to help you break this harmful habit:

◆ Start now to cut down on the amount you chew or dip.
◆ Write down all the reasons you want to quit, and work out a plan for quitting.
◆ Set a date to quit, a week or two from today, and do it.
◆ Ask your family, friends, and doctor to support you.
◆ Throw away all your chewing tobacco or snuff before you quit.
◆ Identify the times when you will most want to use tobacco. Plan to avoid those situations for a while.
◆ Use chewing substitutes such as sugarless gum, sunflower seeds, beef jerky, or hard candy.
◆ Ask your doctor about using nicotine gum or the nicotine patch. If you use three or more tins or pouches a week, use tobacco within 30 minutes of waking up, or swallow tobacco juice, you are most likely to benefit from the gum or patch.
◆ Find healthy activities to keep your mind off smokeless tobacco when you have the urge to use it. Take a walk, relax with a hot shower, lift weights, or do aerobic exercise.
◆ Just as with smoking, if you slip up, don't despair. Make some adjustments to your plan, and you'll be successful next time.

*Source:*
American Family Physician (52,5:1433)

# 13 tips to help you stop smoking

If you really want to quit smoking, you can do it. Hundreds of thousands of people have "walked down this road" before you, and have successfully quit. Most people quit on their own, without a formal program, but excellent programs are available if you would rather use one. Local hospitals are usually a good place to look for them. You should quit when you feel you are ready, and on your own time schedule. Try to pick a time when you won't be particularly stressed by special events, such as a wedding or an important business project.

To successfully stop smoking, you have to have confidence in your ability to quit. Remember that quitting smoking is a process. Don't give up if you don't manage to quit the first time. Most people don't, but at least you've taken that important first step.

If you make it a daily habit to get connected with yourself and other people, manage your stress, and eat a low-fat diet, you'll find it easier to stop smoking. That's because these healthy habits and the unhealthy habit of smoking fill many of the same needs, making you feel less stressed and more in control, helping you keep your weight down, and improving your concentration and performance.

When you are ready to stop smoking, here are some tips to help:

- Read and listen to stories of other people who have successfully quit.
- Write down all the reasons you want to quit on index cards and carry them with you. When you are tempted to smoke, read the cards.
- Tell your family and friends you are quitting, and ask for their support.
- Keep lots of fresh fruits and veggies around to munch on.
- Avoid caffeine and alcohol. Caffeine may increase your craving for nicotine, and alcohol decreases your self-control.
- Indulge yourself in lots of warms baths or showers.
- Get rid of all your smoking stuff, like ashtrays and lighters.
- Have the inside of your car and the inside of your house cleaned to remove the residue of smoke.
- Reward yourself with something special every day.
- Keep your hands busy with a new or old hobby.
- When you feel like smoking, go for a long walk and take breaths of fresh air.
- Place a drop of clove oil on the back of your tongue when you feel the urge to smoke.
- Think of yourself as a nonsmoker.

*Source:*
*Dr. Dean Ornish's Program for Reversing Heart Disease,* Random House, New York, 1990

## It's never too late to quit smoking

There's a common misconception that, once you are older, it doesn't matter if you stop smoking or not; all the damage is already done. Actually, that's not true. All of the health problems associated with smoking in younger and middle-aged people also occur in older people.

In a study of 5,000 adults over the age of 64, doctors found that smoking causes hardening of the carotid artery. This is the artery that carries blood to your brain, so you want it to stay open and flexible. When it hardens and narrows, you have a much greater risk of stroke and heart attack. The risk increases with every cigarette you smoke.

The good news is that if you stop smoking, the situation will improve. Your body may even work to reverse the damage and prevent heart and blood vessel disease.

*Source:*
*Medical Tribune for the Internist and Cardiologist* (36,3:17)

# Caffeine: ways to curb your craving

That dark, steaming cup of morning magic has been brewing controversy since before the 16th century. Do coffee's enticing flavor and rich aroma mask a daily pick-me-up or a wicked addiction? Though research continues, there's no easy answer to this age-old question.

Caffeine is the most widely used mind-affecting drug in the world. One of every three people in the United States consumes at least the caffeine equivalent of two small cups of coffee (200 mg) a day. Caffeine is found not only in coffee, tea, and cola drinks, but also in products made with chocolate and coffee flavors, and many over-the-counter cold and headache remedies.

Dependence on caffeine is certainly not as serious a problem as alcohol, tobacco, or illegal drug addiction. But it is easy to develop a strong physical dependence on caffeine, and the effects can be harmful.

**Caffeine is a stimulant.** It increases your heart rate, respiration, blood pressure, secretion of hormones, elimination, and water loss. Within half an hour after you ingest it, caffeine goes to work on your body. It has a direct influence on your brain and nervous system, thought processes, and muscle coordination. After drinking coffee, you may feel more energetic, type faster, be more alert, be in a happier mood, and have better short-term memory. That all sounds pretty good.

There are some problems, however. When the caffeine wears off, it can leave you feeling more tired and droopy than if you hadn't had it at all. Then you need some more caffeine to feel better, and the cycle of increased energy followed by fatigue continues. Because caffeine stays in your body for three to four hours, it can cause insomnia, adding to fatigue. It also acts as a diuretic, and can lead to dehydration, which contributes to fatigue.

The real problems with caffeine come when you consume too much of it. You can experience nervousness, sweating, shaking, and inability to concentrate. Caffeine has been associated with irregular heartbeats and other heart problems, fibrocystic breast disease, cancer, and birth defects. Drinking one to three five-ounce cups of coffee a day, or the equivalent (300 mg of caffeine), shouldn't cause these problems. It's when you consume much more, as many people do, that the trouble can start.

**Curb your caffeine consumption.** If you are experiencing fatigue, nervousness, or other side effects, you may want to cut down on your caffeine consumption. If you just stop "cold turkey," you'll probably get headaches, fatigue, drowsiness, and depression — not a pleasant prospect. The best way to let go of caffeine is gradually. Here are some tips:

♦ Count the milligrams of caffeine that you are actually consuming each day. Aim for no more than 300 mg daily.

♦ Pay attention to serving size. A five-ounce cup of coffee contains about 100 mg of caffeine. A large mug of coffee may contain twice as much. A 12-ounce cola soft drink has about 38 to 46 mg of caffeine, but a 12-ounce glass of iced tea has approximately 67 to 76 mg of caffeine.

♦ Cut back your consumption of caffeine-containing drinks by one a day. Stay at this level for a while, then eliminate another one.

♦ Switch from brewed coffee to instant coffee, or to an instant blended with chicory or grain. These contain half as much caffeine as brewed coffee.

♦ If you brew your own coffee, make it with half decaf and half regular, gradually shifting the mix toward decaffeinated.

♦ Look for decaffeinated coffees and teas, but avoid ones that have had the caffeine extracted with the solvent methylene chloride, which may cause cancer. If you buy your coffee from a specialty store, you can ask how the coffee beans were decaffeinated.

♦ For an alternative to that second or third cup of coffee, try a grain-based beverage, such as Pero, Postum, or Cafix. If you're a tea drinker, try an herbal tea.

♦ If soft drinks are your source of caffeine, gradually switch to a caffeine-free version.

♦ Check your medicine cabinet for headache or cold remedies that contain caffeine. Substitute other brands that don't contain it.

If you choose to live completely without caffeine, it may take three or four days for the withdrawal symptoms to go away. But once they do, you'll wake up in the mornings with a clear head and a fresh start on the day — and no need for that steaming cup of brew.

*Sources:*
Dr. Dean Ornish's Program for Reversing Heart Disease, Random House, New York, 1990
Food & Mood, Henry Holt and Company, New York, 1995
Hamilton and Whitney's Nutrition Concepts and Controversies, West Publishing, New York, 1994
The Journal of the American Medical Association (272,13:1065)

## Coffee quantity is the key to heart health

Does drinking coffee increase your risk of heart problems? There's new information that should be reassuring if you're a woman whose coffee consumption is limited to just a few cups a day.

Researchers at the Boston University Medical School recently concluded a study comparing heart attack frequency and coffee consumption. This investigation of 858 women, with an average age of 60, found it's quantity that's critical. Drinking less than five cups (assume five ounces each) per day has little impact. After that, risk of heart attack increases significantly with each cup. In younger women surveyed, five or more cups per day led to a 70 percent increase in risk.

Coffee preparation (drip or boiled) was not considered. But researchers did find that women who mix decaf with regular coffee had only a moderately increased risk at even seven cups per day.

***Source:***
*American Journal of Epidemiology* (141,8:724)

# A Safe and Healthy Environment

## How to stay safe in cold weather

If you live in Florida and vacation on the beach, don't worry about frostbite. Otherwise, you need to learn the basics about preventing and treating this cold-weather hazard.

You don't have to be a cross-country skier to be at risk. In mere moments, frostbite can sneak up unexpectedly on outdoor exercisers, on homeowners who rush out barehanded for a quick outdoor repair job, and on motorists stranded on a lonely strip of road.

Take these precautions to protect your fingers, toes, ears, nose, and cheeks:

◆ Some doctors recommend that you smooth a thick layer of petroleum jelly or other ointment over any areas that will be exposed to the cold. That's a bad idea, a new study shows.

When young Finnish military men who trained outdoors in the winter applied protective ointments to their ears and faces, it actually increased their risk of frostbite. Ointments may give you a false sense of security about how well-protected your skin is.

◆ Wear mittens instead of gloves. Mittens allow you to place your thumb alongside your other fingers. That's warmer than having them separated.

◆ Protect your face with a scarf, or even better, a "neck gator" or "turtle fur" — a circle of soft material you can pull up over your mouth and nose. Southerners may have to visit a ski shop or a sports equipment store for special cold-weather clothing.

◆ Don't tie or buckle your boots too tightly. You don't want to block circulation. Wear heavy wool socks and insulated boots.

◆ Wait until you're indoors before enjoying a hot toddy. Alcohol can make you feel warm, but it actually causes you to lose body heat.

◆ Frostbite is painless, so ask a friend to watch your skin for signs. White or grayish-yellow patches mean danger.

◆ Every 15 minutes, check for sensation in your nose, cheeks, ear lobes, hands, and toes. At first, you'll feel a pins and needles sensation. Later, frostbitten areas will feel numb.

◆ Don't forget your ears. When researchers studied 900 soldiers with frostbite, they concluded that wearing scarves and hats with earflaps would have prevented most cases.

*Sources:*
*British Medical Journal* (311,7021:1661)
*U.S. Pharmacist* (21,1:31)

## Frostbite first aid

Have you heard that you should rub frostbitten skin with snow? That old-time remedy can cause permanent damage.

Never rub or massage, but do use your armpits, a warm companion, warm drinks, and warm clothes to thaw your frozen body parts. Remove rings, watches, and anything that is tight. Your goal is to get indoors as quickly as possible, without walking on a frostbitten foot if you can avoid it.

Once indoors, get in a warm (not hot) bath and wrap your face and ears with a moist, warm (not hot) towel. Don't get near a hot stove or heater, and don't use a heating pad, a hot water bottle, or a hair dryer. You may burn yourself before your feeling returns.

Your frostbitten skin will become red and swollen, and you'll feel like it's on fire. You may develop blisters. Don't break the blisters. It could cause scarring.

If your skin is blue or gray, very swollen, blistered, or feels hard and numb even under the surface, go to a hospital immediately.

*Sources:*
The American Medical Association Encyclopedia of Medicine, Random House, New York, 1989
U.S. Pharmacist (21,1:31)

## Winter exercise safety tips

Exercise is an important part of physical and mental fitness for many people, and they're not about to let a little thing like winter get in the way.

But there are a few hazards unique to winter. Remember these tips to keep yourself safe:

◆ Check the weather reports before you go out. Winter weather can change quickly, so pay attention to conditions. If you get stranded, stay in your car or a shelter until the weather clears or help arrives.

◆ When hiking or skiing, know your terrain and stick to established trails.

◆ Dress for the cold, not for fashion. Wear clothes in layers, and consider that the temperature will feel 30 degrees warmer than it is about 15 minutes into a brisk walk or jog. Polypropylene, a synthetic fabric, is best for undergarments. On top of that, you'll need a synthetic or wool sweater or a lightweight fleece jacket. Your outer garments should be windproof and water-repellent, preferably with flaps and zippers to let sweat and extra heat escape.

◆ You're more likely to injure cold muscles in the winter. Warming up, preferably indoors, is more important than at any other time of year.

◆ Buy shoes with treads so you won't slip on ice and snow. You'll need bigger shoes to make room for thick socks.

◆ Try to start out facing the wind. You'll be tired on the way home, but you'll have the wind at your back to help you along.

◆ Take it easy during the first couple of weeks of winter weather. Your body has to work to stay warm, so you don't want to push too hard at first.

Winter exercise has unique advantages, too. Your body burns more calories just staying warm, and you fight off winter depression by getting out in the sunlight. People in many parts of the country get to enjoy cross-country skiing — one of the best strengthening and aerobic exercises. Best of all, you get to eat more during the holidays without fighting the pounds after New Year's Day.

*Sources:*
*The Atlanta Journal/Constitution* (Dec. 23, 1993, E4)
*The Physician and Sportsmedicine* (19,12:19)

## Safer snow shoveling

Snow may look puffy and light, but anyone who's shoveled will tell you that it's hard work. Some experts say that shoveling snow is as strenuous as running 9 miles an hour. Any exercise that strenuous can put strain on your body. While snow shoveling may never be fun, these tips can help you make it safe:

◆ Warm up your muscles. Do a few stretches so that the work doesn't come as a shock to your system.

◆ Wear a hat, since you lose most of your body heat through your head.

◆ Clear snow as soon as it stops falling. Freshly fallen snow is lighter than snow that has melted slightly and become more heavy and dense.

◆ Push the snow out of the way when possible. It's less strenuous to push snow than to throw it with the shovel.

◆ Bend at the knee as you scoop the snow to reduce strain on your back and heart.

◆ Don't eat, drink, or smoke before shoveling. All of these put a strain on your heart.

*Source:*
*The Physician and Sportsmedicine* (21,1:177)

## The silent and deadly winter hazard

Carbon monoxide poisoning can happen at any time of the year, but the danger is greater during winter. Hundreds of people die from carbon monoxide poisoning every year, and thousands of others suffer dizziness, nausea, and convulsions. The gas is frightening because it's odorless and colorless.

One of the most dangerous wintertime sources of carbon monoxide is car exhaust. If you are stranded in your car and you keep the engine on in order to run your heater, make sure that the exhaust pipe is clear. If the pipe is clogged with snow or other material, the exhaust could back up into your car.

Any appliance in your home that burns fuel may emit carbon monoxide. Gas kitchen ranges and kerosene space heaters may emit carbon monoxide if they are not properly ventilated. Be sure to read the instructions on your heater to vent it correctly.

Signs of carbon monoxide poisoning include headache, mental confusion, and extreme tiredness. Get to fresh air and call for help immediately.

If you have several gas appliances, you may be constantly exposed to low levels of carbon monoxide. You may have mild health problems you haven't been able to explain, such as eye, nose, and throat irritation; headaches; fatigue; nausea; heart palpitations; or breathing problems.

If you suspect you may have low-level carbon monoxide poisoning, call the local office of your utility company and ask them to check your gas appliances. Many utilities provide this service for free.

Getting rid of gas appliances may be a wise move for you, especially if you are sensitive to chemicals or if you have asthma, angina, or emphysema. Many people begin to feel much better once they turn off their gas appliances.

*Sources:*
*The Columbia University College of Physicians & Surgeons Complete Home Medical Guide,* Crown Publishers, Inc., 1989
*The Nontoxic Home & Office,* Jeremy P. Tarcher, Inc., Los Angeles, 1992

# Hypothermia: the cold-blooded killer

You may have never heard of *hypothermia,* much less know how to get a handle on it. Here are the bone-chilling facts about this cold-blooded killer.

A body temperature below 96 degrees Fahrenheit is called hypothermia, and it doesn't take arctic temperatures to put you at risk. Even a moderately chilly air temperature of 60 degrees is low enough to trigger hypothermia if you aren't properly clothed.

The National Institute of Aging estimates that of the 28,000 people hypothermia kills every year, the largest percentage are older people. Some medicines, problems with circulation, and certain illnesses appear to reduce the older person's ability to resist hypothermia.

Even though cold temperatures are the most common cause of hypothermia, it may also be triggered by trauma, shock, or cancer. Symptoms can include confusion, low blood pressure, shallow breathing, sleepiness, slow reactions, slurred speech, and a weak heartbeat. Areas of the body that are normally warm, such as the armpits or groin, are cold. A person suffering from hypothermia may appear pale and puffy-faced.

Also, the older you get, the less sensitive you are to cold weather. So, your body temperature could drop to a dangerously low level without you really being aware of it. In addition, older people don't seem to shiver very effectively, which is one of the ways the body warms itself up.

Remember these tips to help prevent hypothermia:

◆ Dress in layers.
◆ Always wrap up well when going outside in the cold.
◆ Set your thermostat to at least a toasty 70 degrees during cold weather.
◆ Avoid extensive exposure to breezes and drafts.
◆ Keep plenty of nutritious food and warm clothes and blankets on hand to help ward off the winter chill. You'd also be wise to always wear a warm hat during these months.

◆ Eat hot foods and drink warm drinks several times during the day.

◆ Ask a family member or neighbor to check on you often.

◆ Ask your doctor if any medicine you're taking increases your risk of hypothermia. Some drugs make it difficult for your body to stay warm. Drugs that may cause a problem include barbiturates, benzodiazepines, chlorpromazine, reserpine, and tricyclic antidepressants.

If your temperature is 96 degrees or less or you feel sluggish or recognize that you're having trouble thinking clearly, see your doctor immediately or go to the nearest emergency room. It's better to be overly cautious than to die of a disorder that doesn't have to be deadly.

To help someone you suspect may be suffering from hypothermia, first call an ambulance. Then, lie close to the person and cover both of you with thick blankets. The hotter you get, the more warmth you can give the other person. Don't rub the person or handle him roughly. That can make things worse.

*Sources:*
*Accidental hypothermia: a winter hazard for older people*, National Institute on Aging, 1995
*Geriatrics* (51,2:23)
*The American Medical Association Encyclopedia of Medicine*, Random House, New York, 1989

# Deadly heat

Hundreds of adults and children get sick and even die when a heat wave hits. Heatstroke can strike quickly, too. At 11 p.m., one overweight 68-year-old woman who lived in a hot apartment complained of feeling ill. Her husband called for an ambulance. When she arrived at the emergency room at 11:38 p.m., she was pronounced dead of *hyperthermia* (high body temperature).

Older people are often more susceptible to heat-related illnesses because of body changes that occur with aging, such as poor circulation and inefficient sweat glands. Most of the people who die of hyperthermia every year are over age 50.

Here are some tips to help you head off hyperthermia:

◆ Ask your doctor if you're taking any medicines that could increase your risk. If you are, and he can't stop or change your medicine, be extra careful not to get overheated.

You should also take extra precautions if you have a heart, lung, or kidney disorder; if you have an illness that causes you to feel weak or have a fever; or if you have a certain condition that requires you to eat a special diet. For example, people with high blood pressure often must eat a low-salt diet, which can increase the risk of a heat-related illness.

◆ Stay out of the sun during the hottest part of the day, from noon until 4 p.m.

◆ Adjust yourself to high temperatures gradually, especially if you're not used to heat. At first, expose yourself to the heat for only short periods. Alternate the time you spend in the sun with some time spent in a cool place. As you adapt, you can adjust the amount of time you spend in the heat little by little.

- Don't take salt tablets even if you are sweating a lot, but do stop and rest often, especially if you're not used to hot weather. In about two weeks, your body will adjust to higher temperatures.

- Take advantage of air conditioning. The woman mentioned earlier had an air-conditioning system but had chosen not to use it. If you don't have air conditioning in your home, consider spending time in public places that provide air conditioning such as libraries, shopping malls, and theaters. For an air conditioner to be beneficial, it should be set below 80 degrees Fahrenheit.

  Fans can help when the humidity is low, but sitting in front of a fan actually can make heat stress worse when the temperature is above 100 degrees or when humidity is high. Instead, take cool (not cold) showers and baths. If you don't have access to air conditioning or fans, keep your home cool by closing your curtains or shades during the hottest part of the day, covering windows exposed to direct sunlight, cross-ventilating your home by opening windows on opposite sides of the house or apartment, and opening windows at night.

- Remember the old saying, if you can't stand the heat, stay out of the kitchen. When it comes to avoiding a heat-related illness, that adage offers some sound advice. Don't overheat your body by eating hot, heavy meals in very warm weather. Also, avoid using the oven as much as possible.

- Keep cool by wearing light-colored, loose-fitting clothes. Cotton fabrics are usually your best choice. Remember to take along a hat or umbrella to provide protective shade when you're outside.

- Drink extra water unless your doctor has instructed you not to. Some people who take *diuretics* (water pills) shouldn't make a change in how much they drink without talking to their doctors. You'll know you're drinking enough if your urine is a clear or very pale color.

- Maintain a normal weight. Being overweight or underweight increases your risk of hyperthermia.

- Don't drink alcoholic beverages or overeat. Alcohol is dehydrating, so cooling off with a cold beer can be dangerous. Choose caffeine-free drinks, juices, and plain water.

- Stay indoors on particularly hot or humid days, especially those days when an air pollution warning is in effect.

- Don't visit popular places when they're likely to be very crowded.

- Never leave anyone, animals included, locked in a hot car. The air gets so hot that the body is unable to cool itself through sweating.

Several days of high temperatures can lead to heat exhaustion, which can then progress to heatstroke. The first signs of heat exhaustion are fatigue; nausea; dizziness; headache; and cramps in the legs, arms, back, or stomach. You may have pale and clammy skin, a fast but weak pulse, and fast and shallow breathing.

If you have any of these symptoms, get in a cool place with your feet propped up. Take tight clothes off, get something to drink, and sponge off with lukewarm water. See a doctor once you are feeling a little better to rule out any risk of heatstroke.

If you have a body temperature above 104 degrees, call for emergency help immediately. You may be suffering from a heatstroke, which is often fatal if not treated quickly.

*Sources:*
*Hyperthermia: A Hot Weather Hazard for Older People,* National Institute on Aging, NIH Publication No. 89-2763, 1989
*Morbidity & Mortality Weekly Report* (44,25:465)
*The American Medical Association Encyclopedia of Medicine,* Random House, New York, 1989

# The big city hazard that strains unhealthy hearts

The stress of big city life may be risky for people with heart disease, but the big city pollution may be even worse. When pollution levels rise, so do hospital admissions for people with congestive heart failure.

In Chicago, Detroit, Houston, Los Angeles, Milwaukee, New York, and Philadelphia, carbon monoxide from car exhaust damages hearts. Pollution accounts for almost 6 percent of the hospitalizations for congestive heart failure in these seven cities.

Like people with breathing problems, people with heart problems should consider staying inside as much as possible on days when pollution is high. Hot, hazy summer days are usually high pollution days.

*Sources:*
*Medical Tribune for the Internist and Cardiologist* (36,21:14)
*Science News* (143,4:52)

# It's no fish tale: Seafood can be deadly

Marybeth Henner works the grocery store seafood counter in a small, inland Georgia town. Her surprise for the day is when anyone orders the catch of the day.

"The limit for most people around here is shrimp. Anything fancier or fishier than that, they don't trust," she says. Some shoppers just don't know how to cook fish, but others are afraid of eating something dangerous.

Striving for a low-fat, nutritious diet, people are eating more fish these days than ever before. But seafood carries its own special set of risks. Some fish is contaminated with chemical pollutants, such as polychlorinated biphenyls (PCBs), mercury, and dioxin. Mercury comes naturally from the earth, but large amounts are also released into the atmosphere and ocean when people burn wastes. High levels of any of these chemicals could cause cancer.

Fish can also be contaminated with deadly bacteria, or histamine can grow on fish that isn't kept cool enough after it's caught. Histamine can cause scombroid fish poisoning, a disease which gives you allergy-like symptoms that usually disappear on their own after a few days.

Fish should be a weekly part of a healthy diet, but only if you follow some precautions.

◆ Don't eat fish more than three times a week.

◆ Don't eat shark or swordfish more than once a week. More than that could give you mercury poisoning.

◆ Alternate between freshwater and saltwater fish.

◆ Eat smaller fish. They will have been exposed to chemical pollution for fewer years.

◆ Pregnant women should eat fish from inland waters only once a month. Toddlers, frail older people, and people with chronic or immune diseases shouldn't eat fish very often either.

◆ Three times a week should be the upper limit on tuna for children.

◆ Toxins collect in the fat, so get rid of as much fat as possible before cooking.

◆ Sportsmen who eat their catch may want to contact the nearest Environmental Protection Agency regional office to find out if they are fishing in polluted waters. You'll find EPA offices in Boston, New York, Philadelphia, Atlanta, Chicago, Dallas, Kansas City, Denver, San Francisco, and Seattle. Fishing is banned in some lakes and rivers, but even small, private lakes may not be safe. A lake near a farm or industrial area can be full of chemicals and fertilizers.

◆ Don't eat raw shellfish. The highest risk of a deadly infection comes from raw oysters and other shellfish. Raw oysters from the Gulf of Mexico can contain *Vibrio vulnificus* bacteria, which can cause diarrhea, serious illness, and even death. Cooking the oysters kills the bacteria. Oysters harvested between April and October are the most likely to be contaminated.

People with certain health conditions should never eat raw oysters. These conditions include:

◆ Stomach problems. You need a healthy digestive system to fight the *Vibrio* bacteria. If you take antacids regularly, don't eat your oysters raw.

◆ Liver disease, diabetes, cancer, or immune disorders, including infection with HIV.

◆ Hemochromatosis, an inherited condition that causes you to absorb too much iron from your food.

◆ Long-term steroid use (as for asthma or arthritis).

◆ Moderate to heavy alcohol use. You shouldn't eat raw oysters if you normally drink two to three alcoholic drinks a day. That much alcohol can cause liver disease, which can have absolutely no signs or symptoms. If you have liver disease, you are almost 200 times more likely to die from a *Vibrio vulnificus* infection.

You shouldn't be afraid of seafood if you keep it cold, clean, and cooked.

Enjoy the health benefits of fish often; just don't go overboard.

*Sources:*
*Archives of Family Medicine* (2,2:210)
*FDA Consumer* (28,7:5 and 29,6:2)
*Medical Tribune* (34,1:21 and 34,3:16)

## The bacterial breeding ground in your kitchen

You'll want to grab your broom handle and scoop your dirty dishcloth into the kitchen trash can after you read these statistics.

When a team from Arizona nabbed dishcloths and sponges from 100 homes in five U.S. cities, they found disease-causing bacteria in 70 percent of them. One out of every five dishcloths and sponges contained *Salmonella* and *Staphylococcus* bacteria — two of the major causes of food poisoning.

If you're like many cooks, you will use a dishcloth to wipe up an area where you've handled raw meat and then simply rinse the cloth out. In a few hours, millions of bacteria can grow in that cloth. When you use it again, you spread the bacteria everywhere.

Your best bet after handling raw meat is to clean up with paper towels and then wash your hands thoroughly. If you use a dishcloth or sponge, put it in the dishwasher along with the dirty dishes. The hot water will kill any bacteria in the cloth.

*Source:*
*Food Safety Notebook* (November/December 1995)

## Overreactions to radioactivity rouse needless fears

First they were zapping chicken and wheat. Now they're exposing strawberries, potatoes, herbs, pork, oysters, and more to radioactivity. Irradiated food is labeled and stamped with an international logo (a circle above two petals), so you could avoid it if you wanted to. However, eating irradiated food just seems to be a shockingly bad idea. It's actually a healthy choice.

Exposing your food to radioactivity is a safe way to get rid of *Salmonella* and other harmful bacteria. The FDA approved food irradiation several years ago because it kills off infection-causing bacteria, worms, insects, and other disease carriers. It also keeps meat, fruit, and vegetables from spoiling as quickly.

X-rays or gamma rays pass through the food and damage the genetic material of any bacteria existing in it. After being zapped, the organisms aren't able to survive or multiply. Medical equipment is sometimes sterilized with the same process.

Of course, the food doesn't become radioactive when it's zapped (just as you don't become radioactive when you are X-rayed), but the rays do break down some substances in the food. The breakdown causes the food to lose a few vitamins and causes a small amount of chemicals to form. That's unfortunate, but you do the same thing when you cook — you create a few chemicals, lose a few vitamins, and kill many, many harmful organisms.

People still get sick and even die from food-borne illnesses, but thanks to processes like pasteurization and irradiation, you're much safer than you used to be.

**Sources:**
*American Family Physician* (47,5:1064) ·
*Food Irradiation: Toxic to Bacteria, Safe for Humans,* a reprint from *FDA Consumer,* Food and Drug Administration, HFI-40, Rockville, Md. 20857
*Journal of Food Protection* (58,2:213)

## Furry friends can be disease-carriers

Little Timmy and the Lone Ranger aren't the only ones who know that pets can be life savers. Case after documented case has shown that pets and people are really good for each other. Nationally, it's estimated that 60 percent of Americans share their homes with a pet of some kind, and many people consider their animals to be part of the family.

But just as children can give parents their contagious diseases, pets can pass along serious — even life-threatening — diseases to their human keepers. Fortunately, most can be easily controlled and treated, and with some common sense and care, you can enjoy years of affection and happiness with your pet.

Since pet-borne infections and parasites are often found in the urine and feces of animals, or on their fur, it's a smart idea to wash your hands after handling your pet or cleaning up their accidents. Don't play rough with pets because they can pass diseases along in bites and scratches.

Also, keep your dog from licking you in the face. Use shampoos and dips to keep your pet free from ticks and fleas that can carry disease.

This is only a sampling of the diseases, microorganisms, and fungi that domestic pets can transmit to humans:

**Roundworm.** Virtually all puppies are born with roundworm, a parasite that passes from the body with their feces. Children tend to pick it up from playing in contaminated dirt. Symptoms include fever, headache, cough, and poor appetite.

**Rabies.** Worldwide, people are most commonly infected with this fatal disease by unvaccinated dogs. Other sources include raccoons, skunks, bobcats, cats, and bats. You can also be infected if you have an open wound that comes in contact with an infected animal's saliva.

If you have been bitten by an animal and you don't know whether it has been vaccinated, clean the wound immediately with running water, soap or detergent, and a solution of iodine or alcohol. Then seek medical attention.

**Strep throat.** Some kids just seem to always have a sore throat that turns out to be *Streptococcal* bacteria. Where's it coming from? Well, if Fido's licking them good-night, he may be the culprit. Dogs can be carriers of the bacteria.

**Scabies.** Dogs can carry the scabies mite, which can show up as an intensely itchy rash. Over-the-counter drugs and lotions can treat the human; the dog will need to be dipped. Wash the infected person's clothes and bedding in hot water and detergent.

**Cat scratch fever.** Rarely serious, cat scratch fever still can be uncomfortable. Symptoms include a sore at the site of the scratch that's slow to heal and swollen, tender lymph nodes one to three weeks later.

**Ringworm.** Ringworm is a skin disease caused by a fungus. It's most often carried by cats, especially long-haired kittens, but it also can be passed on by dogs, horses, and cows.

Children commonly contract ringworm, which typically appears as a red, scaly lesion on exposed skin, particularly the scalp.

**Toxoplasmosis.** Cats usually get this disease from eating small rodents that carry it. They pass it on through their feces, which people may come in contact with in the litter box. Pregnant women and people with weakened immune systems shouldn't risk exposure by cleaning litter boxes because they can get a more severe form of the disease. This is especially serious in pregnancy, because it can cause miscarriage, birth defects, and premature birth. Symptoms of toxoplasmosis include sore throat, cough, congestion, skin rash, fever, headache, and swollen glands.

**Swimming pool granuloma.** This condition comes from contact with tropical fish aquariums, rather than human swimming pools. It usually appears as lesions on the fingers or hands, normally at the site of a cut or scratch.

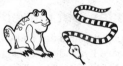

**Salmonella.** Turtles lead the list of animals that can carry salmonella, which can have serious consequences for very young children, the elderly, and people with immune system disorders. Symptoms include vomiting, diarrhea, and severe cramping. Dogs, cats, birds, mice, lizards, snakes, chicks, and ducklings can also carry salmonella.

**Edwardsiella** is an organism similar to salmonella in its symptoms, and it is found in snakes, turtles and toads.

**Plesiomonas,** known as "mouth rot disease" in snakes, can be transmitted to humans, leading to severe intestinal problems.

**Psittacosis** usually is contracted by inhaling contaminated dust from a bird's cage. Birds that can carry it include parrots, macaws, canaries, parakeets, pigeons, turkeys, ducks, and chickens. Symptoms include fever, sore throat, cough, headache, vomiting, loss of appetite, and weakness.

## Tick-borne diseases

**Lyme disease** is transmitted by deer ticks, which pick it up from white-tailed deer, field mice, and other wild animals whose bodies are walking factories for a bacterium called *Borrelia burgdorferi*. If the tiny ticks hop a ride on a passing dog, they and their bacteria can find their way into your home.

Lyme disease can be extremely serious in its later stages. The first sign is usually a small, red pimple that expands to form a ring-shaped rash like a bull's-eye. It may be accompanied by flu-like symptoms, shortness of breath, and a rash. Early treatment with antibiotics is necessary for a full recovery.

**Rocky Mountain spotted fever** typically is transmitted by the American dog tick. Symptoms include headache, fever, and a skin rash. Like Lyme disease, it must be caught early and treated successfully with antibiotics to ensure recovery.

Obviously pet owners the world over love their pets and depend on them for love and affection. But just to make sure you don't get too much of a good thing, you might want to check with your veterinarian about testing and treatment for some of these diseases. And save the kisses for your spouse.

*Sources:*
*American Family Physician* (41,3:831)
*FDA Consumer* (24,3:28)
*Morbidity and Mortality Weekly Report* (41,42:794)
*The Western Journal of Medicine* (158,6:619)

## When this bug bites, get immediate care

If you have come in contact with a tick and you get a rash, fever, headache, or muscle pains, you may have Lyme disease. Go to the doctor immediately.

The longer you wait before taking antibiotics, the more likely you are to suffer long-term effects, like memory loss; difficulty concentrating; constant tiredness; joint pain; and numbness, tingling, and burning pain in your hands and feet. You may be able to avoid these long-term symptoms if you are treated right away.

Some doctors are afraid of "overtreating" for Lyme disease. They don't want to hand out antibiotics if you don't really have the tick-borne illness. That's normally a good attitude, but in the case of Lyme disease, it may be better to be safe than sorry.

*Sources:*
*Annals of Internal Medicine* (121,8:560)
*Arthritis Today* (9,5:9)

# Nature's own pest control

Don't let insects pester you into spending money and putting dangerous toxins in your environment. A sparkling clean house discourages most pests, and for the persistent ones, try safe home remedies.

**Peppermint** turns away mice. They don't like the smell.

**Cloves or red pepper** keeps ants away.

**Salt water** makes fleas flee.

**Fresh bay leaves** in your cupboards will keep pests away for up to a year.

**Beer** knocks out garden slugs and snails. Sink a pie pan or lid of a jar into the ground and fill it with beer.

**Plain boric acid** is the main ingredient in roach-control products.

*Source:*
*How to Pinch a Penny 'Til It Screams,* Avery Publishing Group, Garden City Park, N.Y., 1994

# Nontoxic housecleaning

The most hazardous place in your home may be your cleaning supply cabinet. Ammonia, oven cleaners, furniture polish, scouring powders, disinfectants, glass cleaners — all these carry warning labels that describe the dangers of swallowing the substances or getting them in your eyes.

They don't warn you about the harm you may be causing your body by simply exposing yourself to the toxic substances for years. Some people are sensitive to the fumes and the ingredients, but even if you aren't, your body could react someday with cancer, heart disease, lung problems, or immune system disorders.

To be on the safe side, clean with natural, nontoxic ingredients. These homemade cleansers are less expensive than most commercial cleansers, too. The five basic ingredients you'll need are baking soda, washing soda (also called sodium carbonate or sal soda; available in the detergent section of some stores), borax (a mineral that kills mold and germs), salt, and white vinegar. You'll also need some lemon juice, toothpaste, herbs, and liquid soap (not detergent).

**To kill mold and disinfect surfaces,** mix 1/2 cup of borax with a gallon of hot water. Add some sprigs of fresh thyme. Steep for 10 minutes and strain. After the mixture cools, store it in plastic spray bottles.

**To clean floors,** mix 1 cup of white vinegar with 2 gallons of hot water. Greasy floors may need 1/4 cup washing soda and 1 tablespoon of liquid soap.

**To clean an oven,** sponge a paste of baking soda and hot water onto the stains. You'll have less trouble if you clean immediately after a spill.

**To clean copper pans,** sprinkle pans with coarse salt. Rub the salt into the stains with a lemon cut in half.

**To clean silver**, put a sheet of aluminum foil in your sink, fill it with very hot water, and add a handful of salt. The foil will magnetize the tarnish away. This method works even better if you can put the silver items in a pot on the stove and bring the water to a boil.

**To clean wooden furniture**, dab white toothpaste on water stains. After the paste dries, buff off with a soft cloth. Instead of using toxic furniture polishes, you can use plain mineral oil.

**To clean windows**, mix 1 cup of vinegar with 4 cups of hot water.

**To clean out drains**, mix vinegar and lemon juice with hot water. Freeze vinegar and lemon juice into ice cubes to clean the garbage disposal.

*Sources:*
*How to Pinch a Penny 'Til It Screams*, Avery Publishing Group, Garden City Park, N.Y., 1994
*Martha Stewart Living* (1991,1:32)
*The Nontoxic Home and Office: Protecting Yourself and Your Family From Everyday Toxics and Health Hazards*, Jeremy P. Tarcher, Los Angeles, 1992

# Hidden nursery hazard

Pregnant women living in a home built before 1978 should never, never strip paint or wallpaper in a future nursery unless they are absolutely sure that there's no danger from an old layer of lead paint.

Developing babies are extremely vulnerable to lead poisoning, and the government didn't ban lead paint until 1978. Paint manufacturers removed most of the lead in the 1950s. Test kits you can use at home will reveal the lead content of paint, pottery dinnerware, and water.

*Source:*
*The Nontoxic Home and Office: Protecting Yourself and Your Family From Everyday Toxics and Health Hazards*, Jeremy P. Tarcher, Los Angeles, 1992

# Detoxifying dry cleaning

Did you know that the Environmental Protection Agency lists fumes from slightly damp dry-cleaned items as a common indoor air pollutant?

Dry-cleaned items can be damp because dry cleaning isn't really dry. Clothes are washed with a detergent and a solvent that isn't absorbed by the fabric instead of with detergent and water.

All you have to do to avoid the hazardous fumes is to remove the plastic covering immediately and hang the dry-cleaned item in an unoccupied room with open windows until the solvent evaporates. In cold weather, this could take up to a week for a large item. To speed up the process, put a space heater in the room, open the windows for ventilation, and close the door.

Another way to avoid the fumes is to avoid dry cleaning. Manufacturers sometimes put "dry clean only" on the labels to protect themselves from complaints when people wash an item incorrectly.

Linens and cottons can be washed in the washing machine, dried on medium heat, and taken out while still damp to prevent wrinkles. Even silk can be hand washed in very cold water with mild soap. Don't rub the silk, and let it drip dry. Wash big comforters, sleeping bags, and down jackets in your bathtub with warm water and a mild soap instead of paying a fortune to your dry cleaner. Dry them on low heat.

**Source:**
*The Nontoxic Home and Office: Protecting Yourself and Your Family From Everyday Toxics and Health Hazards,* Jeremy P. Tarcher, Los Angeles, 1992

## Healthier lawn mowing

Concerned about pollution when you mow the lawn? You should be. Mowing for a half-hour typically contributes as much smog to the environment as driving a car 172 miles. And you're right there, breathing it all in.

The government is placing stricter standards on lawn mowers at this moment. That's going to make mower prices jump by the turn of the century.

People with small lawns should consider electric mowers. They are inexpensive (only $100 to $300), lighter, quieter, and easy to start. Two considerations: You'll need a really long, sturdy extension cord, and you'll have to mow your lawn regularly because electric mowers don't have much power. They'll give a slightly uneven cut and even choke down if your grass is high.

Electric mowers give you freedom from fuel and exhaust fumes, and they even have a better repair history than regular mowers.

People with country-club-size lawns who need a riding mower to get the job done should make sure they wear a mask.

**Source:**
*Consumer Reports 1995 Yard and Garden Equipment Buying Guide,* Consumer Reports Books, Yonkers, N.Y., 1995

## Danger in a dome

The next time you catch an event at a domed stadium, make sure you don't also catch an infection.

After the 1991 International Special Olympic Games in Minneapolis-St. Paul, 16 people came down with the measles. Minnesota hadn't had a measles case in four months before the games.

Any time people are gathered in an enclosed area, the risk of a spreading infection is increased. The risk is greater if the event is international since some other countries don't have strict immunization policies.

If you are behind on your immunizations, you are taking a risk when you go to any large gathering. Keep your vaccine shots current and use good hygiene to protect yourself from germs.

**Source:**
*Journal Watch* (15,7:57)

## Sick building syndrome

Do you get sick every time you go to work? It may not be that you hate your job or your co-workers; you may have sick building syndrome. Poor ventilation may contribute to this syndrome, which usually occurs in office buildings.

Symptoms of sick building syndrome include:

◆ Listlessness or fatigue
◆ Headache
◆ Dizziness
◆ Nausea
◆ Sensitivity to odors
◆ Eye irritation and nasal irritation or congestion

These symptoms could be caused by a number of things. However, if the symptoms only occur when you're in a particular building or area, you should suspect sick building syndrome. If others who work in the same building have the same complaints, the problem should be brought to the attention of someone in charge. The building should be inspected for problems with ventilation, heating and air conditioning systems, and indoor pollutants. A very low humidity level in a building can also dry out membranes and cause irritation.

*Source:*
*Indoor Air Pollution, An Introduction for Health Professionals,* American Lung Association, the American Medical Association, the U.S. Consumer Product Safety Committee, and the U.S. Environmental Protection Agency, 1994

## Asbestos and radon dangers

There's no place like home, but the air in your home could be anything but sweet. It may harbor dangerous indoor pollutants. Asbestos and radon, both known cancer-causing agents, may lurk unnoticed in your house.

**Asbestos.** Formerly used for fireproofing, asbestos may still be found in older heating systems, insulation, floor and ceiling tiles, and shingles in some older houses. As asbestos ages, it breaks down into tiny fibers that float through the air of your home, and you inhale them. Over a period of years, these fibers in your lungs can cause lung cancer as well as other respiratory problems. If you smoke, breathing asbestos increases your risk of lung cancer five times, because of the way cigarette smoke interacts with the asbestos. Construction or environmental officials can tell you if there is asbestos in your home and what steps you should take to protect yourself.

**Radon.** This naturally-occurring radioactive gas ranks right behind smoking as the leading cause of lung cancer. Smokers have a 10 to 20 times higher risk of getting lung cancer from radon exposure than nonsmokers. A recent study claimed that low levels of radon didn't cause cancer as much as previously thought. However, according to the National Safety Council, the study was flawed because there were only 1,500 participants, and there should have been at least 10,000 to draw any serious conclusions.

Radon is odorless, colorless, and tasteless, so it is difficult to detect. Test kits may be ordered through the mail or purchased at hardware or department stores. These measuring devices should be state-certified or have the label "Meets EPA Requirements." The EPA estimates that about 6 million homes may have dangerous levels of radon. If you discover that your home is one of them, get a professional to seal foundation cracks and holes and vent the radon-contaminated air from beneath your house.

*Sources:*
*Indoor Air Pollution, An Introduction for Health Professionals,* American Lung Association, the American Medical Association, the U.S. Consumer Product Safety Commission, and the U.S. Environmental Protection Agency, 1994
National Safety Council's radon hotline (1–800–557–2366)

# Electromagnetic fields and cancer scare

Given a choice, most people wouldn't buy a house next to a power line. That's probably wise, but don't be too concerned about the dangers of electromagnetic fields (EMFs). The facts are:

◆ The latest studies of children and electrical workers have not been able to prove a connection between EMFs and cancer.

◆ Recent laboratory studies have not shown that EMFs cause cancerous changes in cells.

Unfortunately, in spite of study findings, some experts are still sitting on the "electrical" fence. They point out that exposure to EMFs hasn't been proven absolutely safe, either.

Most of the worry over EMFs stems from a few studies which link the magnetic fields with leukemia in children. Several other studies show a higher risk of cancer, such as brain cancer, in electric utility workers.

Recently, the world's largest group of physicists, The American Physical Society in Maryland, looked at more than 1,000 papers on EMFs and interviewed magnetic field experts. The Society concluded that fears over EMFs are groundless. They point out that the earth's magnetic field is about 500 milligauss, while a nearby power line can radiate fields of only five to 40 milligauss.

*The Journal of the National Cancer Institute* published a new study that said breast cancer was higher among women working in electrical jobs, but they also published an article pointing out all the problems in the study and calling the EMF/cancer link "unproven."

According to two groups of Scandinavian researchers who recently studied thousands of children, power lines don't pose a threat of childhood cancer.

Some health newsletters you may read try to upset you by claiming that the government is ignoring the dangerous possibilities of EMFs. The newsletters claim that the government of Sweden is regulating EMFs and relocating high tension power lines away from schools. Actually, Swedish officials have clearly stated recently that they are doing neither of these things.

Studies are still being done on EMFs, and researchers may prove someday that exposure to the electricity given off by power lines, appliances, computers, telephones, etc., is hazardous.

A lifetime of exposure to home appliances may turn out to be more dangerous than exposure to power lines. At a distance of one foot, home appliances can radiate magnetic fields from about one to 280 milligauss. However, studies linking home appliances to cancer have also had weak and inconsistent results.

Until we hear more from EMF researchers, it's better to be safe than sorry. There's certainly no need to panic about your exposure to electromagnetic fields, but there's no need to buy a house next to a power line, if you can avoid it.

***Sources:***
*American Family Physician* (4,2:928)
*Cancer Biotechnology Weekly* (May 29, 1995)
*FAQs on Power-Frequency Fields and Cancer,* Version: 3.3.2, Maintainer: jmoulder@its.mcw.edu, Last modified: Dec. 12, 1995
*Journal of the National Cancer Institute* (86,12:885,921)
*Occupational Hazards* (57,3:26)
*Science News* (147,20:308)
*The Atlanta Journal/Constitution* (Feb. 7, 1996, B3)

# First-Aid
# Basics

## When to do CPR before calling 911

If you're certified in *cardiopulmonary resuscitation* (CPR), no doubt you know that in an emergency situation involving injuries you're supposed to call 911 before beginning CPR.

Surprisingly, several recent studies suggest that may not be the best course of action in all cases. According to Seattle researchers, if you are dealing with a child or a young adult under the age of 30, you should spend those first crucial moments trying to clear the airway and resuscitate the accident victim.

Old American Heart Association (AHA) recommendations were based on studies of people age 60 or older who often suffer from *ventricular fibrillation* (uncoordinated quivering contractions of the heart), which can lead to cardiac arrest and sudden death.

Younger accident victims are more likely to have their cardiac arrest triggered by a blocked airway than by ventricular fibrillation. For this reason, researchers suggest that when treating young people it is more important to clear the airway and perform one minute of CPR before calling 911. That one minute of CPR may be all it takes to prevent cardiac arrest and possible damage to the nervous system. Another study revealed that children who receive CPR before reaching the hospital are much more likely to survive than children who don't.

However, a spokesperson for the AHA noted that the organization won't consider changing its official CPR guidelines until more studies are done.

*Source:*
Medical Tribune for the Internist and Cardiologist (36,10:21)

## Better care for burns

Scalding coffee, the shining sun, an iron ready to press — in first aid terms, these all boil down to burns.

Serious burns — a blistering burn bigger than your palm or a deep, dry, white or charred-looking burn — should send you straight to the doctor. Otherwise, you can heal your burn yourself, with the proper care.

Common sense tells you what to do first. As soon as you peel your finger off the red-hot stove burner, cool the burn down (with water, not ice). Hold a wet towel soaked in cool water to the burn for 10 to 30 minutes. The cool compress will help prevent pain, scarring, and swelling and will generally make your burn heal faster. If it's a chemical burn, run tap water over it for several minutes.

After cooling the burn, clean the area with mild soap and water. Leave any blisters alone. They are protecting your skin.

The best ointment to put on the burn is also one of the cheapest — bacitracin (brand name, Baciguent). This antibiotic ointment will help prevent infection. Most people use silver sulfadiazine, but it is more expensive than bacitracin, and it may even slow healing.

Many of the ointments you can buy combine bacitracin with other antibiotics like neomycin, polymyxin, and tetracycline. These are fine, too.

Loosely place a big piece of gauze over the ointment, and hold it in place with some surgical paper tape, such as Dermicare or Micropore. Clean the burn gently and reapply the dressing once a day, or whenever it gets wet or dirty. The gauze shouldn't stick to the burn, but if it does stick, soak it in warm water and remove it very slowly. You don't want to pull off any healing skin.

If the burn is oozing, you'll need some kind of absorbent pad or all-purpose dressing over the gauze. Some drainage is normal, but it should never contain pus or smell bad. Look for redness, swelling, pink fluid, pus, and odor when you change the bandage.

Two new products you can buy to cover burns and wounds cost a little more than your traditional bandages, but they are well worth it. These are *transparent film dressings* and *hydrogels*.

Transparent film dressings can be used by themselves to protect minor burns, and they are waterproof. You can leave the same bandage on for up to seven days. Some brand names are Bioclusive, Tegaderm, Opsite, and Vigilon.

Hydrogels (Nu-Gel, Duoderm, Curasol, Intrasite, and others) are for slightly more serious wounds and burns. They are moist, and they help decrease swelling, speed up healing, and relieve pain. You can store them in the refrigerator for extra pain relief. You'll need a transparent film dressing to hold the hydrogel in place.

Burns tend to heal slowly, but you can speed up the process if you eat a healthy diet, drink plenty of water, and don't smoke. You'll probably know your skin is healing when it starts to itch. Don't scratch it. As soon as the wound is closed, you can use Vaseline Intensive Care Lotion or perhaps a lotion containing urea to help stop the itching.

Newly healed skin is more sensitive to windburn, frostbite, and sunburn, so use plenty of sunscreen on the area. Burning it again could permanently damage your skin.

**Sources:**
*Postgraduate Medicine* (97,5:151)
*U.S. Pharmacist* (20,8:41)

# A deadly dose of poison ivy

*Poison Ivy*          *Poison Oak*

You know how irritating an accidental encounter with poison ivy can be, but did you also know that this plant is a potential killer?

Not many people do, but the fact is that *urushiol*, the irritating oil of poison ivy and poison oak, remains potent once the actual plant has died and dried up.

Not even fire destroys urushiol. In fact, poison ivy becomes so toxic when burned that it ought to carry a warning label.

Three days after burning brush and leaves outdoors, a 22-year-old man was admitted to a hospital in Philadelphia. He was coughing up blood and had a red rash. His condition worsened to the point that he required a respirator to continue breathing. Despite medical treatment, the man died.

Doctors concluded that the man died of *adult respiratory distress syndrome* (ARDS), a lung disorder that was triggered when he inhaled urushiol fumes from some burning poison ivy.

Although this is the first known report linking inhalation of urushiol with deadly lung damage, researchers believe that such a reaction is possible in people who are highly sensitive to the plant.

People suffering with ARDS find it more and more difficult to breathe, which leads to labored and rapid breathing and a dangerous deficiency of oxygen in the blood. Sufferers may turn blue and, if no treatment is given, may eventually die.

To protect yourself, be careful when burning wood or using lawn equipment which may have the dried oil on it. It can cause the traditional rash or the even more dangerous ARDS. Only 25 to 50 percent of the adults who develop this disorder survive. The ones who do survive may be left with permanent lung damage.

Often, people don't link any rashes they develop in winter with poison ivy because the plant is not commonly seen then. However, urushiol can linger on unused fireplace logs, gardening gloves, and tools for many months. People sometimes also develop the poison ivy rash after coming in contact with the family pet after it has wandered through a patch of poison ivy.

You should wash your skin immediately with soap and water if you are exposed to poison ivy. Sponging the affected area with a little rubbing alcohol may also help.

If you develop symptoms of ARDS, especially if you know you've recently been exposed to poison ivy, seek emergency medical care immediately, and let them know that you may be having a severe reaction.

*Sources:*
*Complete Guide to Symptoms, Illness & Surgery,* The Berkley Publishing Group, New York, 1995
*The American Medical Association Encyclopedia of Medicine,* Random House, New York, 1989
*The Journal of the American Medical Association* (274,4:358)

## Stop the itch before it starts

A new lotion looks like it may be able to give gardeners protection from the annoying plant that plagues every outdoor person — poison ivy.

A recent study revealed that a common ingredient in many cosmetic products, called *quaternium-18 bentonite*, may be just what you need to avoid the itchy side effects of an unwanted encounter with poison oak or ivy. As anyone who's ever suffered from poison ivy knows, prevention is a much better solution to this problem than treatment.

The irritating oil responsible for causing the common reaction to poison oak or ivy is called *urushiol*. The new lotion protects people by blocking the absorption of urushiol.

Although quaternium-18 bentonite has traditionally been used as a thickener in sunscreens and lotions, earlier, smaller studies suggested that it might offer protection against poison ivy. The most recent study of this common cosmetic ingredient offers additional support that quaternium-18 bentonite may be a promising poison ivy preventive.

A group of researchers, headed by Dr. James G. Marks, professor of medicine in the division of dermatology at Hershey Medical Center in Pennsylvania, tried a 5 percent solution of the test lotion on 144 volunteers who were clearly sensitive to poison ivy or oak.

All volunteers applied the lotion to one arm and left the other arm bare. They then exposed both arms to poison ivy. All of the unprotected arms developed the characteristic rash reaction to poison ivy. On the arms protected with the lotion, 98 volunteers remained completely rash free, while 46 developed a much milder version of the rash.

Although the lotion is currently under review by the Food and Drug Administration (FDA), it has not yet been approved and is not currently available in stores. Other products, such as sunscreens and regular lotions, which commonly contain quaternium-18 bentonite do not offer the same protection because their formulation is different.

So, while you can't expect to escape problems if you have a run-in with poison ivy right away, the future looks promising. If the poison ivy preventive is approved, you can bet that the present plague of gardeners and outdoorsmen will truly be a problem of the past.

*Source:*
*Journal of the American Academy of Dermatology* (33,2:212)

# Take the sting out of summer

Spring and summer herald the arrival of warm weather, sunny skies, and pleasant picnics. Unfortunately, the party poopers of these almost perfect seasons also swarm out to enjoy the bounty and the beauty, and outdoor lovers everywhere find themselves pestered and bothered by bugs.

Most bugs are more troublesome than life-threatening. However, bees, wasps (hornets), and yellow jackets are responsible for more deaths in the United States each year than all poisonous animals combined. Death occurs when the person stung develops a life-threatening allergic reaction.

If you know you are allergic to insect stings, you should have an *epi kit* handy at all times. An epi kit contains a self-injectable dose of epinephrine, which can help stall an adverse reaction until you get to an emergency room.

However, your best bet if you want to protect yourself from the sting of the sunny seasons is to avoid these insects altogether. The good news is that they usually won't attack unless they feel threatened. The following tips will help you keep the stinging bugs at bay:

◆ Avoid wearing brightly colored clothes or flower prints.

◆ Leave off scented perfumes and other cosmetics, and avoid wearing real flowers.

◆ Protect your arms and legs with long pants and long sleeves.

◆ Don't go barefoot.

◆ Eliminate insect nests in and around your home.

◆ Keep an aerosol insecticide handy.

◆ Be especially cautious in attics and around bushes, leaves, picnic areas, and trash cans.

◆ Gently brush away any stinging insect that lands on you. Slapping at the insect will only irritate it and possibly provoke it to sting. If you are stung and you know you're allergic to stinging insects, remove the stinger if there is one, inject yourself with epinephrine, and hurry to the nearest emergency room. A life-threatening reaction can be prevented if treatment is prompt.

If you aren't allergic, here's how to handle a bee, wasp, or yellow jacket sting:

◆ Remove the stinger from your skin if one is present. Don't attempt to remove the stinger by grasping and pulling it. You'll only squeeze more venom into your body. Instead, scrape the edge of a credit card or a clean knife across your skin to remove the stinger.

◆ Wash your wound with soap and water.

◆ Apply a paste of unseasoned meat tenderizer and water. This helps neutralize the venom.

◆ Use an ice pack or ice cubes wrapped in a clean towel to control pain and swelling. Never apply ice or an ice pack directly to your skin. It could cause frostbite. Soothe your sting with the ice pack for 20 minutes, then let your skin rest for 10 minutes. Repeat the process if pain is still present.

If you don't think you're allergic to stinging insects, but you develop hives or a rash, have difficulty breathing, become dizzy or nauseated, or start vomiting within 30 minutes of being bitten, you should go to the emergency room immediately.

*Sources:*
*Before You Call the Doctor,* Ballantine Books, New York, 1992
*Postgraduate Medicine* (93,8:197)
"The Sting of Summer," Georgia Poison Control Center, 1982

## Natural remedy relieves itchy mosquito bites

Mosquitoes are a major nuisance to mankind. Besides spreading diseases ranging from malaria to *encephalitis* (inflammation of the brain), mosquitoes leave behind an intensely annoying itchy red bump after they bite.

Simply washing the bite with soap and water, applying an antiseptic, and not scratching are enough to keep you from catching a disease in most cases. However, the itchy red bump presents a bigger problem for some people. In most folks, the mosquito bite will disappear in a day or two. On others, it lingers longer than a relative who's worn out his welcome. If you're one of the people who tends to retain traces of mosquito bites for weeks, the *Chinese lycium leaf* may soon have you leaping with relief.

According to a recent report, the juice from young shoots and leaves of the lycium shrub, which commonly grows in China, can completely heal mosquito bites after as few as one to three applications. The juice also apparently prevents any scarring or discoloration from the mosquito bites, which can be problems for people who carry signs of their mosquito bites for a week or more.

If this is a remedy you think you'd like to try, you can obtain lycium leaves and young shoots at most vegetable stalls of major Chinatown areas during the spring and summer. Squeeze all the juice you can from the leaves and shoots and store the juice in a container in your refrigerator. When the bad bug bites, simply apply the juice to the affected area or areas up to three times a day.

At this time, no information is available on how long the stored juice will remain effective or if any preservatives can be used to extend its shelf life. If this remedy works for you the first couple of times you use it, then stops being effective, you'll probably need to make new juice from fresh shoots and leaves.

*Source:*
*HerbalGram (32:25)*

## Don't pussyfoot around with this caterpillar's sting

In its larval stage, its cute teardrop shape and fluffy body may give you the warm fuzzies, but a sting from a puss caterpillar will soon send other less pleasant thoughts swarming through your head.

*Puss Caterpillar Larva*

*Puss Caterpillar Adult*

Commonly found in the southern United States and northern Mexico, the puss caterpillar is capable of causing intense burning and swelling at even the slightest touch. Some people even experience shock and difficulty breathing. Reactions can be especially severe in children.

If you're stung by a puss caterpillar, place a strip of sticky tape on the site of the sting to remove any remaining caterpillar spines or hairs stuck on your skin. Apply ice. If possible, elevate the part of the body where you were stung. If you experience intense itching, take an over-the-counter antihistamine.

Anyone stung by a puss caterpillar who seems to be going into shock should be taken to an emergency room immediately.

*Source:*
*American Family Physician (52,1:86)*

## Do's and don'ts for deadly spider bites

When it comes to dogs, it's often true that the bark is worse than the bite. Spiders, on the other hand, don't bark, and their bites can be pretty painful.

Although almost all of the 100,000 species of spiders have venom and may bite if provoked, only two, the brown recluse and the black widow, pose any serious or deadly threat to humans. Children, because of their smaller size, generally have a worse reaction to spider bites than adults.

**Brown recluse spider.** Brown recluses like to hang out in dark, dry, secluded spots. Although the brown recluse is small, this spider is fairly easy to identify by the violin-shaped marking on its small upper-body section.

You can usually avoid these spiders by being extra careful and observant when rooting around clutter commonly found in attics, closets, garages, storage areas, and wood and trash piles. *Brown Recluse* Wear gloves when rummaging around those areas and when *Spider* doing yardwork.

Take any clothes or blankets you pull from storage outside and shake them thoroughly. This will encourage any brown recluses hiding in those items to move on to a different spot.

A bite from a brown recluse spider can cause a painful, stinging sensation although many times the bite may be painless. However, the site of the bite will quickly turn red, blister, and look blue in the center.

Twenty-four to 48 hours later, the skin around the bite will turn black. Other symptoms include fever, vomiting, and a general feeling of weakness. Get medical treatment immediately if you are bitten by a brown recluse.

Although in some cases, surgery may be necessary to remove the dead skin around the bite area, this is not generally the best treatment to try first. Your doctor should carefully clean the bite site, apply cold compresses, administer antibiotics, and use painkillers before considering surgery. You should not apply any heat to the bite and avoid strenuous exercise.

**Black widow spider.** Of all the spider species, the black widow is the most dangerous. Its very appropriate Latin name, *Latrodectus mactans* means "the murderer." Despite their terrible reputation, black widow spider bites are usually only fatal to children and older adults who do not receive treatment. It's important to seek immediate medical treatment for a black widow bite.

*Black Widow Spider*

Only the female black widow is poisonous. About a half inch long, the black widow sports a shiny black coat with a red hourglass design on her underside.

The good news about black widows is that they are not aggressive and will bite only when disturbed. Black widows prefer protected places such as the angles of doors, windows, and shutters; the undersides of stones and logs; old sheds, garages, and barns; and outdoor toilet seats. Take extra precautions in these areas and you probably won't have any problems. Always wear gloves when doing yardwork.

The bite of a black widow feels similar to the prick of a pin. Symptoms may include a headache, stomach cramps, vomiting, muscle spasms or stiffness, or a rash. These usually develop within an hour of the bite.

Sometimes a doctor will misdiagnose the stomach cramps of a black widow spider bite as a stomach emergency requiring immediate surgery. If you ever find yourself in this situation, be sure to tell the doctor you've been bitten by a black widow.

Even though your first reaction when you suspect you've been bitten by a spider may be to scream and slap wildly at the spot on your skin you last saw it, there are safer, more effective ways of dealing with a spider bite. Here's what to do:

◆ Wash the site of the bite thoroughly with soap and water.

◆ Tie a string around the area just above the bite. The string should be tied tightly enough to cause a slight indention in the skin, but not tight enough to cut off circulation. This tourniquet will help limit the spread of venom.

◆ Apply an ice pack to the bite. This will also help limit the spread of venom. Do not apply ice directly to the skin, which can cause frostbite. If you don't have an actual ice pack, place some ice cubes in a plastic bag, then wrap the bag in a clean cloth before applying it to the bite.

◆ Limit movement of the limb or part of the body where the bite occurred. This also slows the spread of venom.

If you suspect you were bitten by a black widow or brown recluse spider, see a doctor as soon as possible. If you aren't able to identify the spider that bit you but have any of the symptoms discussed above, you should also see a doctor immediately.

*Sources:*
*Before You Call the Doctor*, Ballantine Books, New York, 1992
*Cutis* (56,5:256)

# Key to snakebite first aid

Do you know how to handle a snakebite? Snake breeder and lecturer Dr. Brad Lichtenhan has some firm advice: The only snakebite first aid item you need is a set of car keys, and the only treatment you need to know is how to drive quickly and safely to the nearest hospital.

Cutting the bite, sucking the venom, using a tourniquet, applying ice, drinking alcohol — all these are dangerous and can cause more harm than good.

All you can do is keep the bitten limb still (put it in a splint if you have one), and take off any rings, watches, or items that could be tight or hard to remove later. The snake venom will probably cause the limb to swell.

Some people recommend loosely wrapping an ACE bandage above (not on) the bite to slow the spread of the poison. If you do that, you've got to be very careful to leave it in place until you are in the hospital emergency room. Taking the tourniquet off could release a flood of venom, and you need to have antivenin available to handle it.

Pit vipers, such as copperheads, moccasins, and rattlesnakes, inflict 99 percent of all snakebites. Like all poisonous snakes, they have elliptical eyes instead of round eyes. Their head is triangular and set off from the neck. All snakes have a divided set of scales at the very end of their tails, but poisonous snake scales then become undivided. In other words, you don't want to see scales that go all the way across the tail instead of dividing in the middle.

Every once in a while, someone is bitten by a colorful coral snake. To identify one, remember: "Red and yellow, kill the fellow; red and black, friend of Jack." Coral snakes bite and chew instead of striking and releasing venom immediately, so if you pull them off right away, you may not have been poisoned at all.

*Nonpoisonous Snake Tail*

*Poisonous Snake Tail*

But don't count on a snake's appearance to tell you if it's poisonous. It's almost impossible to tell a nonpoisonous water snake from a poisonous cottonmouth water moccasin, and poisonous rattlesnakes don't always rattle.

There is good news: No snakes in the United States are poisonous enough to kill a person in one to two hours. So, drive safely on the way to the hospital. Take the snake in a bag with you if it is dead, but watch out — dead snakes can bite by reflex. Use a sturdy stick to pick up a dead snake. You'll be best off leaving live snakes alone.

The Southern Arizona Rescue Association, the Organization for Tropical Studies in Costa Rica, and the La Selva Biological Station in Costa Rica will tell you that prevention works where snakebites are concerned. In over one million man-hours in bad snake country, the three organizations reported only one snakebite. Some simple rules:

- ◆ Stay alert — no alcohol or drugs.
- ◆ Wear protective clothes — boots, trousers, slacks, shirts with sleeves.
- ◆ Travel in pairs. A helping hand can be vital in a snakebite situation.
- ◆ Don't reach into holes or under hidden ledges, and watch your step.
- ◆ Leave snakes alone, even if they are sleeping.
- ◆ Don't keep a poisonous pet snake.

*Sources:*
*Emergency Medicine* (27,3:22)
*The Physician and Sportsmedicine* (23,9:72)

## 30-minute solution saves knocked-out teeth

If you want to save a knocked-out tooth, the secret of success is speed. A tooth that is reimplanted within 30 minutes has a 90 percent chance of being saved. After 30 minutes, the likelihood of a successful reimplantation falls 1 percent for every additional minute you delay.

Be careful to only pick up a knocked-out tooth by its crown (the white enamel part of the tooth). Don't touch the tooth's roots. If cleaning is necessary, plug the sink first so the tooth won't accidently slip down the drain. Rinse gently so the roots won't be damaged.

Your best bet is to put the tooth back into its original socket. You can gently bite on a piece of gauze to keep the tooth in place. If returning the tooth to its socket is not an option, carry it in Hank's solution. This specially balanced formula, which comes in the *Save-a-Tooth* kit available at most pharmacies, can keep a knocked-out tooth alive for four to 12 hours. If you don't have any Hank's solution handy, you can store the tooth in a glass of cold whole milk for a short time. However you choose to handle the tooth, just be sure to see a dentist immediately. You may want to head straight to the nearest emergency room. Often, a dentist will be on hand there to treat dental emergencies.

If the tooth has been chipped or fractured, but not completely knocked out, you should still see a dentist within 24 hours. Until you can get to a dentist, eat only soft foods.

The two most common causes of knocked-out teeth are sports injuries and automobile accidents. To protect yourself and your family from a preventable problem, be sure to wear helmets when bicycling, skating, or skateboarding; use mouthpieces when playing contact sports such as football; and always put on seat belts when in a car.

*Sources:*
American Family Physician (52,4:1130)
Before You Call the Doctor, Ballantine Books, New York, 1992

# Ring removal made easy

There's almost nothing as frustrating and painful as a ring stuck on your finger. Try as you might, you just can't get it off. The harder you try, the less progress you make. Dr. Tony G. Pangilinan of West Allis, Wis., has developed a fast, no-mess solution you may want to try the next time you find yourself in this sticky situation.

To remove a ring from a swollen finger, place a strip of adhesive tape on the skin just below the finger knuckle. Push the tape toward your hand while pulling the ring in the opposite direction. This technique helps slide the swollen skin under and behind the ring, making removal easier.

*Source:*
Emergency Medicine (27,5:73)

# Breathing Easy

## Cold comfort

The common cold is aptly named. It is the most common infectious illness in the world. Almost everyone knows the coughing, congestion, and discomfort that a cold can bring.

You know that an ounce of prevention is worth a pound of cure, particularly important since there is no cure for the common cold. Preventing colds may seem like an impossible task, but you can take steps to protect yourself.

◆ Avoid exposure to other people with colds. This can't always be accomplished in the workplace, but try to keep your distance from a sick co-worker.

◆ Wash your hands often. Use a liquid antibacterial soap. Bar soap may harbor bacteria.

◆ Keep your hands away from your nose and mouth. Germs on your hands will spread quickly if they get into your respiratory system.

◆ Take your vitamin C. People have argued for years over whether vitamin C helped prevent colds. New research indicates that, although vitamin C may not prevent colds, it can make the time you suffer from a cold shorter.

Even if you do everything you can to avoid catching a cold, it's probably going to catch up with you sometime. Since the common cold cannot be cured, you can only treat the symptoms to make yourself feel better until the cold goes away. The medication you take depends on what symptoms you have. However, the sheer number of over-the-counter cold medicines can make choosing confusing. Here are some general guidelines:

**Congestion.** Nasal spray decongestants work fast and have few side effects. However, you shouldn't use a spray decongestant more than three days in a row. You may experience a rebound effect, with a worsening of symptoms after prolonged use.

Oral decongestants work more slowly, but they don't produce the rebound effect of nasal sprays. However, side effects, including increased blood pressure, heart rate increase, restlessness, anxiety, and increased blood sugar levels, are more common. For these reasons, people with high blood pressure, heart disease, or diabetes may need to steer clear of them.

**Runny nose and sneezing.** Antihistamines are often used to treat the runny nose and sneezing of a common cold, but they aren't very effective for this purpose. They may also cause drowsiness, dry mouth, low blood pressure, blurred vision, and urinary retention.

**Cough.** Antitussives, the active ingredients in cough medicines, decrease how often and how hard you cough. They also help you sleep and stop throat irritation. Common antitussives include *codeine*, *dextromethorphan*, and *diphenhydramine*. Codeine may not be available over-the-counter in some states because it is a narcotic and, therefore, potentially addictive.

**Expectorants.** Expectorants are supposed to increase the flow of mucus and make it less sticky. *Guaifenesin* is the only expectorant available over the counter, and though it has no side effects, it isn't very effective. Warm fluids, like the chicken soup your mother always gave you when you were sick, and hot tea are actually better expectorants.

**Sore throat.** Local anesthetics for sore throat pain are available in the form of lozenges and sprays. They provide quick but temporary relief. You can also take pain relievers such as aspirin, acetaminophen, and ibuprofen.

Because many cold remedies contain several different medications, check the labels to make sure you're not doubling up on the same medication. For example, don't take a product containing a pain reliever and then take an aspirin, too. Be patient, relieve your symptoms one by one, and your cold will soon be history.

*Sources:*
*Journal of the American College of Nutrition* (14,2:116)
*U.S. Pharmacist* (20,10:16)

# Fleeing the flu bug

Most of us don't think of influenza (flu) as a serious illness, but the flu and diseases related to it claim over 20,000 lives every year.

Influenza is a virus which is usually spread by inhaling droplets in the air that were sneezed or coughed out by an infected person. Symptoms include fever, chills, sweating, sore throat, runny nose, headache, and sensitivity to light. Though many of the symptoms are similar to the common cold, people with colds are usually able to go on with their daily activities. The flu, on the other hand, can interfere with your ability to perform your usual activities.

Vaccines can prevent influenza, but many people don't take advantage of them because they are afraid of the possible side effects. However, flu vaccines cannot cause the flu, and usually the only side effect is soreness at the vaccination site. Less than 5 percent of the people vaccinated experience fever, muscle soreness, and general achiness for one to two days afterward.

People who are the most at risk for suffering severely from the flu are the ones who should get a vaccine. These include:

◆ People with heart or lung conditions.
◆ People who have diabetes, blood disorders, or kidney disorders.
◆ Children with asthma.
◆ People with poorly functioning immune systems, like people with AIDS and people who have had chemotherapy.
◆ People living in nursing homes.

However, you should not get a flu vaccination if you are allergic to eggs, are allergic to the preservative thimerosal, had a bad reaction to a previous flu shot, or are pregnant or plan to get pregnant within three months.

*Sources:*
*The New England Journal of Medicine* (36,21:1)
*U.S. Pharmacist* (21,1:18)

## Gingerly sidestep a sore throat

Soothing your sore throat or laryngitis can be a snap with ginger. This herb has been used for centuries to combat a number of illnesses, including colds and the flu, and may be particularly helpful in reducing mucus. To make a pot of comforting ginger tea, place three or four slices of the fresh root in a pint of hot water. Simmer for 10 to 30 minutes, and sip on the soothing concoction all day long.

*Source:*
*Growing and Using the Healing Herbs,* Wings Books, New York, 1992

## Hands-on healing for sore throat

The next time you have a scratchy sore throat and don't want to take any medication, try reflexology for pain relief. Reflexology involves massaging certain nerve "buttons" that connect to different areas of the body. One reflex button for the throat is on the lower part of the thumb where it fastens to the hand as well as the web between the thumb and hand. Another is on the foot, at the base of the big toe. Search for tender spots by massaging one of these areas, and when you find one, continue massaging that spot until you feel relief.

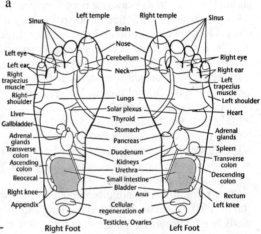

*Source:*
*Body Reflexology,* Parker Publishing Company, West Nyack, N.Y., 1994

## Natural Rx for stuffy sinuses

Millions of people are familiar with the stuffiness and painful pressure of sinusitis, one of the most common chronic ailments.

Your sinuses are air-filled pockets located above your eyebrows, under your eyes, between your eyes, and behind your nose. Normally, mucus from your sinuses drains into your nose and down your throat, where stomach acids destroy it. When your sinuses clog up, the tissues swell, and mucus does not drain properly. This results in a buildup of mucus, which can quickly become infected.

The symptoms of sinusitis include a stuffy or runny nose, painful pressure around your eyes, earaches, and coughing which becomes worse when lying down. It is usually caused by bacterial infection. People with asthma or allergies are more likely to have sinusitis. It may also be brought on by environmental factors such as pollution, cigarette smoke, and weather conditions. Many people find that their sinusitis is worse right before a storm. Some people may have a deviated septum, which means the wall of bone and cartilage between the right and left nostrils is crooked. This can interfere with mucus drainage.

If recurring sinusitis attacks are making you miserable, try the following steps to put a stop to sinusitis.

**Get the right amount of sleep.** Too much or too little sleep may make you more likely to suffer from sinusitis. Sleeping with your head elevated may also help. If you only have sinusitis on one side, try sleeping on the other side. This may help open your nasal passageway.

**Change your diet.** You may have food allergies which could trigger your sinusitis. Try eliminating foods like wheat, milk, or red wine. Spicy foods like garlic, horseradish, and cayenne pepper may help clear sinuses.

**Use a nasal spray.** Saline nasal sprays help moisten and soothe nasal passages. Over-the-counter nasal decongestant sprays should not be used for more than three days in a row. A rebound effect may occur if you use them too much, which means your symptoms will get much worse when you stop using them.

**Exercise.** Most people with sinusitis find that exercise opens nasal passages by increasing the flow of mucus. However, some people may find that exercise makes their symptoms worse.

**Make sure your glasses fit.** Improperly fitting glasses can pinch the bridge of your nose and cause congestion.

**Inhale steam.** Breathing in steam may help. You can add pine oil, eucalyptus, or menthol for a little extra nasal-opening power. A warm facial pack (hot towels) can have the same effect.

**Use a humidifier.** A humidifier may prevent your sinuses from becoming dry and irritated, which could lead to swelling and infection. A humidifier is particularly helpful during the colder months.

*Sources:*
*American Family Physician* (53,3:877)
*The Asthma and Allergy Advance* (January/February 1994)

# Beating a nasal spray addiction

If you've used a nasal spray decongestant, and now think you just can't breathe without it, rest assured that you can. Though it may seem as if you will suffocate if you don't use the spray, discontinue use for six to eight hours and breathe through your mouth.

Until your nose adjusts to not having a nasal spray crutch, you can ease your discomfort by spreading a camphor-menthol-eucalyptus ointment under your nose. A vaporizer or salt-water nasal spray may also help.

You don't want your nose hooked on a spray, so remember, never use a nasal spray decongestant for more than three days in a row. It should provide temporary relief without becoming a lifelong habit.

*Source:*
*Emergency Medicine* (27,2:110)

## A-1 allergy relief

The sniffing, sneezing, and wheezing of allergies can be annoying. The best way to avoid symptoms of allergies is to avoid your allergens (the substances to which you are sensitive) Sometimes you need medication, but knowing what medication to take may be confusing.

**Antihistamines.** Antihistamines block production of a chemical in your body that causes allergic symptoms. They are available over the counter as well as by prescription.

**Decongestants.** Oral decongestants help relieve stuffiness and may offset the drowsy effect that antihistamines can cause. Nasal spray decongestants should only be used in severe cases and for no more than three days.

**Saline.** Saline sprays can moisten and soothe dry, irritated nasal membranes.

**Corticosteroids.** Steroid nasal sprays decrease the swelling of tissues which can lead to infection. When used regularly twice a day, beginning before the allergy season, steroids are very effective in treating allergies.

**Immunotherapy.** Allergy shots help build immunity by exposing you to your allergens a little at a time. They may be needed by people who have been unable to find relief through changing their environments or medication. After two or three seasons of allergy shots, you may be able to discontinue them.

*Source:*
*American Family Physician* (51,4:837)

## Bee pollen's benefits not worth risk

People have been buzzing with talk about the powers of bee pollen. Reports that bee pollen could improve athletic performance led many people to health food stores to stock up. However, a study of swimmers by the National Athletic Trainer Association found no benefit to taking bee pollen. Other claims that bee pollen can increase energy, delay the aging process, and cure a number of other illnesses have yet to be confirmed.

If you have a history of pollen allergies, taking bee pollen could be deadly. Several people with a history of allergies developed severe allergic reactions after taking bee pollen. The amount needed to cause an acute reaction was less than one teaspoonful. On rare occasions, even people with no history of allergies may have a severe reaction to bee pollen.

Be careful if you're considering taking bee pollen, especially if you have a history of allergies. The supposed benefits may not be worth the potential side effects.

*Source:*
*The Lawrence Review of Natural Products,* Facts and Comparisons, St. Louis, Mo., 1995

## Sneeze-free gardening

Do you love to garden but hate to sneeze? Do your allergies make it difficult to enjoy an activity you normally love? Try some of these sneeze-free gardening tips.

**Be picky about what you plant.** If you plant wind-pollinated plants, you'll soon pay the price with your itchy, watery eyes and nose. Wind-pollinated plants include Bermuda grass, juniper shrubs, ragweed, and some herbs. Fruit trees like walnut, pecan, and olive are also wind-pollinated. Bee-pollinated plants, like most colorful flowers, have pollen that is too heavy to blow into your sensitive nose. Most vegetables are also safe.

**Cut your grass short.** If you keep your lawn cut to less than two inches, it will produce less pollen.

**Time your gardening sessions.** Try to avoid gardening before 10 a.m. and near sunset, when pollen counts are high. Warm, sunny days produce the highest pollen counts. The most pollen-free time is on a cool, cloudy day or right after a rainfall.

**Wear a mask.** Disposable masks that fit over your nose and mouth are ideal for keeping out nose-tickling particles during gardening chores.

*Source:*
*The Saturday Evening Post* (267,2:66)

## A cup a day keeps hay fever away

Can drinking coffee help you breathe easier? If you have hay fever, it may.

A study at the Harbor-UCLA Medical Center found that people with hay fever who took caffeine tablets (equal to about 18 ounces of coffee) reported over a 50 percent improvement in their hay fever symptoms. Caffeine has also been found to help asthmatics breathe better by relaxing the bronchial contractions in their lungs. Before you start drinking more java, however, remember that it is a stimulant and still causes side effects like insomnia and increased blood pressure.

*Source:*
*Medical Tribune for the Internist and Cardiologist* (36,23:8)

## A sweet solution to hay fever symptoms

Relief from hay fever symptoms may be as close as the nearest hive. Traces of pollen found in honey may desensitize you the same way that allergy shots do. Eat honey from your local area because it contains traces of the same types of pollen to which you are regularly exposed. For best results, take one to three teaspoonfuls a day over a long period of time.

*Source:*
*The Food Pharmacy,* Bantam Books, New York, 1988

## All-around asthma relief

The breathless, wheezing, chest-squeezing feeling of an asthma attack can make it difficult to enjoy life. You could be at a family picnic or at the theater when an asthma attack strikes. You can help prevent those pleasure-robbing attacks from happening to you.

**Stock up on selenium.** Selenium, a trace mineral, helps lower your risk of asthma. Selenium may be found in meats and shellfish and in vegetables and grains grown in soil rich in selenium. You need about 100 to 200 micrograms (mcg) of selenium a day.

**Get your vitamins.** Vitamin C and vitamin E both protect cells from damage which may help guard against asthma attacks.

**Don't smoke.** Common sense should tell you that smoking can make asthma symptoms worse. Asthma is not only more common among smokers, but also among children of smokers. When you smoke, you inhale damaging oxidants. That's why it's particularly important for smokers to get plenty of antioxidants like vitamin C.

**Get the lead out.** Exposure to lead can make your asthma worse. Though the government regulates the use of lead, you could be exposed to lead through paint in older houses, air pollution, contaminated water, or lead piping. Your doctor can test your blood for lead content, and if it's high, you must track down the source of your lead problem and eliminate it.

*Sources:*
*Journal of the American College of Nutrition* (14,4:317)
*The American Journal of Clinical Nutrition* (61,3S:625S)

# Secrets of safer inhaler use

Since asthma is a lung problem that often requires quick relief, most asthma medicine is taken through inhalers. You just put the nozzle in your mouth, squeeze, and breathe the medicine right into your lungs.

It sounds simple, but there are a few tips you should remember.

◆ Always store your inhaler with the cap on. Small items, like pennies, tablets, and screw caps can get caught in the nozzle. In the rush to get relief from an asthma attack, you might not check the opening for any trash. The force of the inhaler can send these potentially dangerous items right into your lungs.

◆ When it's time for medicine, remove the cap and shake the inhaler well.

◆ Exhale as much air as you possibly can.

◆ Squeeze the bottle while you begin to inhale, and remember to inhale slowly.

◆ After you finish inhaling, hold your breath for five to 10 seconds.

◆ Don't take more than one puff from your inhaler at a time. If you need another dose, wait at least 30 seconds.

◆ Make sure you know about how much medicine is left in the inhaler after each use. Replace if necessary.

◆ Rinse your mouth after using a steroid inhaler.

◆ In cold weather, carry your inhaler close to your body to keep it warm. Using it cold could cause poor distribution of the medication or lung spasms caused by the puff of cold medication.

*Sources:*
*British Medical Journal* (306,6877:575)
*Geriatrics* (48,4:21)
*The Physician and Sportsmedicine* (24,2:21)

## Shooting down asthma shots

Allergy shots may bring relief to people who suffer from hay fever, but if you have allergy-induced asthma, they may not be effective. A study at Johns Hopkins University found that people who had asthma caused by a ragweed allergy were helped only slightly by taking the allergy shots given to hay fever sufferers. This slight benefit decreased even more in the second year. If you're taking allergy shots for your asthma, you may be wasting your time and money.

*Source:*
*The New England Journal of Medicine* (334,8:501)

# 6 ways to stop nighttime asthma attacks

Lots of things can take your breath away — an evening with a special person, an exciting finish at a ballgame, even a car pulling out in front of you. Now add sleep to the list, at least if you are one of the millions of people who have asthma.

People suffering asthma attacks cough, wheeze, feel tight-chested, and have trouble catching their breath. Most attacks are mild, but some people have died from a severe attack.

Most people think asthma attacks are most likely to happen during heavy exercise, and it is true that huffing and puffing can be the culprit. But surprisingly, many attacks happen at night. More than two-thirds of all the people with asthma experience a worsening of symptoms at night.

No one is quite sure why sleep causes asthma attacks. After all, that's when breathing should be easiest. But research on sleep and breathing offers a few clues to this medical mystery.

First, your body has a natural pattern of breathing that has high and low points during a 24-hour cycle. In this pattern, the brain automatically slows breathing during the night. But in people with asthma, the signals from the brain are dramatically enhanced, so the rate of respiration drops too low.

During the day, your body produces chemicals that help your lungs function normally. Two chemicals, cortisol and epinephrine, are especially important to prevent the lungs from constricting. At night, your body cuts back on its production of cortisol and epinephrine. For people without asthma, that doesn't cause a problem. If you have asthma, though, low levels of these chemicals can trigger an attack.

Another factor in triggering nighttime asthma attacks is exposure to things in the air that cause allergies, like dust mites, feathers, and dander. You can find all these things in bed linens. In about half of the people with asthma, there is a delayed reaction to breathing in these allergens, so the things they are exposed to during the day come back to haunt them at night.

While your food allergies may not cause an asthma attack, how your body digests your food can have an effect. Heartburn can worsen asthma, especially at night.

Some people have other problems at night that worsen asthma. One of these problems is sleep apnea, which can cause you to stop breathing for short periods in your sleep.

Finally, your body temperature naturally drops during the night, and that can trigger an asthma attack.

So, now that you are afraid to close your eyes for fear that you will stop breathing, take comfort in these tips to reduce your chances of losing your breath tonight.

◆ Wash your bed sheets often, wrap the mattress in plastic covers, and use pillows and comforters that are made with nonallergenic fillers. This will cut down on the dust mites, dander, and feather particles that make their way into your lungs.

◆ When washing your linens, make sure the water is hot — 137 degrees Fahrenheit or higher — to kill dust mites. You might also replace upholstered furniture in your bedroom with leather furniture and replace your draperies with blinds. An air filter with a fine screen can also cut down on allergens.

◆ Use saline nasal washes to rinse out your sinuses and keep allergens out of your breathing passages.

◆ If heartburn is a problem for you, avoid food and drink several hours before you go to bed. Put 4-inch blocks under the head of your bed to keep your head above the level of your stomach. This helps keep food and stomach acid in its place. Antacids also help, but keep in mind that long-term use of antacids can cause other problems.

◆ Keep your pet out of your bedroom to cut down on allergens around you during the night. Since some people have a delayed allergic reaction, you might even consider keeping your furry pets outside.
Cats seem to cause more problems than dogs. If you can't part with Kitty, then you should at least wash her every two to three weeks.

◆ If you have sleep apnea, talk to a doctor about *continuous positive air pressure*. This is a technique you can learn that will help control your apnea as well as your nighttime asthma.

If these natural methods don't help, it may be time to talk to your doctor about taking medicine that helps control asthma. This is especially true if your nighttime asthma is not triggered by allergens or if your asthma is getting worse.

There are a number of widely prescribed medications for asthma. Many are available as inhalers. Whatever kind of medicine your doctor gives you, be sure to discuss when you should take it if you are concerned about nighttime attacks. You may need more medicine close to bedtime or a special timed-release medicine that will work throughout the night.

As a last resort, your doctor may prescribe a fast-acting drug to open up your airways. You may need to set your alarm clock to wake you about an hour before the time you usually have an attack so you can take the medicine and prevent the attack.

*Sources:*
*American Journal of Medicine* (85S,18:6)
*American Review of Respiratory Diseases* (147:525 and 142:1153)
*Drug Therapy* (23,4:29)
*Lung Line Letter* (7,5:4)
*Postgraduate Medicine* (97,6:83)
*The Western Journal of Medicine* (163,1:49)

## Asthmatics and tranquilizers: a deadly duo

Tranquilizers may help you relax and sleep easier, but if you have asthma, tranquilizers may put you to sleep permanently. A recent study found that people who had used major tranquilizers had over a three times higher risk of death or near-death from asthma complications. If you have asthma, avoid using tranquilizers, if possible. A glass of warm milk and some soothing music might be safer.

*Source:*
British Medical Journal (312,7023:79)

## The food additive that puts asthmatics at risk

Add *sulfites* to the long list of substances a person with asthma may want to avoid. Sulfites are salts used for preserving processed foods.

Sulfite sensitivity occurs in about 5 percent of adult asthmatics or approximately 500,000 people. The symptoms include hives, itching, flushing, tingling, nausea, and asthmatic symptoms such as wheezing and shortness of breath. In rare cases, shock, heavy sweating, and loss of consciousness may occur. Sulfite sensitivity is more common in people who take steroids for their asthma.

If you have a sulfite sensitivity, some foods to avoid include:

◆ Dried fruit (except dark raisins and prunes)
◆ Lemon juice and lime juice (nonfrozen)
◆ Wine
◆ Molasses
◆ Sauerkraut juice
◆ Wine vinegar
◆ Maraschino cherries
◆ Pickled products

*Source:*
Journal of the American College of Nutrition (14,3:229)

## Little-known cause of asthma

If you have asthma, and also suffer from *gastroesophageal reflux disease* (GERD), treating your GERD may cure your asthma. GERD occurs when stomach acids splash back into the esophagus, causing heartburn. About 80 percent of people with asthma also suffer from GERD, which may trigger an asthma attack by spilling stomach acid into your airways, or by making you more sensitive to other triggers.

If you find that your asthma is triggered by reflux, you can either have surgery to prevent the spilling of stomach acid, or take drugs that block the production of stomach acid. In one study of people with asthma and GERD, almost three-fourths of the people improved or eliminated their asthma by treating just their reflux.

People who are most likely to have reflux-related asthma are those who developed asthma as an adult, have no family history of asthma, cough and wheeze a lot at night, and whose symptoms are worse after meals or exercise.

*Source:*
*Medical Tribune for the Internist and Cardiologist* (36,22:6)

# Uncovering an unusual cause of asthma

You could probably use a little help from Sherlock Holmes in tracking down your asthma triggers. However, it's worth the effort if it helps you breathe easier.

One place you might never think to look for a clue to an asthma trigger is right beneath you. The soles of your feet may hold the answer. Molds and fungi are known to cause or aggravate asthma, and athlete's foot is a fungus that you carry with you. Nail clippings or airborne athlete's foot particles could be inhaled, or the fungus could enter your bloodstream directly if your athlete's foot problem is bad enough to cause your skin to crack.

Treatment with antifungal medications and keeping your feet clean and dry might do more than cure your athlete's foot. It might enable you to walk away from your asthma.

*Source:*
*Annals of Allergy, Asthma, and Immunology* (74:523)

# Steer clear of asthma triggers

Allergies and asthma don't always go hand in hand, but most people who have asthma also have allergies. Those allergies can trigger breath-stealing asthma attacks.

Things like pollen, mold, and animal dander can set off an allergic reaction in some people that results in hives, itching, sneezing, and wheezing. When this reaction occurs in the chest, it's called asthma. In the lungs, allergic reactions cause spasms and thick, sticky mucus. When an asthmatic has an attack, his lungs feel clogged and twitchy, and his chest feels tight.

Though not all people with asthma have allergies, those who do should identify their allergic triggers and avoid them. Some of the more common asthma triggers to avoid:

◆ Foods like chocolate, nuts, shellfish, and eggs.

◆ Beverages like orange juice, beer, wine, and milk.

◆ Mold spores and pollen. When pollen counts are high, try to stay indoors as much as possible.

◆ Dander from pets such as cats, dogs, hamsters, and rabbits. If you can't bear to part with your family pet, try to keep it outside and bathe it often.

◆ Feather pillows, down comforters, and wool clothing. Use smooth blankets on your bed.

◆ Dust. Damp dust and damp mop instead of using brooms that raise dust. Use washable fabrics for curtains and rugs.

◆ Cleaning products like bleach and furniture polish.

Avoiding your triggers may help you avoid the chest-squeezing experience of an asthma attack.

*Sources:*
*Allergy and Asthma,* American Academy of Allergy, Asthma and Immunology, Milwaukee, 1995
*Everything You Need to Know About Diseases,* Springhouse Corporation, Springhouse, Pa., 1996

## Essential exam for former smokers

You probably stopped worrying about lung cancer about the same time you stopped smoking. Although quitting smoking does lower your risk of lung cancer substantially, you're not home free yet.

Some risk remains for about 15 years after you quit smoking. A study at Harvard Medical School found that over half the new cases of lung cancer were former smokers.

The good news is that this study suggests an estimated 27,000 lives a year could be saved if former smokers would get yearly chest X-rays. Early detection increases your chances of surviving lung cancer. If you're a reformed smoker, be sure you schedule a yearly chest X-ray. It could save your life.

*Source:*
*Medical Tribune for the Internist and Cardiologist* (36,22:2)

## Newest weapon against cystic fibrosis

An important new use has been found for ibuprofen, that humble, over-the-counter pain reliever. It may prevent lung damage caused by the genetic disorder, cystic fibrosis (CF).

People with CF are plagued by chronic lung infections. Glands in the lining of their bronchial tubes produce excessive amounts of mucus, in which the infections thrive. These chronic infections damage the lungs.

In a four-year study of people with CF, half of the participants took ibuprofen, and half did not. The dosage was 400 milligrams (mg) twice a day for children, and up to 1,600 mg twice a day for adults.

People with CF have to deal with a decline in the function of their lungs over time. This rate of decline was slowed by 59 percent yearly in people taking ibuprofen. For children under the age of 13, the difference was even more dramatic. Those children taking ibuprofen showed an 88 percent smaller decline in lung function than those children not taking it.

In the past, the focus of treating CF was on clearing airways of thick mucus and using antibiotics to control infection. Using ibuprofen to fight the effects of CF is a completely new approach. It reduces inflammation in the lungs without the side effects of stronger drugs such as steroids. Ibuprofen is an economical drug, and it should not add much (under $200 a year) to the cost of treating CF.

People with CF must be monitored carefully by their doctors, and the dosage of ibuprofen should be carefully calculated for each person's height and weight. Ibuprofen does not reverse lung damage that has already occurred, but it can help prevent it, especially in children.

*Sources:*
*Medical Tribune for the Internist and Cardiologist* (36,8:7)
*The American Medical Association Encyclopedia of Medicine,* Random House, New York, 1989

# Headache Healers and Helpers

## Headache danger

Though headache pain can be annoying or even excruciating, nine times out of 10 it isn't dangerous or life-threatening. However, occasionally, a headache may be a symptom of a more serious condition, like meningitis or a brain tumor. When should you suspect that your headache is more than just a pain in the head?

Anything out of the ordinary about your headache should be a red flag. One woman who went to her doctor with a severe headache was told she had a sinus headache. She was given medicine and sent home. The next day, she returned to her doctor for a follow-up visit. The diagnosis was changed to a migraine, and her medicine was changed. When her headache persisted, she went to the emergency room, where it was discovered that she had a blood clot in a sinus that could have led to a stroke. The red flag in her case was the fact that she rarely had headaches, much less one so persistent and severe. She also had no family history of headaches, and she had bumped her head on the headboard of her bed the day before her headache began.

How do you know if a headache is out of the ordinary? If you have a history of headaches, you know what is normal for you. Any of the following symptoms in addition to your headache could be an indication of a more serious problem.

- ◆ Fever
- ◆ Nausea or vomiting
- ◆ Drowsiness
- ◆ Confusion
- ◆ Loss of consciousness
- ◆ Blurred vision
- ◆ Dizziness

If a headache occurs suddenly, follows a head injury, gets progressively worse, or is more severe than usual, see your doctor.

*Source:*
Postgraduate Medicine (98,2:197)

## No more migraine misery

The pain of a migraine can make you feel like you have a bass drummer beating away inside your head. The throbbing, pounding pain can lead quickly to nausea, which is why migraines are often referred to as "sick headaches."

How do you know if your headache is a migraine? Migraine symptoms include pulsating pain which is moderate to severe, becomes worse with routine physical activity like bending over or climbing stairs, and lasts from four hours to three days. You may become more sensitive to light or noise and experience nausea and vomiting

Some people experience a set of warning signs, known as an aura, before a migraine begins. An aura, which usually consists of blind spots, zigzags of light, flashing lights or colors, double vision, or hallucinations, typically occurs about 10 to 20 minutes before an attack begins. Some people also experience numbness, speech or comprehension problems, or paralysis just before their migraines strike.

You may have tried over-the-counter medicine such as aspirin or ibuprofen for your migraines. Sometimes the medicine helps temporarily, but when the headache returns, the pain is even more intense. This is known as the rebound effect. Your doctor can prescribe other drugs to help prevent migraines, most commonly beta-blockers. These work well for stress-related headaches, but they should be avoided by people with depression. However, you can help yourself reduce the frequency and intensity of your migraines.

- Keep a headache diary to help identify and avoid triggers (things that are causing your headaches).
- Avoid oversleeping.
- Reduce your level of stress.
- Eat at regular intervals to avoid low blood sugar.
- Try some fresh ginger. Researchers found that one woman who had suffered from migraines for 16 years was helped by eating fresh ginger daily.
- Take a hot bath and put a cold compress on your head. This may help direct the blood flow to the rest of your body, while constricting swollen blood vessels in your head.

*Sources:*
American Family Physician (51,6:1498)
Emergency Medicine (27,1:45)
Menopause News (6,3:4)

## Turn off migraine triggers

Discovering your migraine triggers could be the key to controlling your migraine pain. Keeping a headache diary will help you identify possible triggers. Then you can experiment by eliminating the possible culprits. Some of the more common triggers include:

- Alcohol — beer, wine (especially red), liquor.
- Artificial sweeteners.
- Bright or flashing lights.
- Caffeine — chocolate, coffee, tea, colas. If you use caffeine, spread it out evenly over the day
- Emotional stress.
- Excessive sleep.

◆ Foods containing tyramine — bananas, avocado, aged cheese, chicken livers, yogurt, sour cream, nuts.
◆ Loud noises.
◆ Meats with nitrites and nitrates — preserved meats and deli meats.
◆ Monosodium glutamate (MSG) — a flavor enhancer.
◆ Premenstrual tension.
◆ Smoke.
◆ Video display terminals.

Try reducing your exposure to these possible triggers to cut back on the severity and frequency of your migraines. If you have serious pain, or if the pain persists, see your doctor.

*Source:*
*American Family Physician* (51,6:1502)

# Fewer migraines with feverfew

When you have a migraine headache, the rest of the world retreats far into the distance. The pulsating pain makes it almost impossible to face your work or your family. Even a walk in the sunshine is out of the question.

Just ask Kristen Yates, a woman of 37 who has suffered with migraines for five years. Her migraines have interfered with her social life, caused her to miss work, and made her fear Saturdays.

"I don't know why, but they always seem to hit on Saturdays," she says of her predictable headaches. "It might only be once a month, or it might skip a few months. But it got so I almost expected to get one the weekend after a big project at work."

Kristen is an avid gardener, but she never knew that the secret to curing her migraines could be as close as her backyard herb garden and the feverfew plant.

Feverfew got its name from the Latin word *febrifugia*, which means fever reducer. It has been used as an herbal remedy for almost 2,000 years. Greek and European herbalists traditionally used feverfew to treat fevers, headaches, menstrual irregularities, psoriasis, arthritis, and stomachaches.

Beginning in the 1970s, scientific studies focused on how feverfew reduces the inflammation and muscle spasms associated with migraines. A special chemical called *parthenolide* in feverfew blocks two of the most active inflammatory agents in the body, *prostaglandin* and *leukotriene*.

To test feverfew's effectiveness in treating migraines, the London Migraine Clinic conducted a six-month study of long-time feverfew users. One group continued taking feverfew and the other took a placebo, but neither group knew what they were taking until after the study was over. The people who took the placebo had a significant increase in the frequency and intensity of headaches as well as nausea and vomiting. Those who were taking feverfew were able to ward off migraines just like they always had.

These positive test results prompted Canadian health officials to grant a Drug Identification Number for a British feverfew preparation. That manufacturer can now claim its nonprescription feverfew product is effective in the prevention of migraine headaches. Any feverfew preparation should contain at least 0.2 percent of the active ingredient parthenolide. The recommended dosage is 125 mg of dried leaves. You can get the equivalent of this by chewing and swallowing one or two fresh leaves each day. You can find feverfew at most health and nutrition stores.

Although a large number of long-time feverfew users have not reported any toxic reactions, toxicity studies have not yet been performed. To be on the safe side, pregnant women and those who are breast-feeding shouldn't use feverfew.

For all of you gardeners, you may want to grow your own feverfew instead of buying it at the store. Plant it in dry, well-drained soil in full sun. The cheery yellow and white daisy-like flowers will add a lively touch to your garden and remind you that your migraine cure isn't far away. Sow seeds in the spring or fall and take stem cuttings in the summer. Divide the roots in the fall. The flowers bloom from July to October. You can harvest the leaves and flowers throughout the blooming season.

If you're a migraine sufferer, you may want to try this time-honored migraine remedy for yourself. Feverfew's powerful anti-inflammatory ingredients will calm your migraines and may keep you from having to take costly prescription drugs.

**Sources:**
*Herbs,* R.D. Home Handbook, The Reader's Digest Association, Pleasantville, N.Y., 1990
*Pharmacy Times* (61,7:32)
*The Honest Herbal,* The Haworth Press, Binghamton, N.Y., 1993
*The Lawrence Review of Natural Products,* Facts and Comparisons, St. Louis, Mo., 1994

# Inexpensive migraine relief

If you are familiar with the pounding pain of a migraine, you'll probably do almost anything to prevent it. Drastic measures may not be needed. Relief could be as simple as a daily vitamin supplement. A recent study of migraine sufferers found that 400 mg of riboflavin daily reduced migraine severity substantially. Though more research needs to be done, riboflavin may provide an easy and inexpensive solution to a very painful problem.

**Source:**
*Nutrition Research Newsletter* (14,2:26)

# A fishy solution for migraines

If you've been fishing around for a solution to your migraines, maybe you should consider fish. In a recent study, researchers at the University of Cincinnati gave fish oil capsules containing omega-3 fatty acids to migraine sufferers. About 60 percent of the people in the study reduced the frequency as well as the severity of their headaches. You can find natural sources of omega-3 in tuna, cod, salmon, and other types of seafood.

**Source:**
*The Food Pharmacy,* Bantam Books, New York, 1988

## Self-control stops headache pain

If you have cold feet (or cold hands), maybe you're afraid of something, but it could be an indication that you have migraines. Researchers find that people who have migraines usually have cold hands and feet. Their finger temperatures tend to be about 70 degrees Fahrenheit, while people without headaches usually have finger temperatures around 85 degrees.

Since migraines are thought to be caused by blood vessels in the head expanding more than they should, researchers theorized that increasing the temperature in the fingers by increasing the blood flow to them might reduce migraines. This technique, called *thermal biofeedback*, proved to be very effective. Up to three-fourths of the people in a study who practiced this twice a day cut migraine attacks in half.

Psychologists can provide professional biofeedback training, but the technique is relatively simple. Find a quiet spot and place a finger thermometer on your index finger. The bulb of the thermometer should be on the fleshiest part of your fingertip. Tape the thermometer securely so it doesn't slip. Write down the temperature.

Put on some soothing music and make sure you're comfortable. Don't cross your arms or legs. Close your eyes and breathe slowly, using your *diaphragm* (the muscle that separates your chest from your abdomen). Breathe in through your nose while counting mentally to four and hold it for four seconds. Breathe out slowly through your mouth for a count of eight. Continue this until you're breathing easily.

Say to yourself, "My hand," as you breathe in and say "is warm," as you breathe out. Concentrate on each part of your body, saying, "My feet are heavy and warm. My legs are heavy and warm, etc." until you feel that your entire body is heavy and warm. Then say "My breathing is calm, and my forehead is cool."

Visualize yourself at a pleasant spot, like a deserted beach or beside a cool waterfall. Picture the sun warming your fingers and feel your heartbeat carrying blood to your fingers. Continue imagining a pleasant scene, allowing yourself to get lost in the soothing music for 20 to 30 minutes.

Record your finger temperature at the end of your session. Practice this method twice a day, and you could see a rise in your finger temperature, as well as a reduction in your headaches.

*Source:*
*Headache Free*, Bantam Books, New York, 1996

## Better breathing, fewer headaches

A breath of fresh air can sometimes clear your head, but learning to breathe properly may prevent your head from hurting in the first place.

You use certain muscles when you breathe, and since you breathe all the time (you'd be in trouble if you didn't), those muscles can get a real workout. If you breathe correctly, from your diaphragm, the neck and upper back muscles aren't used. If you use those muscles with every breath, they can become tense and sore and lead to a headache.

You may think that holding in your tummy makes you more attractive, but it may also lead to improper breathing. Correct breathing involves lowering the diaphragm so the chest cavity above it is enlarged. This causes the lungs to expand by reducing the air pressure around them. If you are constantly trying to hold in your tummy, you can't lower your diaphragm. Instead you probably draw air into your lungs by lifting your rib cage with the muscles of your neck and upper back.

Even if you have been breathing improperly your entire life, you can learn to breathe diaphragmatically in just two to three weeks. A biofeedback therapist can give you the best instructions on breathing properly.

*Source:*
*National Headache Foundation Head Lines* (94:3)

## Relax your way to headache relief

Stress is a way of life. You have work to do, bills to pay, family to take care of, a hundred errands to run, and your juggling act is getting a little shaky. It's no wonder that tension headaches account for almost 90 percent of all headaches.

Tension headaches cause a dull, persistent pain that can last from 30 minutes to seven days. Although they don't usually interfere with your everyday activities, they can still be very uncomfortable. Some people describe the pain as a band tightening around their heads.

The pain of tension headaches is thought to be related to blood vessels in the head as well as stress. Stress can cause muscles to tense up, making the pain worse. Relaxing those muscles can help you get rid of your headache.

In a recent study, researchers divided headache sufferers into three groups. One group used biofeedback techniques to relax their foreheads. The second group concentrated on relaxing their *trapezius muscles* (muscles that attach the shoulder blades to the back of the head) using biofeedback, and the third group practiced relaxation therapy on all their muscles.

Researchers found that half of the people who focused on their foreheads felt relief from their headache pain, a little over a third of the people who relaxed all their muscles felt headache pain relief, but all of the people who concentrated on relaxing their trapezius muscles reduced their headache pain.

Biofeedback techniques involve concentrating on warming the muscles and visualizing relaxing images (see *Self-control stops headache pain* in this chapter). If you can't reduce the stress in your life, maybe you can reduce your headaches by learning to relax.

*Sources:*
*American Family Physician* (51,6:1507)
*Headache* (35:411)
*Headache Free,* Bantam Books, New York, 1996

## Play ball with tension headache

You may be able to relieve stress by slamming tennis balls across a court, but did you know that tennis balls can also help relieve the pain of a tension headache? Simply stuff two tennis balls into the toe of a nonelastic sock and tie it tightly so the balls don't move. Then lie down on the floor with the tennis balls positioned just underneath the spot where your skull meets your neck. The tennis balls will put pressure on the muscles that cause the headache, forcing them to relax. This should eventually ease your tension and end your headache.

*Source:*
*Emergency Medicine* (28,8:46)

## Follow your nose to find headache woes

Do the sunny days of spring with all the lovely flowers blooming give you a headache? If you only get headaches at certain times of the year, or if your headaches are accompanied by a stuffy nose and pressure behind your nose and eyes, sinuses may be the root of your problem.

Most sinus headaches are caused by allergies. Irritants, such as pollen, spark an allergic reaction that leads to stuffy, congested sinuses. This can result in painful head and facial pressure. If your pain gets worse if you bend over or cough, you probably have a sinus headache.

The simplest way to avoid a sinus headache is to avoid your irritants. This may not be as simple as it sounds because you could be allergic to several different things. You can have allergy testing done to identify your irritants or just try to figure them out and eliminate them yourself, one by one.

Because sinus congestion contributes to your headache, relieving your congestion quickly may head off that ache. Warm facial packs, inhaling steam, saline nasal sprays, or decongestants may help. For more information on sinusitis, refer to the *Breathing Easy* chapter.

*Sources:*
*American Family Physician* (53,3:877)
*The Headache Book,* Thomas Nelson Publishers, Nashville, Tenn., 1994

## A fast way to a headache

Unhealthy diet habits will tell on you. Take skipping meals, for instance. Everyone knows that refusing to eat is not an effective way to get rid of excess weight, and it might make you a grouch, too.

A new study has revealed that skipping meals can lead to a nasty headache. The study showed that over one-third of people who chose not to eat (also called "fasting") developed a headache.

Scientists have seen this relationship between fasting and headaches in other studies, but they still don't know why it happens. Maybe it's just your body's way of steering you away from an unhealthy habit.

*Source:*
*The Atlanta Journal/Constitution* (Dec. 26, 1995, B12)

## Clobber cluster headaches

The pain of a cluster headache is often described as the worst pain known to man. More men definitely know about clusters because they strike men six times more often than women.

A cluster headache causes excruciating pain, even more severe than a migraine. The pain is sharp and burning and is almost always located on one side of your head. Your nose may stuff up or run on the affected side. Your eye may water, your eyelid droop, and your face may become flushed.

Clusters are so called because they occur in cycles or "clusters," which may last several weeks or months. During this period, you may have as many as eight attacks a day. The cluster period is followed by a headache-free period until you begin having headaches again.

No one knows for sure what causes clusters, but they may be related to your sleep-wake cycle. Most attacks occur at night and interrupt your sleep. Elevating the head of your bed 8 to 10 inches and sticking to a regular sleep schedule may help prevent clusters.

Many cluster sufferers are heavy smokers and drinkers. Drinking and smoking can trigger a headache during your cluster period but not during your headache-free period.

Some cluster sufferers have found that immersing one of their hands in ice water to the point of discomfort will relieve their headaches.

Because cluster headaches strike so suddenly and severely, most pain relievers don't help. Your doctor can prescribe medicine to help prevent clusters from occurring, and some people successfully use oxygen to stop a cluster headache in its tracks.

*Sources:*
American Family Physician (51,6:1498)
Patient Care (21:71)
The Headache Book, Thomas Nelson Publishers, Nashville, Tenn., 1994

## Headache pain that grinds on you

If you wake up in the morning feeling as though someone slammed your head into a wall, you may suffer from *temporomandibular joint syndrome*, commonly known as TMJ.

Teeth-grinding during sleep is a common cause of TMJ, a joint disorder of the jaw that often leads to severe headaches. Most people will experience *bruxism*, the official name for tooth-grinding or clenching, at some point in their lives. Usually, it is a temporary condition and will go away on its own.

Many people grind their teeth unconsciously in response to stress. The habit may be an outlet for anxiety or anger. If you are very achievement-oriented and compulsively punctual, you're more likely to grind your teeth. Even a stressful event later in life, such as the loss of a spouse, can trigger bruxism.

Teeth-grinding can cause other problems besides TMJ, such as mouth infections, worn-down teeth, and sore necks and backs. That toothache you have may be just a symptom of bruxism. Stopping your bruxism may also stop your headaches.

To help stop the pain, try these tips:

◆ Ask your sleeping partner to wake you if he hears you grinding your teeth.

◆ Close your lips, hold your teeth apart, and relax your jaw. Do this 50 times a day, and then imagine sleeping with your mouth in this relaxed position.

◆ Clench your teeth for five seconds, then relax your jaw for five seconds. Do this exercise five times in a row, six times a day, for two weeks.

◆ Change your sleeping position. Lying on your back with a pillow under your neck and knees may help relax your jaw.

◆ Reduce stress. Try a relaxing bedtime ritual such as reading or a warm bath. If that doesn't work, you may need counseling to help you deal with stress.

One common cause of TMJ is upper and lower teeth that don't fit together properly. If the suggestions to relieve bruxism don't help your headaches, see your dentist. He can probably fit you for an appliance that will realign your jaw and head off your headache pain.

*Sources:*
*American Family Physician* (49,7:1617)
*Pain and the TMJ,* American Academy of Otolaryngology, Alexandria, Va., 22312

## Handling hangover headaches

You have no one to blame but yourself for a hangover headache, but that's little comfort when you're miserable and your head is pounding.

The best way to avoid a hangover is to avoid drinking alcohol. If you decide to imbibe, be careful what you drink and how much. Alcoholic beverages contain ingredients called *congeners*, which help give each beverage its distinctive taste and also contribute to your hangover. Bourbon, red wine, and champagne contain a lot of congeners, which is why they are common headache triggers. Vodka, on the other hand, has hardly any congeners and is less likely to cause a hangover.

Too much alcohol causes a metabolic disturbance in your body, resulting in low sugar in your brain. If you happen to overindulge in alcohol, eating something containing the sugar *fructose* before going to bed may help. Fructose, which can be found in honey and fruits, helps your body metabolize alcohol.

Alcohol can cause dehydration, so be sure to drink plenty of fluids. The old standby of drinking coffee really does help both tension headaches and hangover headaches. It may not sober you up, but it can relieve your headache by tightening up blood vessels the alcohol has enlarged.

*Sources:*
*Food — Your Miracle Medicine,* HarperCollins, New York, 1993
*Postgraduate Medicine* (99,2:38)

## Pain on the rebound

Is your pain reliever giving you a headache? When it comes to curing headaches, the cure may sometimes make the discomfort worse. A recent study of headache sufferers found that over half of them experienced analgesic rebound. This occurs when you take a short-acting pain reliever (aspirin, acetaminophen, etc.) for your headache, and as soon as the effects of the medicine wear off, the pain returns — stronger than before. Almost none of the people in the study were even aware that such a phenomenon existed. Before you pop a pill for your headache, try some nondrug remedies like biofeedback (see *Self-control stops headache pain* earlier in this chapter). Avoid painkillers whenever possible to prevent a continuing chain of headaches.

*Source:*
*American Family Physician* (51,1:203)

# Hold off headaches with hypnosis

Ever been hypnotized?

Think not? Well, think again. Chances are good that you probably have, and you probably hypnotized yourself.

Television serves as a hypnotic tool for some people. Consider the case of Jerry Grover of Atlanta. When the television is on, he becomes so absorbed he neither hears nor notices what is going on around him.

What his frustrated friends and family don't realize when they try to communicate with him while the television is on is that he has fallen into a state similar to a hypnotic trance.

Most people, at one time or another, will recall falling into a similar state, only to come crashing back to current consciousness and realize someone has been trying to attract their attention for several minutes.

Although hypnosis is derived from the Greek word *hypnos*, meaning sleep, hypnosis is actually a state of intense concentration instead of the semiconscious sleep state many people associate with hypnosis.

No one knows for sure how hypnosis works, but it can be a powerful tool for fighting headache pain. The basic process involves concentrating on helpful ideas or images — either from another person, like a hypnotherapist, or from yourself, while you are in a relaxed, hypnotic state.

If you want to try self-hypnosis, sit in a comfortable chair with no distractions and close your eyes. Tense and relax your muscles one at a time until all your muscles are relaxed. Then focus on a pleasant image or concentrate on a helpful suggestion.

For example, you might visualize the blood vessels in your head and concentrate on making them smaller. Another suggestion that might help your headache is to imagine a feeling of coldness in your head which could cause blood vessels to constrict. For a tension headache problem, you could concentrate on relaxing the muscles in your head and neck.

The next time you just can't stand your headache pain, maybe you should put your powers of concentration to good use and practice a little self-hypnotism. If hypnotism can rid you of your headache, your mood should improve, and your family and friends might just thank you instead of becoming frustrated with you.

*Source:*
*National Headache Foundation Head Lines* (96:5)

# Simple Solutions for Common Problems

## Tracking down the cause of your tiredness

Fatigue is a problem that everyone has to deal with from time to time. If you are tired, the cause can be something as simple as too little sleep, or as complex as chronic fatigue syndrome (CFS or CFIDS). To figure out what might be at the root of your tiredness, here is a list of other possible causes of fatigue:

- ◆ Allergies
- ◆ Anemia (caused by low levels of iron or vitamin B12 in your blood)
- ◆ Candidiasis (yeast infection)
- ◆ Heart disease
- ◆ Chronic disease
- ◆ Depletion of your adrenal glands (from stress or overuse of caffeine, alcohol, tobacco, or other drugs)
- ◆ Depression
- ◆ Diabetes
- ◆ Headaches
- ◆ Hypoglycemia (low blood sugar)
- ◆ Infection (a likely cause when fatigue is accompanied by fever)
- ◆ Lack of certain nutrients (sometimes caused by strict dieting)
- ◆ Obesity
- ◆ Premenstrual syndrome
- ◆ Sleep disturbances
- ◆ Stress (excessive or continuous)
- ◆ Thyroid problems (either overactive or underactive thyroid gland)
- ◆ Toxicity (continuous exposure to environmental hazards such as lead, mercury, or aluminum)

If your fatigue continues, be sure to see your doctor. Your problem of tiredness may have a simple solution.

**Source:**
*Alternative Medicine*, Future Medicine Publishing, Puyallup, Wash., 1993

## What to do when you're sick and tired of being sick and tired

Everyone experiences fatigue sometimes; usually it goes away with a good night's rest. But when your fatigue lasts for months, maybe even years, it may be due to Chronic Fatigue Immune Dysfunction Syndrome (CFIDS), commonly called chronic fatigue syndrome.

This condition, which affects almost 2.5 million Americans, has a wide range of symptoms. Besides fatigue, you may experience low-grade fever, night sweats, sleep disturbances, swollen lymph nodes, sore muscles, and mental ailments such as confusion, anxiety, loss of concentration, and memory impairment. The cause of CFIDS is still unknown, but some researchers think chronic fatigue is triggered by viruses such as the *herpes* virus.

The essential amino acid *lysine,* in supplement form, is successfully reducing CFIDS symptoms in some people. Lysine is a popular remedy for cold sores and mouth ulcers caused by the herpes virus. Scientists have found that almost all people with CFIDS carry the herpes virus, but not everyone who is exposed to herpes gets chronic fatigue syndrome.

A California writer, Cameron Stauth, tells his own personal story about how he beat chronic fatigue syndrome by taking large doses of lysine. He now takes lysine for maintenance, along with large doses of vitamin C, and is free of the symptoms of CFIDS.

The theory behind lysine treatment is that people who get CFIDS carry at least one of three herpes viruses: *cytomegalovirus*, *Epstein-Barr virus*, or *human herpes-virus 6*. The viruses remain dormant in your body until some outside factor, such as severe stress, weakens your immune system and triggers them. Lysine helps keep these viruses from reproducing.

Lysine supplements are available in health-food stores. Lysine also occurs naturally in red meat, cheese, eggs, fish, potatoes, soy products, lima beans, and yeast.

The nonessential amino acid *arginine* helps the viruses to reproduce, so if you have CFIDS, don't take arginine supplements and go easy on foods containing arginine. Arginine can be found in cereals, whole-wheat products, brown rice, popcorn, nuts, raisins, pumpkin and sesame seeds, gelatin, and chocolate.

If you think you have chronic fatigue, see your doctor and ask him if lysine supplements might help you.

**Sources:**
*Medical Update* (19,4:1)
*The Saturday Evening Post* (267,6:50)
*The CFIDS Chronicle* (1,1:15)
*The PDR Guide to Nutrition and Health,* Medical Economics Company, Montvale, N.J., 1995

# 4 tips for instant energy

If you think that your lack of energy is due to simple fatigue, here are four little ideas to help you get back on an energetic track:

- ◆ Speaking as loudly as you can, count from one to 10.
- ◆ Stand up, whistle, cheer, stomp your feet, and give yourself a 60-second round of applause.
- ◆ Play some bright, lively music. Sing along, dance, or sway to the beat.
- ◆ Mix a glass of this high-energy drink for yourself: a half teaspoon of vitamin C crystals in a glass filled with half fruit juice, half water.

**Source:**
*Making It On Your Own,* Jeremy P. Tarcher, Los Angeles, 1991

## Dizziness self-defense

Dizziness is a frequent complaint that doctors hear, and it can be a symptom of a number of different illnesses. The most frequently occurring type of dizziness, however, doesn't indicate any underlying disease, and it can often be cured in a few minutes in a doctor's office. It's called *benign positional vertigo* or *BPV*.

If you have moments when it seems the world is spinning around you, possibly with a feeling of nausea, and it occurs when you lie down, sit up, or turn over in bed, you may have BPV. This kind of dizziness is caused by tiny calcium deposits that form in your inner ear. When they are jarred loose, possibly by a blow to your head, they bounce around on the hair cells of your inner ear and are pulled by gravity when you move. Your body gets its signals crossed and dizziness is the result.

Your doctor can diagnose benign positional vertigo by observing the movement of your eyes when you lie down on the "bad" side (the one that seems to cause the dizziness) and then sit up. Once she has diagnosed your condition, the next step should be the cure.

The *Epley maneuver* is a treatment for BPV that is usually effective in 77 percent of cases after just one treatment. Another 20 percent of people are cured after a second treatment. The alternative is to wait for your body to absorb the tiny calcium deposits, which could take as long as 10 weeks or more. The Epley maneuver involves lying down on your affected side, hanging your head down, and turning quickly to the other side, then sitting up, all in a specific sequence. It needs to be directed by your doctor, and it may have to be repeated a couple of times to be sure it worked. After the Epley maneuver, don't lie flat for 48 hours, and try sleeping in a slightly reclining position.

If your doctor doesn't know the Epley maneuver, find one who does. It isn't necessary to suffer through weeks of dizziness when the cure can be so simple.

***Sources:***
*Archives of Family Medicine* (5,3:172)
*British Medical Journal* (311,7003:489)

## Surprising cause of ear pain

If you're suffering from an intense, throbbing pain in your ear, it may not be your ear that's actually hurting. It could be your teeth.

Your head is full of sensitive nerves, and the area in and around your ears is particularly rich in its ability to send messages of pain. By a process called "referred pain," the pain can occur in a molar at the back of your mouth, yet feel as if it's in your ear.

Referred pain from teeth is usually caused by a problem in the pulp of your tooth. This may cause a throbbing, dull, or radiating pain, but it's not easy to pinpoint the specific tooth that's causing the problem. Using local anesthesia, such as Novocain, in different locations may help locate the hurting tooth.

Of course, there is a chance that your ear pain is really coming from your ear.

An infection in your outer ear, usually called "swimmer's ear," or a middle ear infection, such as the kind children often get, could be the culprit.

A good way to tell if you have an outer ear infection is to give a quick downward pull on your earlobe. If this is very painful, you probably have an outer ear infection. This test usually doesn't work for a middle ear infection. You'll need your doctor to diagnose and treat one of these.

Next time you have a bad pain in your ear, keep in mind that it may not be in your ear, but in your teeth.

**Source:**
*Compendium of Continuing Education in Dentistry* (13,8:676)

# Natural treatment for swimmer's ear

"Swimmer's ear," also known as "Hong Kong ear" and "mildew ear," is a bacterial or fungal infection of the outer ear. It usually occurs in warm climates, sometimes as a result of bacteria or fungus getting into your ear when you swim, and it can be very painful. There is no pill you can take to make it go away, and the medicine used to treat it can irritate the inside of your ear.

Doctors at the University of New Mexico in Albuquerque came up with a creative solution. They knew that garlic is an old folk remedy for earache, so they decided to test it scientifically.

When it was used on the two types of fungus that most frequently cause swimmer's ear, a liquid extract made from fresh garlic came up the clear winner. Its antifungal activity was as strong, and in some cases stronger, than the commercial medicines used to treat swimmer's ear. Even at a low concentration, garlic proved to be a potent antifungal substance. In the future, we may be using garlic as a natural treatment for ear infections.

**Source:**
*British Medical Journal* (310,6976:405)

# Exercise for your ears

You know that exercise is good for your health in general, but did you know that it can also help your hearing? Regular exercise that gets your heart pumping and your blood flowing improves your level of physical fitness. A higher level of fitness seems to improve your hearing.

Researchers at Miami University in Ohio studied volunteers at different levels of physical fitness to see whether noise and exercise caused different levels of hearing loss. The people who were the most physically fit had the best hearing. Doctors are not sure of the reason, but it may involve enzymes that work in respiration, the condition of your blood vessels, or the flow of blood to your ears. Whatever the reason, there is clearly a connection between cardiovascular fitness and good hearing.

Walking, stationary biking, or low-impact aerobic dance are good choices for getting your circulation going and keeping your ears in peak condition.

*Source:*
*Medicine and Science in Sports and Exercise* (July, 1994)

## Turn down the ringing in your ears

If you hear a ringing, tinkling, or buzzing sound that no one else hears, you may think it's your imagination or the memory of some music you have heard. But it could be a condition called *tinnitus*. The sound can come and go or be continuous. It can be a high, ringing whine; a squeal; or a low roar. Even if no one else can hear the noises inside your head, you are not alone. Thirty-six million other Americans suffer with the same problem.

The causes of tinnitus can range from a small plug of wax in your ear to a life-threatening aneurysm. Other causes include ear infection, allergy, a hole in your eardrum, high or low blood pressure, a tumor, diabetes, thyroid problems, injury, and a variety of drugs, including aspirin.

The most common cause of tinnitus, however, is damage to the microscopic endings of the nerves in your inner ear. This can be caused by exposure to loud noises. Excessively loud noises can cause hearing loss as well as tinnitus, but many people don't take noise very seriously. Industrial noise, firearms noise, loud music, and stereo headsets can permanently harm your hearing.

If your doctor can determine the cause of your tinnitus, he may be able to give you specific treatment. More often, the cause cannot be identified. Here are some things you can do for yourself that may help your tinnitus:

◆ Avoid exposure to loud noises.
◆ Have your blood pressure checked, and do whatever is necessary to keep it in normal range.
◆ Decrease the amount of salt that you eat. Too much salt impairs good blood circulation.
◆ Exercise daily. This helps your blood circulate properly to all parts of your body, including your ears.
◆ Investigate biofeedback or masking. Biofeedback is a process of learning to relax and control the circulation in certain parts of your body. Masking uses background noise to distract you from the sound in your ears. You may use a radio for this, played on low volume, or purchase a device that goes with a hearing aid to produce constant background noise.
◆ Avoid caffeine and nicotine. They cause blood vessels to constrict, and this impairs circulation.
◆ Get plenty of rest, and don't let yourself get too tired. Your body gets over-stressed and doesn't function as smoothly when you're tired.
◆ Reduce the stress and anxiety in your life as much as possible. Your ears are part of your central nervous system, and they are one of the most delicate mechanisms in your body. Anxiety and upset can affect the whole system.
◆ Stop worrying about the noise of tinnitus. It will not cause you to go deaf

or lose your mind. Learning to accept and trying to ignore the noise may become a necessary part of your life.

**Source:**
*Doctor, what causes the noise in my ears? Ten common questions about tinnitus,* American Academy of Otolaryngology-Head and Neck Surgery, 1993

## Try this simple hearing test

If you aren't sure whether you have lost some of your hearing, take this simple test. Have someone hum the "mmmmm" sound at a mid-range frequency for two or three seconds at a volume slightly softer than casual conversation.

Then you should repeat the sound back. If your humming sounds louder in one ear than another or if you have trouble hearing your friend's humming or your own humming, have your hearing checked by a hearing specialist.

**Source:**
*The Lancet* (346,8967:128)

## Help in choosing a hearing aid

Almost 20 million Americans suffer from some sort of hearing problem. The good news is, hearing aids and other devices can help. If you suspect you have a hearing problem, consult a qualified audiologist. Audiologists are specially trained to evaluate hearing and determine what's causing your problems.

If your audiologist diagnoses a hearing problem, get him to explain what type of hearing loss you have and what type of hearing aid or other devices will be most likely to help. You may also want to ask for his help in selecting a hearing aid. He may either sell hearing aids himself or be able to recommend a reputable shop.

If an audiologist assures you that a hearing aid will help, keep these tips in mind while shopping around:

♦ Look for a company that offers a 30-day trial period to see if the hearing aid meets your expectations. Most reputable hearing aid and audiology offices will offer this service.

♦ Don't be fooled by people who promise that your hearing aid will make all speech clearer or totally eliminate background noise. Hearing aids can help you hear better, but more than likely you still won't be able to understand speech as well as you could when you had normal hearing.

♦ Buy the very best hearing aid you can afford. In a reputable office, a higher price usually means higher quality. The better a hearing aid is, the better it will amplify sounds without distortion.

♦ Consider getting a hearing aid for each ear. That's because hearing loss often occurs about the same time in both ears. If you have hearing loss in both ears, but wear only one hearing aid, you'll probably find it very difficult to distinguish between sounds, especially in noisy places.

♦ Select a style that suits you. You have lots to choose from, including the powerful behind-the-ear style, in-the-ear models, and tiny in-the-ear-canal types. Ask your audiologist to help you choose a hearing aid best suited to your type of hearing loss, lifestyle, ability to work with small objects, and general preferences.

◆ Keep trying. If you bought a hearing aid a few years ago that didn't do anything for you, don't give up. In the past three to five years, hearing aids have improved dramatically in battery life, circuitry, distortion reduction, quality, and style.

◆ Have your hearing tested annually by an audiologist. Continued hearing loss may indicate a medical problem that needs other treatment. This is also a good time to evaluate the effectiveness of your hearing aid.

Keep in mind that it may take some time to get used to a hearing aid. You may feel overloaded by the sound levels at first or experience a high level of background noise. If you're unhappy with your hearing aid, don't hesitate to complain to the company. If you think you've been deceived, contact one of the four agencies with principal regulatory control over hearing aids: the Food and Drug Administration, the Federal Trade Commission, or your state's attorney general or licensing board.

*Sources:*
*American Demographics* (16,11:48)
*Generations* (19,1:47)
*The Exceptional Parent* (25,5:55)
*The Journal of the American Geriatrics Society* (43,8:928)
*USA Today* (123,2597:11)

# Other devices can help your hearing

Along with hearing aids, there are some other ways to make life easier for people with hearing loss. Here are some practical ways to assist your hearing:

**Televised closed captioning.** Most new televisions come equipped with decoding devices built right in. Virtually everything on television is closed captioned, so you can enjoy all your favorite shows — and even some of the commercials.

**Assistive listening devices.** For people who have trouble interpreting sounds that come from some distance away, such as in church or at a movie, assistive listening devices can really help. With the new technology available, a speaker's voice or movie track can be transmitted directly to special headphones you wear.

Under a 1991 federal ruling, theaters and other places where people often assemble are required to stock assistive listening devices for at least 5 percent of the seating capacity. All you have to do to receive one is ask.

**Amplified phone handsets.** These devices, which you can pick up at your local electronics store for about $20, slip over the earpiece of your phone receiver and amplify sounds coming through. Be sure to take your phone with you when you go to purchase this device so the dealer can help match your amplifier to the color and brand of your phone.

Some behind-the-ear hearing aids have a telecoil with a switch which enables the hearing aid to transmit sound directly from the phone into your ear instead of through the phone amplifier. With this option, you're able to tune out background noise.

**Tele-typewriter (TTY)**, also known as a Telecommunications Device for the Deaf (TDD) or Text Telephone (TT). TTYs include keyboards and view screens that attach to telephones allowing you to communicate with other TTYs by typing text.

If the person you're trying to communicate with does not have a TTY, you can use a TTY relay service, which acts as an intermediary between TTY users and users of standard telephones. Most local and long-distance phone companies offer this service.

For more information on TTYs or other listening devices for people with hearing problems, call Telecommunications for the Deaf at (301) 589-3006 or (301) 589-3797 (TTY). If you prefer, you can write to them at 8719 Colesville Rd., Ste. 300, Silver Spring, Md., 20910.

With the technology available today, there's no need to turn your television up so loud it peels the paint off your walls or have to guess what somebody is saying to you. Of course, you won't be able to say you didn't hear your spouse the next time you're called to help with a household project. But that's a small price to pay to have your hearing back.

*Sources:*
*American Demographics* (16,11:48)
*Generations* (19,1:47)
*The Exceptional Parent* (25,5:55)
*The Journal of the American Geriatrics Society* (43,8:928)
*USA Today* (123,2597:11)

## Consumer group helps hard of hearing

If you are experiencing tinnitus or hearing loss due to illness, injury, or aging, you are not alone. It is natural to feel isolated by hearing problems, but you don't have to let them control your life. One group that is doing something about the problem is a nonprofit organization called SHHH, or Self-Help for Hard of Hearing People.

SHHH is a consumer group "dedicated to the well-being of people who don't hear well." Its primary purpose is education. SHHH has a bimonthly magazine, the *SHHH Journal*, and a national organization as well as local chapters all over the country.

If you would like more information, write to: Self-Help for Hard of Hearing People, Inc., 7910 Woodmont Ave., Suite 1200, Bethesda, Md. 20814 or call (301) 657-2248.

*Source:*
*SHHH Journal* (17,1:22)

## See better without glasses

Could you exercise your eyes like you exercise the rest of your body and just throw away your glasses? The belief that exercise can improve your eyesight isn't a new idea. It's been around since the 1920s. The late Dr. William H. Bates, author of the book *Better Eyesight Without Glasses*, said that the root of all eye problems is mental tension. He believed wrong habits of thought, such as a bored stare, or trying to see with too much effort, are at the root of poor eyesight. Bates' ideas remain controversial, but an offshoot of his theories is behavioral optometry.

Behavioral optometrists believe that you can improve your vision, need less correction in your lenses, and make your eyes healthier through a series of exercises like the ones that follow. These exercises, from the book *Seven Steps to Better Vision* by Richard Leviton, should be done without your glasses or contact lenses.

◆ Palming is a method of resting your eyes in total darkness. Rub your palms together briskly to warm them, and place them over your closed eyes without pressing on them. Relax your mind and concentrate on the darkness before you.

◆ Sunning uses natural light to trigger essential physical processes in your body. It is best done for two to five minutes a few times a day before 10 a.m. and after 4 p.m., so you can avoid the hours of brightest sunlight. With your eyes closed, face the sun and slowly move your head from left to right. After about three minutes, stop for a brief session of palming. The contrast between these two actions helps make your pupils more flexible.

◆ Blinking is a natural action that rests your eyes, stretches your eye muscles, massages your eyeballs, and forces your pupils to dilate and contract. Many people don't blink enough, and this can be harmful to your eyes. To do this exercise, make dozens of quick blinks as you turn your head slowly from side to side for about 20 seconds.

◆ Watching a ball improves the shifting of your eyes. Toss a tennis ball into the air and watch it while blinking frequently. Or you can watch a live tennis match, focusing on the back-and-forth motion of the ball.

◆ Thumb zooming exercises your figure and ground focusing. Place your arm out straight in front of you with your thumb up. Relax, breathe, and blink frequently while you focus on your thumb, noting its clear outline against a fuzzy background. Shift your focus to something in the background, at least 10 feet away, and you will see two thumbs. Move your focus back and forth several times between your thumb and the background.

◆ Edging helps your eyes sweep the visual field with rapid shifts and discourages staring. Pick out an object beyond your clear range of vision and use your nose as a pointer to trace the edges of the object. Move your head naturally as you trace the outline, then repeat the process and trace in the opposite direction.

◆ Eye stretching helps the coordination of your eyes by moving them in a systematic manner, as well as stretching the eye muscles and improving circulation. For these exercises, you need to relax, breathe, and blink frequently.

1. Squeeze your eyes tightly shut and hold for a few seconds, then open them suddenly. Repeat several times, closing your eyes as you exhale and opening them as you inhale.
2. With your eyes open, look up as far as you can, then look down as far as you can. Do this without straining, keeping your head facing forward and your neck and shoulders relaxed.
3. Do this exercise only if it doesn't strain your eyes. Look way up while inhaling, then down while exhaling. Do 20 quick blinks. Look as far to the right as you can, then as far to the left as you can, repeating 10 times. Do 20 more quick blinks, then look up to the right, down to the left, up to the left, and down to the right. Repeat 10 times.

*Source:*
*Seven Steps to Better Vision,* East West Natural Health Books, Brookline, Mass., 1992

## Good nutrition clears up cloudy vision

Remember when you were a child, and your mother told you to eat your carrots because they were good for your eyes? Well, it turns out that she was absolutely right. A recent study has shown that eating vegetables high in carotenoids, a yellow pigment found naturally in some fruits and vegetables, can reduce your risk of developing blindness later in life.

Age-related macular degeneration (AMD) is the leading cause of irreversible blindness in people over 65 years old in the United States. It occurs when the retina and other parts of your eye begin to deteriorate and gradually decrease your ability to see. Once it occurs, there isn't much doctors can do to help.

However, it now seems clear that eating lots of healthy vegetables containing carotenoids can help prevent AMD. The theory is that carotenoids prevent the damage that would be caused by scavenging *free radicals* (cell-damaging particles) within the structure of your eyes.

In the study of 876 people, those who ate the most vegetables containing carotenoids had a 43 percent lower risk of developing AMD. Carrots, sweet potatoes, cabbage, cauliflower, and winter squash are high in carotenoids, but dark green, leafy vegetables, such as broccoli and brussels sprouts, seem to provide the best protection of all.

*Sources:*
*Medical Tribune for the Internist and Cardiologist* (36,1:19)
*The Journal of the American Medical Association* (273,21:1703)

## Eye-opening news about vitamin A deficiency

Vitamin A is an essential nutrient for the normal function of the retinas of your eyes. One of the first symptoms of vitamin A deficiency is the loss of your ability to see well at night. Eventually, a severe lack of vitamin A can cause complete blindness.

If you have pancreatic disease, gastrointestinal disease, or have had an intestinal bypass or resection surgery, your ability to absorb nutrients, including vitamin A, is reduced. If you have any type of liver disease, your ability to store vitamin A is impaired. In either of these situations, you may become deficient in vitamin A.

If you have gastrointestinal or liver problems, and you notice that you are also having problems with your eyes, check with your doctor. He can test to see if you have enough vitamin A stored in your body, or if you need to take supplements. Natural sources of vitamin A include beef liver, spinach, carrots, and sweet potatoes.

*Sources:*
British Medical Journal (310,6986:1050)
Complete Guide to Vitamins, Minerals & Supplements, Fisher Books, Tucson, Ariz., 1988

## Scratch that urge to rub your eyes

It may feel good at the end of a long day to rub your eyes, but it's actually a bad habit that can hurt your eyes. A tiny muscle, the *levator*, raises and holds your upper eyelid in place. It is held in place by a tiny band of tissue that can deteriorate with age. Rubbing your eyes can strain this tissue and speed up the process, causing your eyelids to droop.

Eye rubbing is dangerous for people who are nearsighted or who have had cataract surgery. Vigorous rubbing can put pressure on your eyeball and cause detachment of your retina. A detached retina can only be repaired with delicate eye surgery.

If you feel that you must rub your eye, rub just your eyebrow, or the skin over your cheekbone and under your eye. This should provide relief from itching or irritation of your eye. Eye-rubbing may be a tough habit to break, but it's worth the effort to take care of your "windows to the world."

*Source:*
Medical Update (18,10:6)

## Guide to proper use of eye medicine

Most of the time, your eyes function efficiently and without too much fuss. They open for business every morning and get you through the day seeing what you need to see. But occasionally they may need special care, such as eye drops for redness or irritation, or a prescription drug for an eye infection.

Here are some tips to help you use your eye medicine in the safest and best way:

◆ Wash your hands before using any eye medicine.
◆ Check the bottle or tube to be certain the expiration date has not passed. If the eye drops are in suspension (having particles in the liquid), shake the bottle before using.
◆ If you are using ointment and the dosage is once a day, plan to apply it at bedtime. If you must use it during the day, use extra care if you have to

drive or operate machinery. Eye ointments can cause blurred vision.

◆ To administer the medicine, tilt your head backward or lie down and look toward the ceiling. With your finger just below the eyelashes, gently pull your eyelid down and away to form a pouch. This is where the medicine will go.

◆ To avoid contamination and the risk of infection, don't touch the tip of the bottle or tube to your eyelid.

◆ Squeeze one drop of liquid or 1/4 inch to 1/2 inch of ointment or gel into the pouch you have made with your eyelid. Just before releasing the drop, look toward the ceiling. Then look down so that the medicine is distributed evenly over your eye. For ointment or gel, close your eye for one to two minutes and roll your eye around to distribute it evenly. If you need to use more medicine, wait five minutes between drops.

◆ As soon as you apply eye drops, place your finger at the corner of your eye next to your nose and press gently for three to five minutes. This keeps the medicine in your eye and prevents it from draining into your nose.

◆ If you are supposed to use two different types of medicine for your eye at approximately the same time, wait five to 10 minutes between medications. That way, they don't interfere with each other or dilute or wash each other out of your eye.

◆ When you must apply both a liquid and an ointment or gel to your eye, use the eye drops first. Then wait five minutes before using the ointment or gel.

*Source:*
*U.S. Pharmacist* (20,11:58)

## Keep clear of cataracts

Want to steer clear of cataracts? Then be a lean, mean, yogurt-eating machine.

The latest reports from the Physicians' Health Study found that lean men get cataracts less often than overweight or even average-weight men. The study found that lean or average-weight men had the least risk of developing cataracts. Moderately overweight men had a one and a half times greater risk of developing cataracts, and obese men had more than double the risk.

If you decide to go lean to limit your risk of cataracts, be careful not to go to extremes. It's important to get all your essential vitamins and minerals because malnutrition can also increase your risk of cataracts.

Other healthy habits also appear to play a part in preventing cataract development. Most of the men with the least risk of cataracts also took multivitamins, drank little alcohol, and exercised regularly.

Living lean may protect you from cataracts for a while, but it's not a lifelong guarantee. The longer you live, the more likely you are to develop cataracts, which occur as a natural result of aging. It seems that being overweight simply speeds up the process.

While you're becoming lean, you may be able to lower your cataract risk even more by living it up on low-fat yogurt. A French study revealed that yogurt not only knocks out yeast infections, it does a one-two punch on cataracts, too. Researchers aren't sure how this works, but it seems that people who eat the most yogurt are the least likely to develop cataracts.

*Sources:*
*Archives of Ophthalmology* (1995,113:1131)
*Hamilton and Whitney's Nutrition Concepts and Controversies,* West Publishing, New York, 1994
*The Atlanta Journal/Constitution* (Sept. 15, 1994, H6)

# Blinding love

The link between sexual activity and heart attack or stroke is an occasional, unfortunate fact. Now three East Coast doctors have established a connection between sex and temporary blindness. They looked at incidents involving six people, five men and one woman, ages 24 to 53 years, who experienced temporary blindness in one eye. Although they didn't want to admit it at first, it turned out that each person had been engaged in vigorous sexual activity just before his blindness.

The doctors think the cause of the blindness is linked to elevated blood pressure during sexual arousal. Weak capillaries (tiny blood vessels) in your eye can rupture when blood pressure increases dramatically. This rupture can cause a temporary loss of sight, blurring of vision, or a blind spot in one eye.

Men have a higher risk of this happening. One 52-year-old man experienced this kind of vision loss in his right eye 30 times. When his doctor treated him with *nifedipine*, a calcium channel blocker, the symptoms stopped. If you experience any kind of vision problem that doesn't clear up within a few hours, see your eye doctor for a checkup.

*Sources:*
*Emergency Medicine* (29,1:60)
*The New England Journal of Medicine* (333,6:393)

# Neatest way to stop a nosebleed

The best way to stop a nosebleed is to put pressure on the lower cartilage of your nose for at least 10 minutes. Dr. John Ellis of Oakland, Calif., uses common medical supplies to create a simple clamp that can put even pressure on your nose and stop the bleeding. All you need is a tongue depressor and some cloth tape.

Break the tongue depressor in half and wrap tape around the curved ends to pad them. Tape the broken ends together to form a clamp. Place the clamp on your nose, and you can do other things while you wait for your nosebleed to stop.

*Source:*
*Emergency Medicine* (27,4:54)

## When your nose no longer knows

If you couldn't enjoy the sweet scent of roses in the summer or the spicy aroma of pumpkin pie in the fall, life just wouldn't be as nice. But losing your sense of smell, either partially or completely, not only deprives you of pleasure, it's actually dangerous.

Your sense of smell provides your sense of taste, so if you can't smell food, it loses its appeal. If food is spoiled and you can't smell it, you can't tell that it might be dangerous to eat. Without a sense of smell, you may not know when to bathe, change clothes, or clean your house. It's even more dangerous that you can't smell a gas leak, smoke, or some harmful chemical in the air. People who have lost their sense of smell are called *anosmic*. The loss or impairment of smell can be temporary or permanent, depending on the situation and the cause.

A small number of people are born without a sense of smell, but most anosmic people lose their ability to smell either suddenly or gradually. The loss of smell can be caused by a viral infection (mostly affecting older people), trauma to the head (mostly affecting younger people), or inflammation in your *olfactory* (aroma-sensing) system.

One woman who had gradually lost her sense of smell tried everything to regain it, including medicine and surgery. It was finally discovered, after her dog died, that she had been having an allergic reaction to her pet for a number of years. Her allergy caused inflammation and swelling in her olfactory system, and she lost her sense of smell.

If you have no sense of smell, you need to take extra precautions to make up for the lack of one of your five senses. You should have several smoke detectors installed in your home; use an electric rather than a gas stove, if possible, or at least have a gas detector installed; and get someone else to check that food is not spoiled before you eat it. If you are in doubt about any food, throw it out.

If you have lost your ability to smell, see your doctor. He may be able to pinpoint the cause and give you back the scent of roses.

*Source:*
*Postgraduate Medicine* (98,1:107)

## Cold sore cure

It's aggravating and humiliating to have an ugly cold sore pop up on your lip just before an important occasion, but it can happen if you're a person who routinely suffers from cold sores. Also known as fever blisters, cold sores are caused by the *herpes simplex* virus. The virus can lie dormant in a nerve of your face, then travel down the nerve to cause an outbreak at a most inconvenient time, often when you're under stress.

Now there's help in the form of *lysine*, an essential amino acid which actually seems to counteract the herpes virus. Lysine is an "essential" amino acid because it can't be manufactured in your body, so you have to get it in the foods you eat or in supplement form. In our bodies, lysine plays an important role in the repair of damaged tissue and in the production of antibodies, hormones, and enzymes.

Lysine supplements seem to be the most successful way to treat a cold sore. The late Dr. Richard Griffith, professor of medicine at Indiana University, suggested treatment of cold sores with a daily dose of 500 mg (milligrams) of L-lysine per 22 pounds of your weight. If you are a 122-pound woman, you would take six 500-mg tablets, or 3 grams daily. If you are a 185-pound man, you would take nine 500-mg tablets daily, or 4.5 grams of lysine. To prevent outbreaks, Dr. Griffith recommended taking a 500-mg tablet daily. If you want to try these megadoses of lysine, talk with your doctor first. If you prefer to get lysine from your diet, choose lean red meat, cheese, milk, eggs, fish, lima beans, potatoes, soy products, and yeast.

To enjoy the healing properties of lysine, it may be even more important to avoid foods which contain the amino acid *arginine,* which blocks lysine's action. Foods such as peanuts, walnuts, seeds, whole grains, rice, and gelatin are very high in arginine. To avoid a cold sore attack, don't eat large servings of these foods, especially before an important occasion.

*Sources:*
*Medical Update* (18,12:6)
*The PDR Guide to Nutrition and Health,* Medical Economics Company, Montvale, N.J., 1995
*The Saturday Evening Post* (267,6:54)

# Make your teeth last a lifetime

People used to think that losing your teeth was just a natural part of aging, but dentists now know that, with proper care, your teeth can last a lifetime. To prevent diseases of the bone and tissue supporting your teeth, called *periodontal disease*, pay special attention to your teeth and gums.

*Gingivitis*, an early form of gum disease, is caused by bacteria. If your gums are red and swollen, and they bleed when you brush your teeth, you may have gingivitis. Left untreated, gingivitis can develop into periodontal disease.

To keep the bacteria from thriving in your mouth, brush and floss your teeth at least twice a day. Over-the-counter and prescription mouth rinses help prevent receding gums, too.

If you have arthritis or a neurological disease such as Parkinson's, you may not be able to wield a toothbrush or floss. Look for specialized tools such as electric toothbrushes, mouth-irrigating machines, special picks, and tiny brushes that slide between your teeth.

Arthritis and some medications can cause you to have a dry mouth. Saliva has an important role in keeping your teeth healthy. If your mouth isn't producing enough, it's a good idea to drink more liquids to keep up the moisture level in your mouth.

Eating a healthy diet of fresh foods and getting enough calcium is an important part of keeping your teeth healthy. Smoking robs your body of nutrients, and it also increases your chance of getting gum disease, so don't smoke.

Seeing your dentist regularly is a must for keeping your teeth healthy. If you have gum disease, twice-a-year dental visits may not be enough. However, the daily care you give your teeth is really the deciding factor in keeping them for a lifetime. If you aren't sure about the most effective way to brush and floss, your dentist can show you how.

**Source:**
*The Atlanta Journal/Constitution* (Oct. 4, 1995, B3)

# Orange juice and sensitive teeth

If you have sensitive teeth, you've probably noticed an odd thing about brushing your teeth right after breakfast. If orange juice was part of the meal, brushing can hurt your teeth. This phenomenon is not a figment of your imagination.

Your teeth have microscopic tubes leading from the surface to the nerves inside. Brushing your teeth helps to clog these tubes so your teeth don't feel so sensitive. The acid in the orange juice counteracts this effect. To decrease tooth sensitivity, don't brush right before or after consuming orange juice or other foods or drinks high in acid.

**Source:**
*Medical Abstracts Newsletter* (15,9:5)

# Expert help for relieving varicose veins

Some people get varicose veins in their 20s, and their short skirts and pants go to the bottom drawer of the dresser permanently. They may do nothing about the condition, accepting it as a sign of aging. But relief can be as simple as a new pair of stockings or regular walks around the block.

Veins have one-way valves to keep the blood from being pulled back down into your legs by gravity. Varicose veins are caused by a weakening of these valves, which become distorted and visible through the skin. They can also be extremely painful. Varicose veins have recently been linked to "restless leg" syndrome, a condition that causes severe discomfort when the legs are still and is a major contributor to insomnia.

In some cases, heredity plays a big role. If one of your parents or grandparents had varicose veins, the chances are pretty good that you could get them, too. Although men sometimes get varicose veins, women get them two to four times more often, especially during pregnancy.

Varicose veins may get worse after long periods of standing in one place or sitting with legs bent or crossed. Other factors that contribute to varicose veins are being overweight, going through menopause, aging, and frequent heavy lifting that causes abdominal strain.

Varicose veins can be treated by outpatient surgery. Another treatment option involves drug injections that cause the veins to be reabsorbed into the body. But there are noninvasive treatments available, too. Here are the three best ones:

**Exercise and rest.** Mild varicose veins can be relieved by walking on a regular basis, avoiding standing for long periods, and resting with your feet raised higher than your hips. Walking helps to keep the blood flowing and increases the tone of muscles that support the veins.

**Support hosiery.** These can provide immediate relief from the itching and aching that is often associated with varicose veins. Standard ready-to-wear support stockings are made so that the most pressure is exerted at the ankle, with somewhat less pressure at midcalf and even less at midthigh. This helps keep the blood flowing back toward the heart. Many styles of support stockings can be purchased in drugstores and department stores.

**Compression stockings.** If your varicose veins are more severe, your doctor may prescribe custom-made compression stockings, available for both men and women. These are designed to deliver precise amounts of pressure in specific areas of your leg, according to your particular needs. Your doctor can recommend a qualified fitter who will ensure that you get the right style and design for your symptoms. Both support and compression stockings should be put on first thing in the morning, before blood has pooled in your feet and ankles.

While many people with varicose veins enjoy good health, they may be a sign of more serious problems with your blood vessels. If you think you're at risk, take steps to improve the health of your veins and prevent problems before they start.

*Sources:*
*Medical Tribune* (36,15:2)
*Postgraduate Medicine* (98,1:200)
*U.S. Pharmacist* (20,7:S11)

# Fend off foot fungus

If you're troubled by itchy athlete's foot or nail fungus, your doctor can prescribe medicine to get rid of it. But how do you keep it from coming back? Here are three tips for preventing the recurrence of foot fungus:

◆ Periodically, apply an antifungal cream to prevent the fungus from getting reestablished. Apply it to your toes, nails, the skin between your toes, and the bottom surface of your foot.

◆ Be sure to discard any old shoes that you wore without socks when you had the fungus. It might seem wasteful to throw away a pair of shoes, but it's worth it to avoid getting the fungus again.

◆ Don't go barefoot in public showers or bathrooms. Places that stay constantly moist are breeding grounds for foot fungus.

*Source:*
*Emergency Medicine* (28,11:25)

# Defeat your sweaty feet

If you're troubled by excessively sweaty feet and hands, also known as *dyshidrosis*, relief may be as close as your kitchen. Here are two remedies to try if excess moisture on your feet or hands is causing you some embarrassing moments.

A simple bath of good, old-fashioned tea can dry out your feet, according to Dr. J. Mark Knopp of Indianapolis. He recommends making a strong solution of two or three tea bags per quart of water and pouring the cooled solution in a shallow pan. Then soak your feet for 20 minutes at a time. Soak every night the first week, three nights the second week, and then as needed. Presumably, the same thing should work for hands, but you might want to put a sealer of clear nail polish on your fingernails before soaking so they don't get stained.

If tea is not enough to dry those tootsies, you might want to ask your pharmacist for a solution of aluminum chloride. Apply to hands and feet at bedtime, then wrap them in a layer of plastic kitchen wrap to improve the absorption.

For really stubborn cases, your doctor can prescribe a battery-operated device that sends an electric current through your skin to temporarily close your sweat glands. After a few days of treatment, you may get up to six weeks of relief.

Don't forget the simple old standby remedies for sweaty feet: antiperspirant sprays, wearing shoes and socks made only of natural materials, and changing socks frequently. Also, try going barefoot or wearing open sandals around the house, dry your feet thoroughly before putting on shoes after a bath or shower, store your shoes where they can get lots of ventilation, and don't wear the same shoes two days in a row.

*Sources:*
*Emergency Medicine* (28,8:46)
*Medical Update* (18,10:6 and 19,6:6)

## Calluses call for a soft approach

If your shoes feel uncomfortable because you have corns and calluses on your feet, your first reaction is probably to file off that bumpy skin. Unfortunately, this kind of friction is not helpful. It was friction that caused the thickening of your skin in the first place, and filing just aggravates rather than helps it. The best approach is to use skin-softening cream to help keep corns and calluses flexible and soft. For removal of these skin problems, see your dermatologist or podiatrist.

*Source:*
*Postgraduate Medicine* (97,1:35)

## Top healers and helpers for heel pain

If it feels as if a knife is sticking into the bottom of your foot when you first stand up in the morning, you may have *plantar fasciitis*, a common form of heel pain. The *plantar fascia* is a band of tissue similar to a tendon that stretches along the bottom of your foot. It works like a rubber band between the heel and ball of your foot to form the arch, and it determines whether you have high arches or flat feet. When the plantar fascia is damaged, it can cause intense pain in your heel.

Plantar fasciitis is a repetitive strain injury caused by overexercising, changes in your foot due to aging, or a combination of both. Walking, running, and other sports that require you to push off from your feet, such as tennis and basketball, can strain and injure the plantar fascia. A pad of fat covers your heel and protects the plantar fascia by absorbing the shock of walking and running. As you age, the fat pad thins and provides less protection. The plantar fascia itself also becomes less flexible and more prone to injury.

If your heel pain is due to plantar fasciitis, here are some steps you can take to ease the pain:

◆ If you're a very active walker or runner, cut back temporarily. Also, be sure that your shoes provide the proper support and padding for your feet.

◆ If you are overweight, lose weight. It can make your heels feel better.

◆ If you have either high arches or flat feet, ask your doctor about *orthotics*, which are arch supports that fit into your shoes. They must be individually fitted to your feet.

◆ If your work involves standing in one spot for long periods of time or standing on a hard surface, put some type of padding on the floor where you stand.

◆ Take a mild over-the-counter pain reliever to help relieve the heel pain.

◆ Do stretching exercises at least twice a day. With both knees slightly bent, place one foot flat on the floor behind you. Bend your front knee more, straightening your back leg and keeping your back heel on the floor. Move your heel gently up and down to feel the stretch in your back foot. Repeat with the other leg.

Another stretch is done next to a wall. Place your heel on the floor and your toes up on the wall. Gently stretch your heel and the bottom of your foot as you push against the wall.

◆ Strengthen the muscles of your foot by scrunching up a towel with your toes as if you're going to pick it up.

◆ To strengthen your calf muscles and help hold your heel in place, try this exercise: In a sitting position, hold one leg out straight in front of you. With an old bicycle inner tube or any long, flexible piece of rubber, hook the toe part of your outstretched shoe and pull gently back toward you as you push against the tubing.

If your heel pain doesn't improve, see your doctor. He may suggest trying a removable splint that you can wear at night to keep your heel stretched out. If the pain continues after all other treatments, there are some drug and surgery options still open. However, a good program of stretching and strengthening therapy should have you feeling better in a flash.

*Sources:*
American Family Physician (52,3:901)
The Physician and Sportsmedicine (23,6:77)

## Booster shot beats up bacteria

Tetanus vaccines have been so successful since the 1940s that most people no longer think of the disease as a serious threat. However, lately, hundreds of people older than 60 have died from tetanus.

By the time people are age 60 or older, fewer than half of them are protected from tetanus, and by the time they are 70, fewer than one-third of people are sufficiently protected.

Tetanus is caused by bacteria that live in rusty metal, soil, street dust, organic garden fertilizers, and pet poop. Any injury can expose you to the tetanus bacteria. If you had your last tetanus vaccine many years ago, your body may not now have enough antibodies to fight the bacteria.

The current recommendation for adults is one tetanus booster shot every 10 years. If you never had tetanus shots as a child, you should take the original series of three shots. If you haven't had tetanus shots for many years, ask your doctor about getting a booster shot.

*Sources:*
*Medical Update* (19,4:6)
*The New England Journal of Medicine* (332,12:81,761)

## Caffeine may heighten hypoglycemia

You ate a big plate of pasta for lunch, along with a salad and some toasted garlic bread. Now it's 2:30 and you're feeling a little droopy, so you reach for a cup of coffee. The weak, trembling feeling you had after your second cup of coffee isn't really hypoglycemia. It's a reaction to the caffeine.

Researchers at the Yale University School of Medicine tested people who had just eaten high-carbohydrate meals by giving them varying amounts of caffeine. They measured the glucose levels of the people studied and found that the levels were within the normal range and shouldn't have caused the hypoglycemic reaction. However, the addition of caffeine made the people feel as if their blood sugar was much lower than it actually was.

You might want to keep this in mind next time you feel an afternoon slump in energy after a lunch high in carbohydrates. A caffeine-free drink might be a better choice.

*Sources:*
*Annals of Internal Medicine* (119,8:799)
*Journal Watch* (12,10:73)

## After-dinner dizziness cure

Here's some news on the flip side of caffeine. This good news is about how caffeinated beverages help stabilize blood pressure after meals.

It's common for older people to experience a drop in blood pressure after meals. The medical name for the condition is *postprandial* (after-meal) *hypotension* (low blood pressure). You can become lightheaded and dizzy when you stand up, and you may faint. Even if you have high blood pressure, you may experience these symptoms.

Studies of healthy older people show that drinking coffee or tea right after a meal can prevent this drop in blood pressure. Caffeinated beverages raise the blood pressure just enough to hold off those potentially dangerous symptoms.

Younger people also experience this drop in blood pressure after eating, but they can usually combat it by getting up from the dinner table and taking a walk. The exercise will raise their blood pressure enough to keep away symptoms. But the safe option for an older person is drinking a caffeinated beverage, then taking a walk once you feel stable on your feet.

*Sources:*
*Archives of Internal Medicine* (155,9:945)
*Medical Tribune* (36,13:16)

# Hidden causes of incontinence

She's been your best friend for years. She's seen you through countless problems and shared all your secrets. But even she doesn't know that you suffer from incontinence.

Urinary incontinence is the uncontrolled leakage of urine which can occur at any time. It affects 10 million Americans and yet, the idea of "wetting your pants" is so embarrassing, most people won't mention it to their best friends, and less than half will discuss it with their doctors.

Incontinence mainly affects people over 40, although younger people can also be affected, and more often affects women than men. It can be caused by a variety of factors including illness, surgery, being overweight, childbirth, certain drugs, and urinary tract infection. Weak bladder muscles and nerve disorders are among the more serious causes. Men who have enlarged prostates or have had their prostates removed due to cancer may also experience loss of control.

Dietary habits may also affect incontinence. Experiment by eliminating these items from your diet one at a time for seven to 10 days:

◆ Caffeinated beverages like coffee and tea
◆ Carbonated beverages
◆ Citrus fruits
◆ Tomatoes and tomato-based foods
◆ Highly spiced foods
◆ Chocolate
◆ Sugar and honey
◆ Milk and milk products

You need to find out the cause of your incontinence because it could be a symptom of another problem or a side effect of medication. Tell your doctor about it, even if you can't tell your best friend.

*Sources:*
*Family Urology* (Spring 1995)
*Journal of the American Society of Geriatrics* (42,12:1257)
*The Atlanta Journal/Constitution* (Dec. 7, 1995, B3)

THE BIG BOOK OF HEALTH TIPS

## Preventing incontinence during exercise

Up to a third of women experience *stress incontinence* when they exercise. This uncontrollable leakage of urine, even if it's just a dribble, can keep you from exercising, especially around other people. But you don't have to limit your life and your favorite activities. Researchers have found some new ways to help solve the problem.

A tampon provides the simplest method for handling mild incontinence during exercise. Worn in the lower part of the vagina, a tampon supports the *urethra*, the canal through which urine leaves the bladder. Moisten the tip of the tampon with water to make it easier to insert and remove.

Though many women have never heard of it, a *pessary* is a device inserted into the vagina to help support the weight of the uterus. Pessaries specially made to prevent stress incontinence also elevate the urethra to prevent leakage. They can be worn for short periods of time while you exercise, and they don't cause any weakening of your muscles. The cost of this type of pessary is around $50.

A new device has been designed especially for active women. It's called the *bladder neck support prosthesis (BNSP)*. This device is extremely flexible, it supports the urethra effectively, it helps reinforce the muscles of the pelvic floor in a way similar to surgery, and it comes in 25 different sizes for a perfect fit. It performed effectively when tested on runners, hikers, and other active women. The only negative aspect of the BNSP is its $300 price tag. However, if active sports are an important part of your life, and you have stress incontinence, you may want to ask your doctor about this new device.

*Sources:*
*Medical Abstracts Newsletter* (15,6:8)
*The Physician and Sportsmedicine* (24,1:16)

## Drugs that can cause incontinence

It is almost impossible to know every side effect that a drug can have, and different people will react differently to the same drug. However, it's a good idea to be as informed as possible about any medicines that you are taking. If you are having problems with incontinence and don't know the cause, it's possible that it could be caused by a drug you are taking. Here is a list of seven drugs that can cause incontinence in some people:

### Antipsychotic agents
Chlorpromazine HCl (Ormazine, Thorazine); Thioridazine HCl (Mellaril); Thiothixene (Navane); Haloperidol (Haldol)

### Antihistamines
Diphenhydramine HCl (Benadryl, Diphenacen, Wehdryl); Hydroxyzine

### Antidepressants
Amitriptyline HCl (Elavil, Endep, Enovil); Doxepin HCl (Adapin, Sinequan)

### Decongestants
Ephedrine

148

**Diuretics**
Furosemide (Lasix); Bumetanide (Bumex)
**Antihypertensives**
Methyldopa (Aldomet); Clonidine HCl (Catapres); Prazosin (Minipress)
**Sedative-hypnotics**
Benzodiazepines

If you are taking one of these drugs and cannot find another reason for your incontinence, ask your doctor if your medicine might be the cause.

*Source:*
*Postgraduate Medicine* (97,5:109)

# Stop kidney stones before they start

If you've ever felt the pain of a kidney stone, you probably did everything you could to make the pain stop. Kidney stones are a problem of metabolism involving calcium, a chemical called *oxalate*, and *uric acid*, a component of urine. The average person eats foods that contain calcium and oxalates every day, and getting a bit extra usually isn't a problem. But in people who have the tendency to get kidney stones, too much calcium or oxalates can spell disaster.

Kidney stones can attack anyone, at any age, but they show up most often in white males. For most people, the first attack occurs around age 35 in men and 30 in women. Others may not get their first attacks until age 55. If you've had one kidney stone episode, your chances of having another are higher. Half of the people who get one kidney stone will have another one within eight to 10 years. What's worse, the period between attacks gets shorter each time.

Doctors have traditionally treated kidney stones with medications to help dissolve them or surgery to remove them. More recently, *lithotripsy* (sound wave) therapy has been used to blast stones apart while they're still inside the body. Lithotripsy is especially effective when dealing with large stones that can cause infections. In most cases, though, when the stones are small, dietary control is often the first line of defense.

According to researchers, these simple dietary changes can go a long way toward preventing stones from forming:

**Fill up on fluids.** How much is enough? You need to drink at least 10 10-ounce glasses of liquid per day and reduce your salt intake. The more urine you produce, the more stone-causing minerals you flush out.

**Cut back on foods that are rich in oxalates.** Red meat contains proteins that actually promote the formation of oxalates in the body. Other foods rich in oxalates include chocolate, black tea, beets, figs, ground pepper, parsley, rhubarb, spinach, and poppy seeds.

**Drink cranberry juice.** It can help reduce urinary tract bacterial infections, which seem to play some role in stone formation. Studies have not yet revealed whether cranberry juice can actually prevent stones from forming.

**Watch your consumption of dairy products.** They're loaded with calcium.

More than two quarts of milk or six ounces of cheese a day is too much. Just stick with the recommended daily allowance (RDA) of 800 mg of calcium, since it's critical to other body functions.

*Sources:*
*Patient Care* (29,11:22)
*Science News* (143,1:196)
*The Saturday Evening Post* (267,5:36)

# Tea troubles kidneys

If you have a history of kidney stones, you probably know that drinking regular black or green tea is not good for you. These teas contain oxalate, one of the building blocks of kidney stones. A recent study shows that herbal teas are a better choice, since several varieties tested contain lower levels of oxalate than regular tea. Coffee is also low in oxalate, so if you really miss your afternoon cup of tea, you can enjoy a tasty substitute.

*Source:*
*Medical Abstracts Newsletter* (15,6:4)

# Healthy Digestion

## Wash away bad bacteria with this popular beverage

Remember when your sometimes tipsy but always proper Aunt Agnes said she was drinking a little wine with dinner to "aid digestion"? Great excuse, Aunt Agnes, because the scientists have proved you right.

In a recent experiment, scientists set up test tubes filled with red and white wine, bismuth salicylate (the active ingredient in Pepto-Bismol), tequila, or water.

They then added three types of bacteria that normally invade and upset your stomach — *Escherichia coli*, salmonella, and shigella.

Within a half hour, the wine had nearly wiped out all three types of bacteria. The Pepto-Bismol ingredient also knocked out the *E. coli* within 30 minutes, but it took over an hour to kill the salmonella and shigella.

The tequila and the water had almost no effect on the bacteria. Obviously, it's not the alcohol that kills the infection-causing bacteria, but other substances in the wine. The bacteria-fighting substance may be a *polyphenol* that is freed when the wine is fermented. Polyphenols are powerful protective compounds found in apples, grapes, strawberries, wheat bran, tea, and other foods.

The study also revealed that wine aged for 10 years works better against bacteria than older and younger wines.

Wine can apparently be a more powerful antibacterial than Pepto-Bismol, especially against the bacteria that causes traveler's diarrhea.

No more laughing allowed at Aunt Agnes' excuse for a dinnertime nip.

*Source:*
British Medical Journal (311,7021:1657)

## The spice that aids digestion

Cinnamon fires up more than your taste buds. It warms your digestive juices, too. The spicy sprinkle in cakes, pies, and cookies may help your stomach break down fatty desserts.

Chinese researchers say that cinnamon has both a pain-relieving and a "warming" effect in the stomach and spleen. The warming effect stimulates the liver to release bile, which is necessary in the digestion of fats. Bile also helps set the muscles in the digestive system in motion.

Cinnamon oil has been used for centuries as a folk medicine for upset stomach and diarrhea. It's usually called "cinnamon drops."

Cinnamon doesn't have to go hand in hand with fat. A sprinkle on toast and in oatmeal adds flavor and may aid digestion, too.

*Source:*
The Lawrence Review of Natural Products, Facts and Comparisons, St. Louis, Mo., 1995

# 8 ways to halt heartburn

Pizza, enchiladas, spaghetti with meatballs ... mmmm. The mere mention of these foods usually causes mouths to water and eyes to light up. However, if you suffer regularly from heartburn, eating spicy foods like these can mean paying for it later with a burning pain in your chest.

Heartburn, which is also called acid indigestion, actually has nothing to do with your heart. It occurs when stomach acid flows upward into your windpipe, causing a burning sensation. Normally a ring-like "door" separates the two areas, keeping the acid out, but when the door becomes weak, it loses its ability to stay closed.

One common cause of heartburn is a *hiatal hernia*. This is a condition where the stomach pokes upward into the chest through an opening in the diaphragm. Research suggests, however, that some people have heartburn symptoms simply because they are just more sensitive to the activity in their stomachs.

**Be careful how you spell relief.** Many heartburn sufferers automatically turn to antacids for relief without realizing that antacids do have some side effects. Seltzer-type products contain a lot of salt and shouldn't be taken by people who are on low-salt diets. Antacids that are high in calcium shouldn't be taken by people with kidney problems. The calcium antacids can also cause a rebound effect, resulting in even greater acid production.

Antacids that contain magnesium may cause diarrhea. Many antacids will include aluminum along with the magnesium. The aluminum tends to cause constipation, so the two ingredients balance each other out.

**Keep juices in their place.** Simple changes in your lifestyle may be all you need to get relief. By making these techniques part of your daily routine, you may be able to reduce, and even prevent, your episodes of heartburn.

- Avoid these common foods: fatty and spicy dishes, citrus fruits and juices, chocolate and chocolate drinks, peppermint, and spearmint. A survey of 400 heartburn sufferers showed that grapefruit juice causes more heartburn than any other beverage, followed closely by orange juice and tomato-containing juices.
- Eat small, frequent meals and avoid eating just before bedtime. You shouldn't lie down for four hours after eating.
- Give your jaws a workout. The more you chew, the more acid-neutralizing saliva you produce. Chew your food slowly and thoroughly, and chew on something like sugarless gum after a meal.
- Cut down on coffee, tea, alcoholic beverages, and whole milk.
- Drink liquids about an hour before or after meals to keep your stomach from bloating.
- Never bend over immediately after eating.
- Use good posture when eating — sit up straight and don't stand or lie down to eat.
- Avoid wearing clothes and belts that fit tightly around your stomach. If you

are overweight, losing those extra pounds may help relieve your symptoms.

◆ Give up smoking.

◆ Use 4- to 6-inch wooden blocks or bricks to raise the head of your bed. Or, you can try putting a foam wedge beneath your upper body. Extra pillows usually don't do the trick.

If your heartburn is ever severe and is accompanied by nausea, sweating, weakness, fainting, or breathlessness, or pain that extends from your chest to your arm or jaw, you may have something much worse than a pepperoni pizza that didn't digest well. These symptoms could be indications of a heart attack. Contact your doctor immediately or call for emergency help.

*Sources:*
*Before You Call the Doctor*, Fawcett Columbine, New York, 1992
*Environmental Nutrition* (18,2:1)
*Food Safety Notebook* (6,3:28)
*Medical Update* (15,8:5 and 17,6:1)
*The Merck Manual, 16th Edition*, Merck & Co., Rahway, N.J., 1992

# Don't take heartburn lightly

Since you can usually stamp out heartburn's blaze with changes in your life-style, it isn't often considered a "serious medical condition." That doesn't mean you should take it lightly.

The stomach acid and juices that rise into your windpipe can do damage. The esophagus can begin to bleed regularly and become permanently narrowed because of scar tissue. See the ***Complementary Cancer Care*** chapter for one of the worst consequences of daily heartburn.

See your doctor if you're a regular heartburn sufferer. He may do an endoscopy, which means he will look at your esophagus through a tube with a light at the end.

You may need a prescription drug, or if your esophagus is very damaged, you may need to have it surgically dilated. Hiatal hernias, one of the causes of heartburn, sometimes need repair, too.

*Sources:*
*American Family Physician* (52,3:965)
*The Merck Manual, 16th Edition*, Merck & Co., Rahway, N.J., 1992

# How to get maximum mileage from your antacid

When you suffer from heartburn, the image of a soothing liquid antacid coating your innards is comforting. Most people, including doctors, have always thought that liquid antacids work better against heartburn than tablet antacids.

But Oklahoma researchers were surprised recently to find that tablets actually provide greater and longer-lasting relief than liquids. Sixty-five heartburn sufferers concluded that Tums E-X tablets and Mylanta Double Strength tablets controlled heartburn better than the liquid Mylanta II and Extra Strength Maalox.

The tablets did a better job of lowering acid levels in the esophagus and reducing the number of times stomach juices flowed back into your windpipe. In fact, two hours after taking the medicine, only people who had used the liquid antacids were still having heartburn.

The tablets mix with your saliva to form a gummy substance that sticks to your esophagus better and longer than the liquid medicine. Plus, the act of chewing the tablets may bring out the natural antacids in your saliva.

*Source:*
*Medical Tribune for the Internist and Cardiologist* (36,21:6)

## Convincing evidence closes *H. pylori* case

One doctor wanted so badly to convince everyone that *H. pylori* bacteria, not stress and spicy foods, cause stomach pain and ulcers that he deliberately swallowed the germs. Sure enough, he developed the stomach pain and inflammation doctors call chronic gastritis.

A recent study looked at people who had been treated for an ulcer. Some people took antibiotics to wipe out *H. pylori* bacteria in their stomachs. Less than 13 percent of these people were troubled by ulcers again.

As for the people who did not receive *H. pylori* treatment, their ulcers almost always returned. Almost three out of four of the stomach ulcers came back, and close to 100 percent of the ulcers that were in the duodenum (the part of the small intestine that connects to the stomach) returned.

Pretty convincing evidence, doctor.

*Source:*
*American Family Physician* (52,6:1717)

## New test makes ulcer cure easier

You have a one in two chance of having *H. pylori* bacteria in your stomach if you're over age 60. These wicked little bacteria cause stomach ulcers, pain, and inflammation. Up to 95 percent of people with stomach ulcers are infected with *H. pylori* bacteria.

No one is sure exactly how you get the germs, but you probably swallowed them at some point in your life.

Fortunately, a patent has been granted for a very simple test that can detect the bacteria. The Food and Drug Administration recently approved a new breath test to detect H. pylori. The simple procedure takes only 30 minutes and is 95 percent accurate.

If you have the bacteria, your doctor can prescribe an antibiotic that will kill them. Getting rid of the *H. pylori* germs usually gets rid of any ulcers that may be forming.

*Sources:*
*American Family Physician* (52,6:1717)
*Pharmacy Times* (61,8:4)

## Your medicines may mix up ulcer test

If you have an ulcer or the beginnings of one, you probably take antacids like Pepto-Bismol and Pepcid AC regularly. If you do, you should be tested for the *H. pylori* bacteria to see if they have invaded your stomach and are causing your ulcer.

Before you go in for the test, stop taking your antacids for a few days. These medicines can cause you to get false-negative results on your *H. pylori* test. Antacids temporarily lower the number of bacteria in your stomach so that their presence doesn't show up on the test.

You may wonder what the big deal about *H. pylori* is if you can control it with Pepto-Bismol. It is easy to lower the number of bacteria temporarily, but actually curing yourself of the infection takes antibiotics. You will probably need to take more than one type of antibiotic for one or two weeks, possibly longer.

Getting rid of the *H. pylori* bacteria with antibiotics is very likely to completely cure your ulcer. Not only will your stomach pain improve or disappear, but you may also be able to quit taking those daily antacids — a positive move for your health.

*Source:*
*The Journal of the American Medical Association* (275,8:622)

## Avoid this deadly duo: *H. pylori* and heartburn drugs

Living with *H. pylori* bacteria in your gut puts you in the high risk category for stomach cancer. You boost your risk even higher if you add heartburn drugs to the scenario, a new study shows.

Heartburn drugs, such as the widely used Prilosec, decrease the amount of stomach acid you produce. The low-acid environment is good for your heartburn, but it apparently allows *H. pylori* to cause additional damage to your stomach lining.

Researchers knew that the common *H. pylori* infection was a stomach cancer risk factor, and they knew that many people with the infection took heartburn drugs. That's why they took a five-year look at almost 200 people who suffered from heartburn.

After five years of taking acid-lowering drugs, one out of three heartburn sufferers who were infected with *H. pylori* were on their way to stomach cancer. They had destructive inflammation and precancerous changes in their stomach linings. Because of the drugs, the *H. pylori* had damaged their stomachs much more than usual.

The acid-lowering drugs were harmless in the heartburn sufferers who weren't infected with *H. pylori*.

This study provides more convincing evidence that you should be tested for

*H. pylori* if you suspect you may be infected. It's especially important to be tested and treated with antibiotics if you take or plan to take acid-lowering heartburn drugs.

*Source:*
*The New England Journal of Medicine* (334,16:1018)

## Good gas, bad guess

You get little sympathy when you complain about a bloated stomach. Most people just write off that uncomfortable feeling as "too much gas."

Actually, a bloated stomach isn't related to gas at all. You can have a bloated stomach and produce a perfectly normal amount of gas, a new study shows.

This discovery is going to turn some old medical advice on its ear. In the past, everyone offered the same solutions for bloating and for gas — like eating less cabbage and beans. Avoiding these foods may help if you have excessive gas but won't necessarily help with bloating.

Most people who regularly suffer with bloating have irritable bowel syndrome (IBS). If you have this digestive problem, you often have to put up with stomach pain and cramping and with loose, diarrhea-like stools. IBS is hard to treat and often means trying out different dietary changes to see what works for you.

People who have bloating every once in a while may be eating more fiber than they are used to. Fiber in supplements like Metamucil and Citrucel, vegetables, wheat bran, and whole-grain wheat bulks up your fecal matter. That can make you feel bloated, but try not to worry about it. Bulky fecal matter that is easy to eliminate is exactly what you're striving for.

Don't let anyone tell you that your bloated stomach is "just gas." It isn't. More likely than not, either you need to search for a solution to your IBS or you need to think good thoughts about what all that fiber is doing for your health.

*Source:*
*Annals of Internal Medicine* (124,4:422)

## Do you really pass too much gas?

You may just think you're gassy. On average, men in the United States pass gas 13 to 14 times a day. That's normal. Passing gas over 20 times a day is considered excessive.

Passing too much gas may be related to the healthy foods you eat.

♦ Milk and dairy products can cause gas for people who don't digest lactose well.

♦ "Fermentable" foods can cause gas. These include cabbage, beans, broccoli, apple and grape juice, bananas, nuts, and raisins. These foods usually aren't completely digested and absorbed. When the undigested sugars reach the colon, they are fermented by bacteria, resulting in gas.

Swallowing air can cause gas. Eating too fast, chewing gum, and smoking can cause you to swallow air, or it can simply be a bad habit. To break the air-swallowing habit, hold a pencil or another object between your teeth whenever possible.

You shouldn't be too concerned about how much gas you produce. Your health isn't at risk, and things could be worse: Researchers report one study participant who passed gas an average of 141 times a day, including 70 times in one four-hour period. Now that's gas.

*Sources:*
*Annals of Internal Medicine* (124,4:422)
*The Merck Manual, 16th Edition*, Merck & Co., Rahway, N.J., 1992

# Conquering constipation

Many men are quite proud to be "regular as a clock" with their bowel movements, and rightly so. Their daily habit is the envy of every constipated man and woman in the world.

Although most people know when they are constipated, some people just think they are. A daily bowel movement isn't essential to good health or even good humor. You can call yourself constipated if you meet two or more of the following:

◆ You have fewer than three bowel movements a week.
◆ About a quarter of your bowel movements require straining.
◆ You feel like you still need to go after at least a quarter of your bowel movements.
◆ A quarter of your bowel movements produce hard, pellet-like stools.

Usually, you can overcome constipation without medicine or a doctor's help. Here's what you need to do:

**First and foremost, eat more fiber.** Start off the day with a high-fiber breakfast cereal — one with more than six grams of fiber per serving. Some cereals, such as General Mills Fiber One, have at least 12 grams per serving.

Eat plenty of whole-wheat bread, vegetables, and whole fruits. Add beans to your menu several times a week. Broad beans, lentils, baked beans, black beans, lima beans, and pinto beans all have seven grams or more of fiber per cup. Look for high-fiber snacks, such as popcorn, raisins, and nuts.

If you think you need a fiber supplement, try adding raw, unprocessed wheat bran to your cereal and soups or buy a high-fiber preparation such as Citrucel, Fiberall, Metamucil, or FiberCon.

**Exercise.** The more you move your body, the faster food and waste will move through your intestines.

**Schedule an appointment for your bowels.** Establish a pattern for your bowels by sitting on the toilet at the same time every day. Bowels work best in the morning and after a meal, so pick a time 10 minutes to one hour after breakfast.

Spend several minutes in the bathroom, but don't strain. Propping your feet on a small step stool may ease bowel movements.

**Don't ignore the urge to go.** A history of ignoring your bowels' urges may contribute to constipation. This is one interruption you should welcome.

**Drink six to eight glasses of liquids a day.** Water will help keep your stools soft. Caffeine and alcohol cause you to lose water, so they will make you more constipated instead of less.

**Massage your belly?** Some natural healers recommend massaging your lower stomach in a clockwise motion.

**Soften stools with an enema.** You shouldn't use enemas often, but you may want to begin your new constipation-free lifestyle with one if you have hard stools that are difficult to expel. Your stools could be impacted.

Don't give up on these measures too early. Give yourself several weeks of making all these changes before you call yourself a hopeless case. Very, very rarely does someone need surgery for constipation.

Remember, a change in bowel habits is a warning sign of cancer. If you've only recently become constipated, see your doctor for a checkup.

*Sources:*
*Inside Tract: Maintaining Your Digestive Health,* Glaxo Institute for Digestive Health, P.O. Box 899, West Caldwell, N.J. 07007–0899
*Medical Abstracts Newsletter* (15,10:6)
*Postgraduate Medicine* (98,5:115)

## Sweet cure for constipation

The Greeks have a sweet cure for constipation. They mix one to two tablespoons of honey in a glass of water to get things moving again.

This cure works for many people because honey contains more fructose than glucose. Both of these are natural sugars. When foods are higher in fructose than glucose, you often aren't able to absorb and digest the fructose very well. Your body has to get rid of the undigested sugar, so you have a bowel movement.

Honey contains higher amounts of fructose in excess of glucose than any food except apples, pears, apple juice, or pear juice. Apples and pears are known to be natural laxatives, too. Apples and pears also have the advantage of being low in calories, so you can eat as many as you want.

As for the honey cure, if you can afford the calories (one tablespoon has 64), you may want to try three tablespoons of honey instead of one or two. Three tablespoons seems about twice as effective in bringing on a bowel movement.

Unfortunately, this constipation cure won't work for everybody. Some people are excellent fructose digesters, so honey won't have a laxative effect for them. But even excellent fructose digesters should have some success with apples and pears. They are high in fiber, and a high-fiber diet is the most effective treatment that exists for constipation.

*Source:*
*The American Journal of Clinical Nutrition* (62,6:1212)

## Apples control constipation and diarrhea

Anything that controls constipation should promote diarrhea, and vice versa, right? The logic usually holds true, but apples are an amazing digestive aid that break the mold. Apples contain a fiber called pectin, which absorbs water in your stomach and intestines then swells into a gummy lump.

That bulky mass improves constipation because it helps get your bowels moving and softens hard stools. It also helps with diarrhea because it bulks up stools that are too watery.

*Source:*
*The Lawrence Review of Natural Products,* Facts and Comparisons, St. Louis, Mo., 1995

## Laxative warning: This kind may cause cancer

If you have a box of laxatives in your medicine cabinet, check the list of ingredients. If you see *phenolphthalein*, you may want to throw the medicine away.

Many common laxatives, such as Ex-Lax, contain phenolphthalein, and a recent government study revealed that the chemical causes cancer in rats and mice.

Of course, the amount fed to the animals was far more than you would get in a normal laxative dose. Nevertheless, the U.S. Food and Drug Administration believes the chemical could be hazardous to humans.

As soon as the study results came to light, manufacturer Schering-Plough Corp. removed phenolphthalein from two of its laxatives, Correctol and Feen-A-Mint.

Even if the drug didn't increase your risk of cancer, you shouldn't use laxatives unless absolutely necessary. Phenolphthalein works by stimulating the muscles that force food and waste through your intestines. Your muscles can become dependent on the drug, until you can't have a bowel movement unless you take a laxative. This dangerous situation is hard to correct.

Try to correct your constipation naturally before turning to a potentially harmful and habit-forming drug. If on a very rare occasion you feel you must use a laxative, the safest option is an osmotic laxative. Common brands are Lactulose and Milk of Magnesia.

Osmotic laxatives contain ingredients (like magnesium) that your body can't absorb well. These ingredients stay in your intestines and draw water there. The bulky, watery mass gets your bowels moving and usually brings you relief within three hours. These laxatives aren't addictive, but they could have dangerous side effects, such as upsetting your fluid and electrolyte balance, if you used them too often.

*Sources:*
*American Family Physician* (53,4:1229)
*Medical Abstracts Newsletter* (15,10:6)
*The Atlanta Journal/Constitution* (March 23, 1996, A6)

## Help for hemorrhoids

Every third American suffers from hemorrhoids, so don't be embarrassed by the problem. A hemorrhoid is simply an enlarged vein in your lower rectum.

The ones on the inside can bleed (you'll see the blood in your stools), but they don't hurt. They can make you feel as though you still need to use the restroom when you just went. If the hemorrhoids fall out of your rectum (prolapse), they may begin to ache and itch. With the help of a little lubricating jelly, you can gently push prolapsed hemorrhoids back into the anal canal.

Hemorrhoids that form outside of your rectum can become very painful, swollen, and itchy.

The best way to prevent and treat both the internal and external hemorrhoids is to eat more fiber and drink more water. Water and fiber soften your stools so you don't have to strain to pass them.

Exercising every day will also improve your hemorrhoids for two reasons. Moving around instead of sitting takes pressure off veins in the rectum, and exercise helps prevent constipation, one of the main causes of hemorrhoids.

Sitting in several inches of warm water with your knees raised can bring relief for hemorrhoids. Do this for 15 minutes three times a day, if possible.

You may find bowel movements less irritating if you gently lubricate the area, inside and out, with nonpetroleum jelly. Another soothing tip for after a bowel movement: Try wiping with a baby wipe instead of regular toilet tissue.

As for over-the-counter hemorrhoid products, their basic ingredient is a lubricant to relieve irritation. Nonpetroleum jelly would do the same job. Some products do contain other helpful ingredients such as:

◆ Hydrocortisone — relieves inflammation and itching.
◆ Anesthetics (benzocaine, pramoxine) — slightly deaden pain.
◆ Vasoconstrictors (ephedrine, phenylephrine) — reduce swelling and relieve itching.
◆ Astringents (witch hazel, zinc oxide) — help shrink blood vessels.
◆ Counterirritants (camphor) — soothe and comfort area.
◆ Aloe vera gel — reduces irritation.

You may find many other ingredients listed, such as wound-healing agents and antiseptics, but some of these have not been proven useful.

If your hemorrhoids are very painful and you get little relief from these methods, you should have your doctor treat them. Hemorrhoid treatment once meant surgery and a hospital stay, but times have changed.

One option is a fairly painless but slightly uncomfortable procedure called rubber band ligation. The surgeon slides a rubber band around your hemorrhoid, then you wait about a week for the hemorrhoid, along with the rubber band, to drop off.

Your doctor can also zap your hemorrhoids with infrared light, electrical current, or a laser beam, causing them to shrink and dry up. Another method is injecting the hemorrhoid with a liquid that glues the vein walls together. The hemorrhoid shrinks and disappears.

Whichever treatment you and your doctor choose, you'll be glad you took this step. Hemorrhoids may not be a life or death situation, but there's no reason to live in pain or discomfort.

Of course, after your treatment, you'll need to exercise, eat a high-fiber diet with lots of water, and avoid straining on the toilet so your hemorrhoids won't come back.

*Sources:*
*Drug Facts and Comparisons,* Facts and Comparisons, 111 West Port Plaza, Suite 400, St. Louis, Mo. 63146–3098
*Environmental Nutrition* (18,2:1)
*Medical Update* (18,2:3)

# Dealing with diverticular disease

Chances are, you're going to have *diverticulosis* someday. You may have it now. Half the people over age 60 have the pea-sized pouches along the large intestine walls called *diverticula.*

You can have diverticulosis and never know it. But when the diverticula become infected and inflamed, you may begin to regret the diet habits that gave you those pouches. Infected diverticula can cause cramps, pain, tenderness in the left side of the stomach, gas, and blood in your stools. That's called *diverticulitis.*

You can keep the pouches from growing in the first place with a diet high in fiber and low in fat and red meat. Researchers figured out the connection between diet and diverticular disease by sending questionnaires to over 50,000 male health professionals over a six-year period. They found that the men who ate the most fatty red meat and the least fiber were the most likely to be troubled by diverticulitis.

High-fiber fresh fruit is the most important addition you can make to your diet. The fruits stimulate the growth of helpful microbes in your intestines. The microbes increase bowel movements and keep food waste moving through your system. Waste that sticks around can cause pouches to form or can irritate existing pouches.

Red meat, on the other hand, causes intestinal bacteria to produce substances that weaken the colon, allowing diverticula to form.

Preventing diverticular disease is easier than treating it. You'll usually need bed rest, antibiotics, and a clear liquid diet to allow your bowels to heal.

When your diverticula are inflamed and painful, some doctors recommend that you avoid popcorn, nuts, and seeds. These foods can get stuck in the pouches and cause more irritation.

*Sources:*
*Environmental Nutrition* (18,2:1)
*The American Journal of Clinical Nutrition* (60,5:419)

## What you can do about irritable bowel syndrome

When you have irritable bowel syndrome, you might as well leave out the "bowel." A stomach that's always upset gives you plain "irritable syndrome."

You'll be glad to hear that as irritating as IBS is, it doesn't progress to anything worse. As Johns Hopkins Professor Marvin M. Schulster says, "This syndrome won't kill anyone, although some victims occasionally wish it would."

Don't resign yourself to being a victim, though. No new cures have been discovered for IBS, but don't give up on the diet and lifestyle changes that have been recommended for years.

Your goal is to get your stomach to react more normally to food and stress. Most people's intestines squeeze gently and steadily to move food along the digestive path· Food is broken down and absorbed or eliminated as waste.

If you have IBS, your intestines either squeeze too hard or not hard enough. Sometimes undigested food is rushed painfully through your system, causing cramps, diarrhea, and the strong urge to find a restroom.

Other times, sluggish intestines let food sit in place, leading to constipation and bloating. Symptoms also include gas, mucus-covered stools, stomach gurgling and feeling like you still need to have a bowel movement when you just had one.

Anyone over 40 with these symptoms should rule out digestive diseases like *colitis* (inflammation of the colon). Your doctor should examine your colon with a flexible tube known as a sigmoidoscope. Once you've determined that you do have IBS, take these tried-and-true steps to control the syndrome:

◆ If a certain food seems to bring on your symptoms, avoid it. This tip seems obvious, but in a recent study, over half the people who had trouble digesting milk hadn't made the connection between having a bout of IBS and eating dairy products like cheese, butter, milk, and ice cream.

Fatty foods trouble many people; and spicy, fried, and sugary foods are common culprits. Foods with the artificial sweetener sorbitol can cause diarrhea, so check the ingredient list on your sugar-free candy and gum. If you have too much gas, watch out for beans, cabbage, nuts, onions, and apple juice.

◆ Caffeine stimulates your bowel muscles as well as your brain, so it can cause diarrhea. Watch yourself for side effects from caffeinated coffee, tea, or cola. Nicotine and alcohol can cause digestive problems, too.

◆ High-fiber fruits, vegetables, and whole grains will help keep your colon working smoothly, as long as you also drink plenty of water. A psyllium fiber supplement such as Fiberall or Metamucil produces good results for most people.

Eating more fiber is one of the best things you can do for your digestion, but some types of fiber may make you feel worse instead of better. A large amount of wheat bran or high-fiber citrus fruits don't agree with some IBS sufferers.

- Exercise will help your intestines work better. It also relaxes you, and you've probably figured out that stress and tension have a direct effect on your stomach.
- Your tummy will appreciate any steps you take to reduce stress and find happiness. Some people who take antidepressants find that their stomach troubles almost disappear. Buy cassette tapes to help you learn to relax or meditate.
- A typical and embarrassing time for symptoms to appear is early in the morning when you've rushed to an important meeting or appointment. Try waking up an extra 30 minutes early so that you can have a relaxing morning. Build in time to listen to a stress reduction tape or go for a short walk.
- You can have stomach problems and be the most emotionally stable and mentally healthy person on the planet. If you're happy, don't feel that you need to find a connection between your stomach and your mind.

However, one study has shown that almost half the people with IBS have a history of verbal or sexual abuse. If you think counseling would help you improve your mental or emotional state, get it. Your digestion is almost sure to improve as well.

*Sources:*
*American Family Physician* (53,4:1229)
*Irritable Bowel Syndrome: Answers to Your Questions,* Procter & Gamble, P.O. Box 171, Cincinnati, Ohio, 45201
*Postgraduate Medicine* (98,5:248)

# Enjoy milk without troubling your tummy

Would you like to be able to enjoy a bowl of cereal or a cup of ice cream without dealing with an upset stomach later? A new study says you probably can, and you don't have to buy expensive tablets to help you digest the dairy products.

About one out of every four people don't have enough of the enzyme lactase they need to digest milk sugar. When these people eat too much dairy food, the undigested milk sugar moves through the digestive system, causing bloating, cramps, gas, diarrhea, and nausea.

In the past, those people have been advised to avoid milk completely or to use lactose-reduced products and lactase tablets.

Now, a new study says that most of these people can drink up to 8 ounces of milk a day without experiencing any symptoms of lactose intolerance.

Minnesota researchers found 30 people who said they had severe lactose intolerance. Tests showed that only 21 of the 30 really couldn't digest lactose. The researchers gave all these people 8 ounces of milk daily for one week. Then they had them drink lactose-free milk for one week. No one could tell which type they were drinking.

The people in the study were astonished to discover that they had no more stomach problems when drinking regular milk than when completely avoiding dairy products.

The researchers realized that people have digestive troubles all the time and many people found it easy to blame dairy products for those troubles. Actually, dairy products cause stomach problems much less often than you'd think, even for people who can't digest it very well.

The results of this study don't mean that people with lactose intolerance can now drink several glasses of milk a day. But they do mean that almost everyone can enjoy a small amount of any dairy product without having stomach problems later.

If you thought a morning bowl of milk and cereal wasn't an option for you, try it again. Start with a cup or less of milk a day. The best news is that once you start drinking milk, it usually becomes easier for you to digest. After a week or so of drinking less than one cup a day, you may be able to drink more with no discomfort.

*Sources:*
*The American Journal of Clinical Nutrition* (58,6:879)
*The New England Journal of Medicine* (333,1:1)

# Fatal food allergies: Are you at risk?

Hay fever sufferers and those prone to hives, take heed: You could be rushed to the emergency room someday for an allergic reaction to a food you eat. You need to be prepared.

Foods you may be allergic to include flaxseed, pepperoni, apples, and carrot juice. In the past, when a person with allergies was hurried to the hospital suffering with severe symptoms, nobody ever knew why. No one could explain the sudden, dangerous allergic emergency.

Finally, a few observant doctors made the connection between allergies like hay fever and food allergies. Certain people can have a reaction to a food that sends their everyday allergies into overdrive.

For instance, one little boy regularly reacted to the sun by breaking out in small hives. But twice, he began wheezing, his throat started closing, and he had to be rushed to the emergency room. On both occasions, the boy had eaten a pepperoni pizza before going outside. The nitrates in the pepperoni had made his usual minor allergic reaction to the sun much, much worse.

In Europe, almost three out of four people who have hay fever also have allergies to fruits and vegetables. Allergies to apples are so common that a researcher in the Netherlands looked for a way to make them edible. He sliced some apples, microwaved them for one minute, and fed them to people with apple allergies. Eight out of 10 had no allergic reaction at all.

Apparently, you can be mildly allergic to raw apples but not allergic at all to cooked apples. It's really true that you can enjoy applesauce and apple pie when you can't enjoy a raw apple.

If you have allergies, you should watch yourself for allergic reactions to food, especially to flaxseed, pepperoni, apples, and carrot juice. If you do have to make an emergency trip to the hospital or to your doctor, be prepared to tell the people in charge what you've been eating. It's important that you figure out what your food triggers are so you can avoid them.

Try this easy recipe for a healthy "apple pie" that may not trigger your allergies. Bring orange juice and a little sugar or honey to a boil in a nonstick pan, add apple slices, and sauté until apples are tender and the liquid is gone, stirring occasionally. Delicious warm or cold.

*Source:*
*Medical Tribune for the Internist and Cardiologist* (36,6:17)

## How to avoid diarrhea when you take antibiotics

Finally, researchers have come up with a cure for digestive troubles caused by antibiotics, and you should make sure your doctor knows about it. It comes from lychee nuts.

Diarrhea and other serious stomach problems are a dangerous possible side effect of taking antibiotics. Some people who take antibiotics to cure an infection get diarrhea that continues to trouble them for years. Long-term antibiotic therapy leaves some people with digestive illnesses such as *colitis* (inflammation of the colon) and *toxic megacolon* (an extremely dilated colon that may rupture).

Taking antibiotics can cause stomach problems because it upsets the balance of organisms in your body. While the drug kills the bacteria that caused the original infection (the one that made you sick), other bacteria or fungus can overgrow and cause a new infection. An organism first recognized in the 1980s called *Clostridium difficile* causes most stomach infections.

Recently, researchers trying to cure antibiotic-related diarrhea got promising results from a yeast made out of lychee nuts. You take the lychee-nut yeast along with a new antibiotic to kill your stomach infection. The combination worked much better than just taking an antibiotic alone.

If you have a stomach infection caused by taking antibiotics, ask your doctor about the lychee nut cure. The yeast was undergoing investigational clinical trials in the United States in 1994.

*Sources:*
*Emergency Medicine* (27,5:32)
*The Journal of the American Medical Association* (271,24:1913)

## Is your kitchen making you sick?

The Rogers are a very healthy family. Mom, Dad, and kids all play sports and exercise, eat vegetables from their huge garden, and even get enough sleep. But every once in a while, the whole family suffers together through a night of diarrhea and vomiting. Nobody escapes the flu.

Or is it the flu?

The five-person family can't afford to let food go to waste, so leftovers are always eaten, sometimes after they sit on the counter for three or four hours.

When Mom cooks desserts, the family converges on the kitchen to lick cake batter off beaters and to eat the raw cookie dough. And, the big cuts of meat that never thaw fast enough in the refrigerator usually end up defrosting on the kitchen counter.

Outbreaks of food poisoning from fast-food restaurants often make the evening news, but far more common are the small cases of food poisoning that crop up in your kitchen at home.

People like the Rogers usually don't see a doctor for the stomach flu or a "24-hour bug," so they never find out that food-borne illnesses are causing their symptoms. Some 7 million Americans will suffer from food poisoning this year, because at the right temperature, bacteria you can't see, smell, or taste can multiply to the millions in a few short hours.

Here are the basic rules that will keep you and your family safe:

**First of all, shop for food in good condition.** Refrigerated food should be cold to the touch and frozen food should be rock-solid. Canned foods should have no dents, cracks, or bulging lids. Check the use-by date, and don't eat the food when the date has passed. Keep meats separate from your other food.

Finally, never leave food in a hot car. Grocery shop right before you go home.

**Keep your refrigerator at 40 degrees Fahrenheit or less.** Many people's refrigerators are set at over 50 degrees — warm enough to allow bacteria to multiply. Put a thermometer in your refrigerator to make sure the temperature is safe.

**Throw away any meat that's been at room temperature for more than two hours.** You may have heard that you shouldn't put hot leftover food in the refrigerator. That's not true. Large amounts of leftovers should be divided into small containers for quick cooling. Store any stuffing separately from the bird.

Refrigerated leftovers are usually safe for three to five days. When you reheat, bring to a boil or microwave with a lid.

**Pour a mixture of bleach and water down your sink every few days.** Bacteria can grow on food particles trapped in the drain, disposal, and connecting pipe.

**Clean cutting boards well.** Wash first with warm, soapy water, then with a bleach solution.

**Eat hamburgers well-done.** Cooking them until they are brown instead of pink is a good start, but not good enough. Press the burger with a spatula to squeeze the juices out. Juices should be yellowish or clear.

**After microwaving, let food stand for a few minutes.** Microwaving creates pockets of heat in food. The heat will spread when the food stands.

**Don't eat raw eggs.** Homemade raw cookie dough, eggnog, and cake batter can give you a salmonella infection. Fried eggs shouldn't be runny. If you don't want to cook your homemade ice cream, use pasteurized eggs instead of raw eggs. Eggs shouldn't be left unrefrigerated for more than two hours, and they shouldn't be stored in the refrigerator door.

**Clean kitchen counters with hot water and soap, then a bleach solution or a commercial sanitizer.** Wet dishcloths and sponges harbor bacteria. Keep them clean. Wash the can opener blade every time you use it.

**Wash dirty dishes in hot water right away, then air-dry.** An automatic dishwasher is sanitary, too. If you must let a dish soak for several hours, pour the dirty water out before cleaning.

**Wash hands with warm water and soap for at least 20 seconds before and after handling food.** Wash hands especially well after handling raw meat, poultry, and fish. If you wear rubber gloves, wash them.

**Thaw foods in the refrigerator or the microwave.** Put raw meat on a plate so juices won't drip. You can also put food in a water-tight plastic bag and thaw it in a sink filled with cold water. Change the water every 30 minutes to keep it cold enough.

**Cook large meats, like roasts or turkeys, at 325 degrees Fahrenheit or above.** Cooking at lower temperatures allows bacteria to grow.

**Don't serve food with the utensils you used to cook it.** And never put grilled meat back on the platter that held the raw meat.

**At parties, remember the two-hour time limit for leaving food out.** Keep food refrigerated until you're ready to warm it or serve it.

Following all these rules can feel time-consuming and unrewarding. If you or your family get food poisoning, you may never know what caused it. Symptoms can develop a half hour or several weeks after you eat contaminated food. Try to remember the possible consequences — mild or severe cramps, nausea, vomiting, diarrhea, and dizziness — and handle your food as safely as possible.

*Sources:*
*A Quick Consumer Guide to Safe Food Handling,* HG Bulletin No. 248, U.S. Department of Agriculture, Food Safety and Inspection Service
*FDA Consumer* (29,8:14)
*Food Safety Notebook* (September 1995)
*Medical Update* (19,6:6)
*The Unwelcome Dinner Guest: Preventing Food-Borne Illness,* a reprint from *FDA Consumer,* Food and Drug Administration, HFI-40, Rockville, Md. 20857

## Food poisoning from your pet

Don't keep Iggy the Iguana in the kitchen, and wash your hands after petting him. Around 90 percent of pet turtles, iguanas, rattlesnakes, and other reptiles may carry salmonella, the bacteria that's the culprit behind many cases of food poisoning.

Pregnant women, small children (age 5 and under), and other people who are vulnerable to infection shouldn't touch reptiles at all.

*Source:*
*Medical Update* (19,2:6)

## Digestive problems that demand a doctor's care

Keeping your 25-foot-long digestive tract in good working order usually requires simple, basic maintenance. You'll see the same advice over and over for heartburn, indigestion, gas, diarrhea, constipation, and hemorrhoids:

♦ Eat a variety of vegetables, fruits, and grains.
♦ Drink plenty of water.
♦ Avoid getting too much alcohol or caffeine.

When these steps fail and digestive damage goes beyond your ability to control, you'll probably know it. Here are some sure signs that should send you running to a doctor:

♦ Severe stomach pains occurring with shaking and chills.
♦ Frequent vomiting or blood in your vomit.
♦ Blood in your stools or tarry-black stools.
♦ A sudden change in your bathroom habits that lasts for at least several days.
♦ Painful or difficult swallowing.
♦ Yellow skin or whites of your eyes (jaundice).
♦ Dark, tea-colored urine.

*Source:*
*Medical Abstracts Newsletter* (16,2:1)

# Heart-Smart Living

## A grape way to prevent heart attacks

You may have heard that drinking alcohol can help prevent heart attacks. If alcoholic beverages aren't usually in your cupboard, please, don't rush out to the package store. Researchers have discovered exactly why there seemed to be a connection between alcohol consumption and a decreased risk of heart disease, and it has little to do with alcohol.

The first studies on heart disease and alcohol revealed a lower incidence of heart disease in people who drank alcohol on a regular basis. Then it was discovered that wine lowered risk, while beer had no effect, and spirits actually increased the risk of heart disease. Taking that information one step further, researchers found that red wine lowered risk, while white wine didn't. In processing, the skins are removed from the grapes to make white wine, but the skins are left on to make red wine. Could grape skins contain something that helps fight heart disease?

Researchers soon discovered that grape skins contain *flavonoids*. Flavonoids provide powerful antioxidant protection, which helps keep cholesterol from damaging your artery walls, and they also help prevent blood clots. Nutritionists have been thrilled to discover these natural disease-fighting compounds in many types of fruits and vegetables.

You already know that you can find flavonoids in grapes and red wine. Other sources include:

| | | |
|---|---|---|
| ▸ Strawberries | ▸ Apples | ▸ Garlic |
| ▸ Grapefruit | ▸ Tea | ▸ Ginger |
| ▸ Onions | ▸ Kale | ▸ Oregano |
| ▸ Eggplant | ▸ Ginger | ▸ Black pepper |

Drinking red wine can indeed decrease your risk of heart disease. However, you don't have to drink alcohol. Grape juice will do.

*Sources:*
Archives of Internal Medicine (155,4:381)
British Medical Journal (310,6988:1165)
Food Safety Notebook (January 1996)
Geriatrics (50,4:14)
The Journal of the American Medical Association (273,16:1249)

## Aspirin heads off heart attacks

Those little white pills pack a powerful punch. They relieve your worst headaches, muscle aches, and arthritis pains. But their power doesn't stop there. Now researchers say aspirin can even stop a heart attack in progress.

Leading cardiologists recommend that you keep some aspirin in your first aid kit. If you experience the symptoms of a heart attack (crushing chest pain which may extend down your left arm or up into your jaw and back or feeling breathless, restless, or nauseated), call for emergency help and then take one regular aspirin immediately.

To get the quickest benefit from the aspirin, chew it, crush it, or suck on it, rather than swallowing it whole. However, you should not take aspirin if you are allergic to it. That could make an already bad situation much worse. Many emergency rooms now use aspirin as the first line of treatment for people suspected of having a heart attack.

Taking aspirin after you've had a heart attack aids recovery and helps prevent future attacks. The clotting of blood platelets in arteries thickened by cholesterol is what usually causes a heart attack or stroke. But aspirin keeps the platelets in your blood from forming dangerous clots.

Some experts believe that as many as half of all strokes and heart attacks can be prevented by the regular use of aspirin. In a study of 22,000 doctors over a five-year period, those who took one aspirin tablet every other day lowered their risk of heart attack by 44 percent.

Several Massachusetts hospitals kept track of their heart attack patients for three years. They found that the people who had been taking aspirin regularly had smaller, less severe heart attacks than those who had not.

Evidence from another recent study suggests that even very low doses of aspirin may benefit people at risk for heart attack.

Ask your doctor if daily aspirin therapy could help you. A beginning dose of 200 to 300 mg is needed to ensure your body stores enough of the drug. Then daily doses can be lowered to 75 to 100 mg, about the dosage of a "children's" aspirin.

Be sure to give aspirin, the undisputed king of over-the-counter drugs, a spot of honor in your throne room. You never know when it might play a leading role in a serious human drama — your life.

**Sources:**
*American Family Physician* (51,5:1280)
*Archives of Internal Medicine* (155,13:1386)
*Cardiac Alert* (15,12:4)
*Drug Therapy* (23,6:53)
*Geriatrics* (48,9:93)
*Medical Tribune* (34,9:1)
*The Journal of the American Medical Association* (270,20:2502)
*The New England Journal of Medicine* (330,18:1287)
*U.S. Pharmacist* (19,3:116)

# High fiber, low heart disease

Do you love eating cold cereal for breakfast? Then you may be just a kid at heart ... literally. A new study has shown that a high-fiber diet can cut your risk of heart disease substantially, and your breakfast cereal can be the biggest dose of fiber you get all day.

Researchers found that men who ate the most fiber had a risk of developing heart disease about a third lower than men who ate the least amount of fiber. The high-fiber group also had about half the risk of death from heart disease.

This study led experts to conclude that adding 10 grams of fiber a day to your diet can reduce your risk of having a heart attack by one third.

The type of fiber you eat also makes a difference. Though fruits and vegetables are also a good source of fiber, the most protective benefit comes from cereal fiber. Most people in the study got the bulk of their fiber from cold breakfast cereal. Maybe cereal isn't just for kids, after all.

*Sources:*
*Health News* (2,5:1)
*Journal Watch* (16,6:46)

# Healing from the sea

A fatty fish may save your life. No, Tubby the Tuna isn't going to rescue you from drowning, but eating tuna may keep you from having a heart attack.

Certain seafood contains omega-3 fatty acids, which have been shown to reduce the risk of heart disease. These fatty acids reduce the clumping of platelets in the blood and lessen the risk of coronary spasms. Experts say that eating just one three-ounce serving of fatty fish a week cuts your risk of heart disease.

Salmon is a great source of omega-3, and you can also find it in tuna, cod, and many other types of fish and shellfish.

*Sources:*
*Medical Tribune for the Internist and Cardiologist* (36,22:7)
*The Journal of the American Medical Association* (274,17:1363)

# A dime's worth of heart attack protection

A dime may be worth more than you think. A British study recently concluded that a dime's worth of vitamin E a day can slash your risk of heart attack by 75 percent if you have heart disease.

Vitamin E protects against heart disease by acting as an antioxidant and lowering LDL cholesterol levels in the blood. High levels of LDL cholesterol are a risk factor for heart disease.

Vitamin E may also help keep platelets from sticking to blood vessel walls and forming clots which can lead to strokes and heart attacks. Platelets clutter arteries with clots by sending out anchor strands to attach themselves to blood vessel walls. Vitamin E prevents the platelets from sending out these strands. Taking vitamin E along with a low daily dose of aspirin provides an even more powerful anti-clotting effect.

The U.S. recommended daily allowance of vitamin E is 15 international units (IU) for men and 12 IU for women. However, in order to get the most heart protecting benefits, the British researchers recommend 400 IU daily.

Check with your doctor before taking vitamin E supplements. Vitamin E may not be advisable for people with very high blood pressure or people taking blood thinning medication.

*Sources:*
*Medical Tribune for the Internist and Cardiologist* (36,18:13)
*Postgraduate Medicine* (98,1:175)
*The American Journal of Clinical Nutrition* (62,6S:1315S)
*The Lancet* (347,9004:781)

## How to bypass heart surgery naturally

Want to lose weight without dieting, reverse your heart disease without drugs or surgery, feel better than you ever have in your life, and get your insurance company to pay for it?

Dr. Dean Ornish has been so successful in his quest to reverse heart disease without drugs or surgery that insurance companies want to cash in on the benefits.

Both Mutual of Omaha and Blue Cross and Blue Shield of California are just two of the several insurance companies who've agreed to help cover the costs for qualified participants in Ornish's Lifestyle Heart Trial program.

Of course, you can always practice Ornish's principles at home without having to go anywhere.

Insurance companies are on the right track. Ornish's program just makes good economic sense. Bypass surgeries typically cost $50,000 to $60,000 per person. In contrast, Ornish's program costs $5,000 to $6,000 per person. That's a savings of at least $45,000 in money alone. In addition, you'll save yourself the emotional turmoil of heart surgery and time spent recovering.

If feeling great sounds good to you, give Ornish's program a try. And think big — big changes, that is. Contrary to popular opinion, Ornish believes that starting with small changes in your diet and lifestyle is not your best option.

Ornish finds that people are more frustrated by small changes than they are with sweeping ones. The reasons? Sweeping changes, like the ones Ornish recommends, make you feel better fast, often in as little as seven days.

Small changes often take much longer to make you feel better, leaving you feeling deprived with nothing to show for it. And Ornish says that making big changes are actually easier than making small changes. Ornish suggests five steps to feeling better fast:

- ◆ Get connected with yourself and others. Ornish contends that people develop self-destructive habits like smoking, drinking alcohol, overeating, and putting themselves under constant stress to help them cope with isolation, from themselves and from others.

  Getting connected with yourself means taking time to listen to your feelings. Ornish finds that meditation is often the most effective method for helping people connect with their inner selves.

  Getting connected with others means learning effective ways to communicate. To communicate well, express your wants and needs clearly without appearing judgmental toward other people.

- ◆ Manage your stress. Take some time every day to regularly stretch and relax your body. Two quick and easy stretches you can do anytime, anywhere, include shoulder shrugs (raising and lowering your shoulders several times) and forward stretches. You can do a forward stretch either sitting in a chair or standing up. Simply bend over and try to touch your toes. Reach as far as you can, but remember not to bounce.

  To relax your entire body, work your way from the tips of your toes to the top of your head, tensing and relaxing all muscles.

- ◆ Eat a low-fat, low-cholesterol diet. If you've been diagnosed with heart disease or want to lose weight, Ornish recommends that no more than 10 percent of your calories come from fat.

But you don't have to worry about constantly counting calories or fat grams. Just center your meals around fruits, vegetables, grains, legumes (such as beans and peas), and soybean products. Stay away from high-fat vegetarian foods like avocados, olives, coconut, nuts, seeds, and cocoa concoctions.

You should also avoid all animal products with the exception of egg whites and 1 cup of nonfat yogurt or milk a day. Limit alcohol to 2 ounces per day or less. Try to avoid caffeine, which may worsen irregular heartbeats or provoke stress.

Don't eat when you're distracted by a good book or television show. Stop eating when you feel satisfied. If you stuff yourself, even on this slimming fare, you'll still gain weight.

◆ Stop smoking. If you make it a daily habit to get connected with yourself and other people, manage your stress, and eat a low-fat diet, you'll find it easier to stop smoking. That's because these healthy habits and the unhealthy habit of smoking fill many of the same needs, making you feel less stressed and more in control, helping you keep your weight down, and improving your concentration and performance.

To successfully stop smoking, you have to have confidence in your ability to quit. And remember that quitting smoking is a process. Don't give up if you don't manage to quit the first time. Most people don't, but at least you've taken that important first step.

Here are five tips to keep your body's craving for nicotine under control:

▶ Keep lots of fruits and veggies around to munch on.

▶ Indulge yourself in lots of warms baths or showers.

▶ Get rid of all your smoking stuff, like ashtrays and lighters.

▶ Reward yourself with something special every day.

▶ Place a drop of clove oil on the back of your tongue when you feel the urge to smoke.

◆ Exercise regularly. For the best results from Ornish's program, be sure you exercise regularly. Since you eat so little fat on this food plan, you don't need to exercise yourself silly to see results. Walking 20 to 60 minutes a day at a pace that feels good to you will probably be plenty. To keep yourself motivated, choose fun activities that make you feel good.

Ornish recommends you follow these guidelines for at least three weeks. That's how long it takes to establish new habit patterns. But many people are feeling so much better after just seven days that it's not even a question whether to continue the program or not. The only question they have is why they waited so long to start in the first place.

Some experts feel that Ornish's strict guidelines may be too daunting for most people. Dr. Ornish contends that people on his program feel so much better, so quickly that they're naturally self-motivated to continue. You be the judge.

*Sources:*

*Dr. Dean Ornish's Program for Reversing Heart Disease,* Random House, New York, 1990
*Eat More, Weigh Less,* HarperCollins, New York, 1993
*The Journal of the American Medical Association* (274,11:894)
*The Lancet* (336,8708:129)

## Fight heart disease with folic acid

In our ongoing war against heart disease, a new weapon could be leading the battle. A simple vitamin deficiency could be responsible for 40 percent of heart attacks and strokes suffered by American men. The vitamin is folic acid.

Dozens of studies have shown that folic acid reduces the level of homocysteine in the blood. Homocysteine, an amino acid, can cause narrowing of the arteries, leading to an increased risk of heart disease and stroke.

Homocysteine could be responsible for many unexplained deaths in people who are otherwise healthy. When all the studies are added together, researchers estimate that if people would increase their daily intake of folic acid to 400 micrograms, as many as 50,000 deaths a year from heart disease could be prevented.

Mom was right when she told you to eat your spinach. Folic acid is a B vitamin found mostly in green leafy vegetables. Though folic acid and other important B vitamins are available in supplements, it is best to get your vitamins from food. Good sources of folic acid include:

| | |
|---|---|
| ► Spinach | ► Green leafy vegetables |
| ► Orange juice | ► Lentils |
| ► Kidney beans | ► Black beans |
| ► Lima beans | ► Peas |
| ► Tomato sauce | ► Fortified cereal |
| ► Romaine lettuce | ► Leaf lettuce |

*Sources:*
*Hope Health Letter* (XVI,2:1)
*The Journal of the American Medical Association* (274,13:1049)
*The Saturday Evening Post* (267,3:40)

## Warm baths help heart health

Soaking in a warm bath can be very relaxing. Doctors now say it can also be very helpful for people with congestive heart failure. A new study found that people with congestive heart failure who took short baths (about 10 minutes) in warm water improved their heart function and decreased congestion in their lungs. This could be a safe, drug-free, and fun way for people with congestive heart failure to help themselves. So, find your rubber ducky and dive in.

*Source:*
*Medical Abstracts Newsletter* (15,12:2)

## Coffee drinkers, take heart

Do you need just one cup of coffee to get motivated in the morning or do you guzzle it all day long? Either way, there is now reason to rejoice. New information shows that drinking coffee does not increase your risk of heart disease.

A recent study of over 85,000 women found a strong correlation between coffee drinking and smoking. Among women who drank six or more cups of coffee a day, 58 percent were smokers. This connection between smoking and coffee drinking may account for the previous finding that coffee contributed to heart disease. However, after taking the smoking factor into account, even women who drank six or more cups of coffee a day did not have a higher risk of developing heart disease.

*Source:*
*The Physician and Sportsmedicine* (24,4:18g)

# Chase away chest pain

Do you ever feel like an invisible python is squeezing your chest? If your pain is dull and constant, not brief and sharp, you're probably experiencing *angina*. The pain of angina may make your chest feel tight or heavy, or you may feel a burning or squeezing sensation. Sometimes the pain may start in the chest, but then spreads to the rest of the upper body.

Clogged arteries (*atherosclerosis*) which interfere with the blood flow to the heart can cause angina. You are more likely to experience angina during vigorous exercise, after heavy meals, during sex, or when you're under emotional stress. People with angina actually have a low risk of heart attack, probably because the angina serves as a warning that they may be overexerting themselves. However, if your angina suddenly increases in intensity, length, or frequency, it could mean that your atherosclerosis may be getting worse. This puts you at an increased risk of heart attack.

Though strenuous exercise may trigger angina, a regular program of moderate exercise will improve your heart rate and blood pressure, which reduces angina symptoms. Changing your lifestyle will improve your angina. Lose weight, stop smoking, try to limit stressful situations, and eat healthy meals.

*Source:*
*The Physician and Sportsmedicine* (23,7:79)

# The heartbreak of hair loss

When Samson awoke to find his locks had been shorn, he knew it was going to be a bad day. Sudden hair loss could be a warning signal to you, too. Evidence indicates a link between balding and heart disease.

One study found that the connection between hair loss and heart disease seems to depend upon how fast you lose your hair. Men who experienced slow balding did not have an increased risk of heart disease. However, among men who were examined at six-year intervals, those who lost moderate amounts of hair were almost twice as likely to develop or die from heart disease. Those who lost all or most of their hair in six years were two and a half times as likely to develop heart disease, and four times as likely to die from it.

Though no one believes that balding causes heart disease, it may be a side effect of a developing heart condition. Therefore, hair loss (especially rapid hair loss) may serve as a warning to men that they may be at increased risk for heart attack. Since forewarned is forearmed, they can then be more careful about their diet and lifestyle.

If you experience rapid hair loss, you may need to take steps to protect your heart. Perhaps if Samson had been warned, he would have protected his.

*Source:*
*The Journal of the American Medical Association* (269,8:998)

## Common home appliance can cause chest pain

If you have unexplained chest pain, a faulty heater could be responsible. Carbon monoxide poisoning or exposure can trigger unstable angina, or chest pains. Faulty kerosene heaters, blocked chimneys, defective furnaces, or improperly ventilated fireplaces or wood stoves could all cause carbon monoxide buildup in your home. Carbon monoxide testers can warn you of dangerous levels of gas. One of these inexpensive detectors outside each sleeping area could protect your family and help you breathe easy.

*Source:*
*The New England Journal of Medicine* (332,13:894)

## Heart attack or breast implant?

You suddenly experience crushing chest pain, shortness of breath, and pain in your left arm. Your first thought is that you're having a heart attack. If you have a breast implant, however, your self-diagnosis could be wrong. A group of Texas doctors studied 11 women with silicon breast implants who experienced severe chest pain but had no sign of heart disease. The attacks happened six weeks to seven years after the breast implant surgeries and were apparently caused by silicon leaking into the surrounding tissue. All the women had their implants removed and reported a considerable or complete reduction in pain.

*Source:*
*Emergency Medicine* (27,5:78)

## Heart-safe sex

If you've suffered a heart attack and fear that having sex could trigger another one, here's heartening information. Researchers conclude that although sexual activity can trigger a heart attack (as any vigorous physical activity can), the risk of increase is very small, only one chance in a million. This risk is not any greater for those with heart problems. Regular exercise decreases this risk even more, so perhaps instead of avoiding sexual activity, you should engage in it more often.

*Source:*
*The Journal of the American Medical Association* (275,18:1405)

## Healing a 'broken' heart

Once you've been through the trauma of a heart attack, chances are you'll do anything to avoid another one. Here are some things you can do to prevent a second attack:

**Take your vitamins.** Vitamins E and C both show great promise in treating people with heart disease. One study found that men who took a supplement of 100 IU (international units) of vitamin E daily after a heart attack developed significantly less artery blockage than men who took less than 100 IU. Another study found that heart attack survivors who ate foods high in vitamin C, such as citrus fruits, broccoli, cantaloupe, and green pepper, had low levels of an enzyme which indicates heart damage.

**Remain active.** You probably won't feel like sprinting out the hospital doors immediately following a heart attack. However, mild exercise improves blood flow and artery dilation. You can start slowly and increase your activity level until you exercise for 30 minutes at least three or four times a week.

**Don't ignore depression.** Among people who have suffered a heart attack, those with severe depression were more likely to die from their heart condition. Sometimes depression following a heart attack goes untreated because symptoms may be confused with side effects from the heart attack. If you feel depressed, ask your doctor for help.

**Practice prevention.** All of the things which could have prevented your first heart attack can still prevent your second. In other words, stop smoking, lose weight, eat less cholesterol and fat, and limit your alcohol and salt intakes. Make a decision to change your lifestyle for the better, then stick to it ... for life.

*Sources:*
*Geriatrics* (50,4:16 and 50,8:16)
*Journal of the American Dietetic Association* (48,3:65)
*Medical Tribune for the Internist and Cardiologist* (36,13:24 and 37,3:19)

# Home heart rehabilitation

Home is where the heart is. When you're recovering from a heart attack, that's especially true.

Only 15 percent of the people who could benefit from cardiac rehabilitation actually participate. This may be because some people live too far from a rehabilitation center or are unable to travel. Others may be uncomfortable exercising in front of strangers. Home rehabilitation may provide an alternative for many people.

New home rehabilitation programs use heart monitors that hook into telephone modems so that a nurse or therapist can observe the patient's heart rate as he exercises. They also provide headphones for communicating with therapists, as well as exercise equipment. In a recent trial run of a home-based program, people improved their fitness levels as much as those who went to a hospital rehabilitation center. Doctors view this as an exciting option that may increase the number of people who participate in rehabilitation.

If you'd rather rehabilitate where you habitate, maybe a home rehab program is right for you.

*Source:*
*Medical Tribune for the Internist and Cardiologist* (37,3:1)

# 6 ways to lower your cholesterol

Confused about cholesterol? Join the club. Most of us know that we need to control our cholesterol levels, but don't understand how or why.

Cholesterol makes up the main part of the plaque that sticks to blood vessel walls, clogging arteries and contributing to heart disease. Cholesterol combines with two forms of lipoproteins to travel in your body, high-density lipoprotein (HDL) and low-density lipoprotein (LDL). Both contain fat and protein. However, LDL is mostly fat, but HDL is mostly protein. They also perform different functions in the body. HDL takes excess fat and cholesterol from tissues to the liver to be dismantled. LDL carries fat and cholesterol to the body tissues. High levels of LDL forecast a high risk of heart disease, while high levels of HDL indicate a low risk.

Here are some tips for controlling your cholesterol:

**Eat more fiber.** Adding water-soluble fiber to your diet can lower your LDL cholesterol. Water-soluble fiber is simply fiber which dissolves easily in water. Grains like oatbran and buckwheat lower cholesterol effectively. Cereal enriched with psyllium, another water-soluble fiber, reduces LDL in children as well as adults.

**Try some soy.** Consider substituting vegetable protein like soy for animal protein as much as possible. Researchers found that a low-fat, high-protein diet lowers LDL and does not result in decreased production of HDL as a high-carbohydrate diet can. One study found adding soy to the diet resulted in as much as a 24 percent drop in LDL and recommended substituting half your animal protein with vegetable protein. You can easily find many soy products including tofu, soy milk, soy flour, and soy meat.

**Lose weight.** In a recent study, people who lost 5 pounds or more on a low-fat diet and kept it off for six months reduced their cholesterol levels by 10 percent. Those who didn't lose weight only reduced their cholesterol levels by 4 percent, even though they were also on a low-fat diet.

**Cut the fat.** Avoid saturated fat as much as possible. The more unsaturated a fat, the better it is for your cholesterol level. The more saturated a fat, the more solid it is at room temperature. Animal fats are the most saturated fats, while most vegetable oil is unsaturated.

**Get moving.** Changing your diet can lower LDL cholesterol, but it doesn't raise HDL cholesterol. However, exercise can raise the levels of HDL in your blood. Jogging or walking briskly for 30 minutes three to five times a week will significantly raise your HDL.

**Add some niacin.** This miracle B vitamin lowers LDL cholesterol and raises HDL cholesterol significantly. Despite its obvious benefits, doctors have avoided recommending niacin because of its side effects. Itching, flushing, rash, and stomach pain commonly occur with increased niacin intake. Ask your doctor if niacin therapy could help you lower your cholesterol level.

*Sources:*
*Archives of Internal Medicine* (155,4:415)
*Medical Tribune for the Internist and Cardiologist* (36,16:2 and 37,4:19)
*Nutrition Research Newsletter* (14,2:20 and 14,5:60)

## Cholesterol testing tips

Keeping an eye on your cholesterol level? If you're going to have a cholesterol test, don't eat anything or drink anything but water for 12 hours before being tested. You should also avoid vigorous exercise for 24 hours before being tested. Exercise can temporarily lower levels, which makes the results of the test inaccurate. If you truly want to know what your cholesterol levels are, don't let yourself be cheated out of an accurate report.

*Sources:*
*American Family Physician* (53,3:978)
*Medical Update* (18,11:6)

# Put some spring into your arteries

A little spring in your step usually means that you're feeling pretty snazzy. Some spring in your arteries means that they're doing a pretty snazzy job circulating your blood. This elasticity allows your arteries to expand or contract in response to your body's need for blood. If stiff arteries can't get the blood where it's needed quickly, like to your heart during exercise, you may end up with chest pains. Reducing cholesterol returns the spring to hardened arteries and helps prevent heart attacks in the future. However, it can also make you feel better now by pumping your blood more efficiently and preventing chest pain. Putting some spring into your arteries may also put some spring into your step.

*Source:*
*Circulation* (91,12:2898)

# Good news about salt

Have you been passing up the salt shaker to keep your blood pressure down? Well, shunning the seasoning may mean more to your body than just disappointing your taste buds. New evidence shows that drastically limiting your intake of salt may result in an unwanted surprise.

Although considered by many to be a nutritional no-no, a daily seasoning of salt is necessary for your body to function. The body needs salt to retain water, keep up your blood volume, and help your kidneys function normally. The American Heart Association recommends that you limit your sodium intake to 3,000 mg a day, or about one and a half teaspoons of salt. Most Americans consume an average of 4,000 to 5,800 mg of sodium a day, which is too much. That's why there has been a concentrated effort by doctors and public health officials to encourage Americans to cut back on salt.

However, not everyone reacts to salt the same way. Researchers found that people are either "salt sensitive" or "salt resistant." After eating a large amount of salt, the blood pressure in salt-sensitive people rises. When they cut back on salt, their blood pressure falls. Older people and people with high blood pressure seem to be the most salt-sensitive. People who are salt-resistant don't experience much of a rise or fall in blood pressure when they eat salty foods.

So, if limiting salt lowers blood pressure in salt-sensitive people, why not just put everyone on a low-salt diet? Several studies have indicated that less is not always better. Some researchers say that when people who are salt-resistant reduce their salt intakes, their blood pressures actually rise.

Many factors besides salt are thought to worsen high blood pressure. Smoking, obesity, drinking too much alcohol, and a lack of exercise are often culprits. The Intersalt study, a famous salt study which looked at blood pressure and salt intake in 32 countries, found little relationship between salt intake and blood pressure. In fact, of all the possible lifestyle changes to lower your blood pressure, reducing calories has the biggest overall impact.

Both sides of the salt argument agree that too much salt in anyone's diet is not healthy and that an average person is safe within the recommended guidelines of one and a half teaspoons of salt a day. If you are concerned about your blood pressure, check with your doctor before you ban the salt shaker. Find out if you are salt-sensitive and what guidelines are best for you.

*Sources:*
American Journal of Hypertension (4,5:416)
Environmental Nutrition (13,3:1 and 14,8:1)
Journal of the American College of Nutrition (14,5:428)

# 10 diet tips help you get a grip on blood pressure

High blood pressure increases your risk for many serious diseases, including stroke, artery disease, kidney failure, and blood vessel damage. You may be able to control your blood pressure without drugs by following a few dietary recommendations.

**Salt.** Over half the people with high blood pressure are salt sensitive. For these people, particularly the elderly, reducing salt intake lowers blood pressure significantly.

**Calcium.** In salt sensitive individuals, increasing calcium intake lowers blood pressure as effectively as reducing salt intake. Increasing calcium intake to 1,500 mg a day may provide great protection against high blood pressure.

**Alcohol.** Reducing excessive alcohol intake (three or more drinks a day) can substantially lower your blood pressure.

**Fiber.** Increased fiber intake may prevent high blood pressure. Doctors recommend a diet containing 25 to 30 grams of fiber a day. Grains, fruits, and vegetables are good sources of fiber.

**Magnesium.** This mineral may help reduce high blood pressure and improve overall heart health.

**Potassium.** High potassium intake may reduce the risk of high blood pressure, particularly in blacks. However, people with kidney problems should consult their doctors before increasing their potassium. These people have a greater risk for potassium overload, a potentially fatal condition. If you are trying to reduce your salt intake, be aware that many salt substitutes contain a high amount of potassium.

**Fat.** Weight reduction lowers blood pressure, and a low-fat diet certainly contributes. However, certain types of fats actually help protect against heart disease. Omega-3 fatty acids, or fish oil, may lower blood pressure.

**Carbohydrates.** In order to keep your blood pressure under control, you should try to eat more complex carbohydrates, (starchy foods like pastas, potatoes, and rice) and limit your simple sugars (cane sugar, syrup, honey, molasses, and brown sugar).

**Caffeine.** Though caffeine intake usually does not directly affect blood pressure, people who have high blood pressure may be overly sensitive to caffeine. Also, high caffeine intake can cause calcium loss, which could contribute to high blood pressure.

**Garlic.** Garlic may do more for your blood than keep vampires from sucking it. Studies show that garlic can reduce blood pressure in people with high blood pressure.

These dietary measures can all help to reduce your blood pressure. Which are the most effective? The three best bets for reducing your blood pressure without drugs:

◆ Less salt
◆ Less weight
◆ Less alcohol

*Sources:*
*Archives of Family Medicine* (4,8:709)
*British Medical Journal* (311,7018:1486)
*Journal of the American College of Nutrition* (15,1:21)
*Journal Watch* (16,3:24)
*The Saturday Evening Post* (267,4:20)

# Exercise control over high blood pressure

If you have high blood pressure, you may have been advised to avoid exercise. People with high blood pressure have an increased risk of suffering a heart attack. Concern about exercise-induced heart attacks led many doctors to tell their patients to toss their tennis shoes.

Though strenuous exercise can cause a temporary increase in blood pressure, a regular exercise program will eventually lower blood pressure. Exercise helps you lose weight, and weight loss contributes to lower blood pressure. The key is to exercise correctly.

If you have severe high blood pressure, you should try to lower it with diet and medication before attempting any strenuous exercise. Once your blood pressure is under control, ask your doctor if you can begin aerobic activities, such as jogging or walking. Three to five sessions per week for 20 to 60 minutes should soon produce results.

People who have high blood pressure should avoid weight training because lifting heavy weights can cause a sharp rise in blood pressure. However, circuit training, which uses lighter weights with more repetitions, may be a good alternative. The most effective circuit training program consists of 10 to 15 repetitions in 30 to 45 seconds with a 30 to 50 percent resistance load. The resistance load is a percentage of the maximum weight that you can lift in a single repetition. You should rest 15 to 30 seconds between exercises and perform about 10 to 12 exercises two or three times per session.

Caffeine and exercise may not mix well for those with mild high blood pressure. Be aware that caffeine can temporarily cause a sharp increase in blood pressure, just as exercise can. Mixing the two at the same time may be asking for trouble.

Don't let high blood pressure keep you from the gym or the tennis courts. Just exercise a little common sense, and enjoy the benefits exercise can bring.

**Sources:**
*Medical Abstracts Newsletter* (16,2:8)
*The Journal of the American Medical Association* (273,24:1965)

# Hidden danger in licorice

Everyone knows by now that too much salt may raise your blood pressure, but did you know that a seemingly harmless piece of black licorice can send your blood pressure skyrocketing? Though many people think that black licorice containing *glycyrrhizic acid* is no longer available in the United States, many types of imported licorice still contain this flavoring. Glycyrrhizic acid may cause salt retention and potassium loss, which can lead to high blood pressure. Certain kinds of chewing tobacco also contain licorice flavor. Some skin ointments, anti-hemorrhoidal creams, eye drops, and nasal sprays also contain ingredients which can have the same effect as licorice.

In searching for blood pressure culprits, you may need to look no farther than your medicine cabinet. *Diuretics*, or water pills, which commonly appear in weight loss products, may also affect your blood pressure. Some over-the-counter painkillers, such as aspirin, ibuprofen, and naproxen could make your blood pressure medication worthless. Some types of birth control pills could also counteract the effects of your blood pressure medication.

Since many innocent items may elevate your blood pressure, you should discuss all possibilities thoroughly with your doctor.

**Sources:**
*Archives of Internal Medicine* (155,5:450)
*Emergency Medicine* (77,6:18)

# Finger monitors unreliable

Put your finger in and get your blood pressure reading out. Simple, but not very accurate. A recent study found that automated finger monitors were accurate less than one in four times. Doctors warn that these finger monitors can give false readings that are positive or negative. Therefore, these readings may cause needless alarm in some people and give false reassurance to others. Home cuff monitors do give reliable readings, which makes them a better bet for keeping your finger on your blood pressure level.

**Source:**
*Medical Tribune for the Internist and Cardiologist* (36,20:8)

# Can music and fast talk kill you?

Your blood pressure can shoot through the roof for the oddest reasons. A recent study found that the faster people talk, the higher their blood pressures rise. One doctor even found that playing a french horn can be dangerous. The doctor monitored one man's blood pressure while he was playing the french horn and discovered that the man's blood pressure rose dramatically when he played high notes. Does this mean fast talk and music will kill you? Probably not, but if you play a horn, maybe you should consider switching to the guitar

*Sources:*
*Psychosomatic Medicine* (44,6:545)
*The New England Journal of Medicine* (333,5:327)

## Unequal treatment for high blood pressure

Women have fought long and hard for equality. However, high blood pressure does not affect men and women equally. Women more often develop high blood pressure, particularly after menopause. Oral contraceptives and pregnancy also may raise blood pressure.

Though they are less likely than men to suffer heart damage from their high blood pressure, women also do not respond as well to blood pressure medication. In fact, except in cases of extreme high blood pressure in women, the risks of taking blood pressure medicine outweigh the benefits. Women can lower their blood pressures more effectively by making a few lifestyle changes, like losing weight, exercising, and cutting out cigarettes and alcohol.

*Source:*
*Archives of Internal Medicine* (155,6:563)

## 5 warning signs of stroke

Stroke strikes terror into the hearts of many elderly people. Nearly three-fourths of all strokes occur in people over age 65. Strokes cause more disability than any other factor, and they take the lives of hundreds of thousands each year. A stroke deprives the brain of oxygen and damages brain cells. Receiving immediate medical attention can determine whether or not you survive a stroke. However, most people don't know how to spot the warning signs of a stroke. The most common symptoms are:

◆ Sudden dimness or loss of vision in one eye
◆ Weakness or numbness of the arm, leg, or face on one side of the body.
◆ Slurred speech, loss of speech, or trouble understanding speech.
◆ Sudden unexplained headache.
◆ Dizziness or falling for no reason.

If you experience any of these symptoms, seek help right away. Getting help quickly could save your life.

*Sources:*
*Medical Tribune for the Internist and Cardiologist* (36,15:20)
*The American Medical Association Family Medical Guide*, Random House, New York, 1982

## Self-defense against stroke

Prevention holds the key to fighting strokes. Stroke, the third leading killer in the U.S., leaves more than half its survivors mentally or physically impaired. Protect yourself from this killer by taking some preventive measures.

**Exercise.** Even moderate levels of exercise can reduce your risk of stroke.

Yale researchers found that men who walked just three to 12 blocks every day reduced their risk of stroke by almost one-third. Men who walked over a mile (more than 12 blocks) cut their risk of stroke in half. The protective benefits of exercise apply to women as well.

**Stop smoking.** The nicotine in cigarettes contributes to stroke incidence. Smokers who kick the habit reduce their risk of stroke substantially.

**Cook with canola.** A diet high in certain types of oil may help you avoid strokes. *Alpha-linolenic acid*, a fatty acid found in canola, walnut, and soybean oils, reduces the risk of stroke in middle-aged men, according to a recent study. This study found that even a small increase of alpha-linolenic acid in the blood decreased the risk of stroke substantially. Canola oil also has the added benefit of containing monounsaturated fatty acids, which also help protect against heart disease.

**Eat your fruits and veggies.** Harvard researchers found that three half-cup servings of fruits and vegetables lowered stroke risk by 22 percent over time. Vegetables seemed to provide more protection than fruits.

**Vitamin E and aspirin.** A daily dose of vitamin E and aspirin can reduce the stickiness of your blood by more than half. This can prevent clotting which can lead to a stroke or heart attack.

**Vitamin C.** Elderly people who have a high intake of vitamin C are much less likely to suffer a stroke.

**Guard against infection.** If you've had a recent infection, be aware that your stroke risk rises. Bacterial infections make you almost six times more likely to suffer a stroke.

*Sources:*
*American Family Physician* (51,8:1977)
*British Medical Journal* (310,6994:1563)
*Geriatrics* (50,7:14)
*Medical Tribune for the Internist and Cardiologist* (36,5:9, 36,8:17 and 36,15:20)
*The Journal of the American Medical Association* (273,14:1113)
*The Journal of Nutrition* (125,4:1003)

# Monday morning stroke

Do you have the Monday morning blues? If you just hate facing the stress of work on Monday morning after a great weekend, you may be more likely to suffer a stroke. A recent study found that more strokes occur on Monday morning than any other time of the week. People who had strokes on Monday were more likely to smoke and drink alcohol. Working men were twice as likely to suffer a stroke on Monday as men who didn't work. Researchers speculated that changes in physical activity and increased smoking and drinking over the weekend contributed to the risk of stroke. Add that to the sudden return of job stress on Monday morning, and the results could be deadly. If you want to lower your risk of Monday morning stroke, consider limiting your smoking and drinking over the weekend (or better yet, cut them out altogether), and try to reduce your stress level, particularly on Monday mornings. Otherwise, Mondays may make you more than blue.

*Source:*
*Medical Tribune for the Internist and Cardiologist* (36,16:5)

# Diabetes Self-Defense

## Carbohydrates get canned in favor of fat

"Move over carbohydrates; make way for monounsaturated fats." If that's a meal plan you could enjoy sinking your teeth into, read on.

**Favoring fat.** Anything in favor of fat may sound more like advertising for a cooking oil than a health book article. However, doctors and researchers are actually investigating the theory that more monounsaturated fat and fewer carbohydrates may be a heart healthier alternative to the traditional diet for managing noninsulin-dependent diabetes (NIDDM).

This news rocked the diabetic health community which, until 1994, had generally recommended a high-carbohydrate diet for NIDDM.

**When fat fights fat.** However, several recent studies seem to indicate that a high-carbohydrate, low-fat diet may cause higher triglyceride levels than a lower-carbohydrate, higher-fat diet.

High triglyceride levels may cause hardening of the arteries, which can raise your risk of heart disease, especially if you have diabetes. If you have kidney disease, high blood pressure, or a weight problem, high triglycerides can increase your heart disease risk even more.

Researchers speculate that a high-carbohydrate diet leads to increased levels of insulin after meals, which causes your liver to produce very-low-density lipoprotein (VLDL) cholesterol. Then, the VLDL cholesterol leads to higher triglyceride levels in your blood.

**New fat/carbohydrate combination.** One study found that diabetics whose diets were made up of 55 percent carbohydrates and 30 percent fat, with 10 percent of the fat being monounsaturated, had higher insulin and triglyceride levels than did diabetics whose diets were made up of 40 percent carbohydrates and 45 percent fat, with all additional fat being monounsaturated.

Although more research remains to be done to determine the exact effect that the ratio of fats to carbohydrates has to do with diabetes and heart disease, consider asking your doctor or nutritionist to design a diet for you that draws 40 percent of your daily calories from carbohydrates (instead of the typical 55 to 60 percent) and 25 percent of your calories from monounsaturated fats. Olive oil is one of the most popular sources of monounsaturated fats.

**Common mistakes.** However, you will have to be very careful if you decide to try this approach. One common mistake is increasing monounsaturated fats without decreasing carbohydrate intake, which defeats the whole purpose of the diet change and can lead to unwanted weight gain as well. You also need to be careful not to let more than 10 percent of your total fat intake come from saturated fats, such as animal fat and coconut, palm, and palm-kernel oils.

**Calories still most important consideration.** In addition, you should keep in mind that reducing the amount of calories you eat is more important for diabetic control than what combination of carbohydrates and fats you eat. If you're still struggling to keep your calorie count down, you may not need the additional strain of trying to do a balancing act with carbohydrates and monounsaturated fats.

*Sources:*
*Hamilton and Whitney's Nutrition Concepts and Controversies,* West Publishing, St. Paul, Minn., 1994
*Journal of the American College of Nutrition* (14,4:369)
*Medical Tribune for the Internist and Cardiologist* (36,4:1)

# Salmon slams the brakes on diabetes

Eskimos eat lots of fish. Pima Indians of the Southwest rarely do. Even though the two groups are genetically similar, Eskimos have a much lower diabetes risk than the Pima Indians.

The Eskimos' secret? Eating salmon.

A recent study at a Seattle veterans' hospital revealed that eating salmon slashes the risk of developing diabetes in half. Researchers studied 666 people age 40 or older. Those who ate salmon every day were 50 percent less likely to develop diabetes or a prediabetes condition than the people who didn't eat salmon daily.

Eating a little salmon every day may help reduce your risk of developing diabetes, even if you have a long history of this disease in your family. It seems that some salmon each day helps keep diabetes away.

*Source:*
*Diabetes Care* (17,12:1498)

# The vital vitamin for clearing up diabetic complications

To supplement with vitamin C or not to supplement with vitamin C — that is the question diabetes researchers are debating these days.

Not surprisingly, several studies seem to indicate that supplements may be helpful.

Doctors know that vitamin C is vital to good health. Normal levels of vitamin C are needed to help your body produce *collagen* (the protein needed to make muscles and bones), keep teeth and gums healthy, help your body absorb iron, and boost your immune system.

**The disease-fighting vitamin.** On the disease-fighting front, previous studies have demonstrated that extra vitamin C seems to help lower cholesterol levels and help destroy cell-damaging free radicals, which may speed up the aging process as well as cause arthritis, cancer, cataracts, and heart disease.

Interestingly, several studies have also indicated that noninsulin-dependent diabetes appears to increase the formation of these damaging free radicals while decreasing the number of antioxidants (such as vitamin C) that can protect your body against free radical destruction. Scientists reasoned that it would just make sense for extra vitamin C to provide extra protection to diabetics.

A recent study of diabetics over age 70 lends support to that theory. The 40 study participants were given 500 milligrams (mg) of vitamin C twice a day for four months. (The recommended daily allowance for vitamin C is 60 mg.) Tests following the supplement period showed that cholesterol levels dropped significantly as did the number of free radicals. The participants also had better blood sugar control.

**Increases blood vessel strength.** A 1992 study found that 1,000 mg of vitamin C taken daily increased the strength of blood vessels in the feet, hands, kidneys, and retinas of people with diabetes. That's great news for diabetics since most of the health problems they experience result from diseased or damaged small blood vessels.

**Improves blood circulation.** More recently, a small study conducted by Harvard researchers suggested that vitamin C may even be able to improve circulation in people with noninsulin-dependent diabetes. In this study, participants were injected with a combination of vitamin C and methacholine, a vasodilator used to make veins open a little wider than normal. The combination increased blood flow through the participants' veins by 36 percent.

The results from this study seem to suggest that extra vitamin C may actually be able to prevent diabetes-related eye damage, kidney damage, and hardening of the arteries. However, researchers say that more studies need to be done to determine if vitamin C injections are really safe, helpful, and effective.

**Best natural "C" sources.** In the meantime, you can help protect your body from damage caused by diabetes by filling your diet with lots of luscious vitamin C foods. Good fruit sources of vitamin C include citrus fruits, raspberries, strawberries, mangoes, cantaloupes, honeydews, and papayas. Good vegetable sources of vitamin C include asparagus, broccoli, brussels sprouts, cabbage, cauliflower, kale, greens, spinach, tomatoes, and turnips.

Keep in mind that vegetables containing vitamin C are very fragile when it comes to cooking. They may lose up to half of their vitamin C during boiling, blanching, or steaming. The best way to cook vegetables containing vitamin C is in the microwave. At most, microwave-cooked vegetables only lose 15 percent of their vitamin C. Many microwaved vegetables retain all their vitamin C.

**A multivitamin makes sense.** You may also want to take a multivitamin. In addition, some researchers suggest taking vitamin C supplements, although recommended doses vary. Dr. John Cunningham, professor of nutrition at the University of Massachusetts at Amherst, says he sees no harm in taking 250 to 500 mg of vitamin C a day. Dr. Stuart M. Berger, author of the bestseller *How to be Your Own Nutritionist*, recommends 1,000 to 2,000 mg of vitamin C a day.

Since vitamin C can cause uncomfortable side effects, such as diarrhea and vomiting, if taken in large doses, and may interact adversely with certain medicines, you should discuss taking extra vitamin C with your doctor.

He can tell you how vitamin C may interact with any medicines you're taking, as well as monitor how your liver and kidneys respond to the extra vitamin C. It's also important to let your doctor know if you're taking supplements because large doses of vitamin C can affect the accuracy of urine tests used to check blood sugar levels.

*Sources:*

*Diabetes: Questions You Have...Answers You Need,* People's Medical Society, Allentown, Pa, 1993
*How to Be Your Own Nutritionist,* Avon Books, New York, 1987
*Journal of the American College Of Nutrition* (14,4:387)
*Medical Tribune for the Internist and Cardiologist* (37,2:2)
*The Diabetic's Book: All Your Questions Answered,* G.P. Putnam's Sons, New York, 1994
*The Doctor's Complete Guide to Vitamins and Minerals,* Dell Publishing, New York, 1994

# Miracle mineral helps defeat diabetes

Although *chromium* is commonly advertised as a weight loss aid, it also helps control diabetes.

Chromium is a mineral which helps your body produce and use insulin. Insulin transports sugar from foods you've eaten out of your blood and into your body's cells. There it's converted into energy. By helping your body keep a steady supply of insulin, chromium helps keep sugar moving out of your blood at a steady rate. This prevents your blood sugar from going too high (as in diabetes) or too low (as in hypoglycemia).

Several studies have shown that adding chromium to diabetics' diets helps their insulin do a better job of getting sugar from the blood. Diabetics can use all the help they can get in this process. In many cases, they were able to reduce or eliminate the amount of insulin they had to inject each day to function normally.

In addition, chromium appears to lower LDL or "bad" cholesterol and total cholesterol in the blood. It also raises HDL or "good" cholesterol. This significantly lowers your risk of heart disease, a common health problem many diabetics must eventually face.

However, as important as chromium appears to be for good health, about 90 percent of Americans don't get enough chromium in their diets. Recent surgery, a severe burn, a chronic wasting disease, or alcohol or drug abuse may increase your need for chromium.

In addition, food manufacturing often removes chromium from foods. Since Americans tend to eat a lot of prepackaged, highly processed foods, such as sugar and white flour, this could be the reason why so many people don't get enough chromium. Heavy exercise, such as long-distance running, can also cause your body to lose chromium faster than usual.

Plus, chromium is sometimes hard for your body to absorb. Some scientists think that less than 1 percent of the chromium in foods you eat is actually absorbed by your body. Taking calcium carbonate supplements can also limit how much chromium your body can absorb. Because it's so hard to absorb, some manufacturers add picolinate acid to chromium. This results in chromium picolinate, which is more easily absorbed.

However, one recent study found that a normal dose of chromium picolinate damaged chromosomes in the ovary cells of hamsters. Researchers noted that the type of chromosome damage they observed can eventually cause cancer. Chromium nicotinate, another popular form of chromium supplement, did not have this effect.

If you're curious about your chromium level, ask your doctor for a serum chromium test. Always talk to your doctor before taking chromium (or any other supplement), especially if you have diabetes or a lung, liver, or kidney disease.

If you would rather get your chromium from the foods you eat, there are lots of delicious natural sources of chromium. They include:

◆ Brewer's yeast
◆ Oysters, fish, and other seafoods
◆ Mushrooms
◆ Liver
◆ Apples with skins
◆ Prunes
◆ Nuts
◆ Asparagus

Even though chromium can't cure diabetes, it can help control it. Talk with your doctor about making chromium part of your battle plan for beating diabetes.

*Sources:*
*FASEB Journal* (9,1643)
*Hamilton & Whitney's Nutrition Concepts and Controversies,* West Publishing, New York, 1994
*Medical Tribune for the Family Physician* (35,10:19)
*Nutrition Health Review* (1990,53:14)
*The Complete Guide to Vitamins, Minerals, and Supplements,* Fisher Books, Tucson, Ariz., 1988
*The Doctor's Complete Guide to Vitamins and Minerals,* Dell Publishing, New York, 1994
*The Physician and Sportsmedicine* (22,8:30)
*The Real Vitamin and Mineral Book,* Avery Publishing Group, Garden City Park, N.Y., 1990

# New diet is sweet news for diabetics

Deciding what to eat can be a problem for everyone, and it's even worse if you're dealing with diabetes.

The good news is that the latest research offers new hope for those with the diabetic-diet doldrums.

For years, doctors recommended a standard, very strict diet to everyone who had diabetes. Now, researchers have learned so much about the effects of carbohydrates, proteins, and fats that the American Diabetes Association (the ADA) revised its guidelines in May of 1994 for the first time in 10 years.

The new guidelines let you create an individual diet, using advice from a registered dietitian. Your ideal diet will depend on what type of diabetes you have, your lifestyle, and your health profile.

**Satisfy your sweet tooth sometimes.** The ADA is relaxing its restrictions on sugar, the simple carbohydrate once considered to be a diabetic's biggest no-no. Experts used to believe that simple carbohydrates like sugar entered the blood more quickly than the complex carbohydrates in breads and vegetables.

They thought that, because diabetics can't process sugar efficiently, eating too many simple carbohydrates caused a sugar surge.

But the truth is that all sugars enter your blood at nearly the same rate. Moderate amounts of sugar are no more damaging for diabetics than other carbohydrates.

However, the total amount of carbohydrates you consume is important, say the experts. While you used to keep track of how much complex and simple carbohydrates you were eating, now you just have to be sure carbohydrates make up only 55 to 60 percent of your total calorie intake.

So, satisfy your sweet tooth every now and then, but be sure to adjust your diet accordingly. Cut back on calories from starches by a corresponding amount and watch your fat intake, since many sweets contain large amounts of fat.

**Unlike Jack Sprat, you can eat some fat** although you must keep track of the kind of fat you're eating, similar to the old way of monitoring your carbohydrates.

Stay away from saturated fats, which are found in animal products and in coconut, palm, and palm-kernel oils. They're more likely to increase the amount of cholesterol and triglycerides in your blood.

Instead, choose one of the two types of unsaturated fat. The first type, polyunsaturated fat, is found in corn, safflower, sunflower, and soybean oils. Monounsaturated fat, now thought to be the healthier of the two, is found in olive and canola oils and in some deep water fish.

Whether you're diabetic or not, you should get no more than 30 percent of your daily calories from fat. No more than 10 percent of these should come from saturated fat, no more than 10 percent from polyunsaturated fat, and no more than 10 percent from monounsaturated fat.

Some researchers believe that fat isn't so bad for you after all. One study found that a high-fat diet low in saturated fats can lower LDL (bad) cholesterol levels just as much as a high-carbohydrate diet.

**Fill up with fiber.** Researchers say fiber helps you regulate your blood sugar and possibly decreases your need for insulin.

Apples, berries, figs, oranges, pears, prunes, broccoli, brussels sprouts, carrots, cauliflower, lettuce, and potatoes are a few of the many natural sources of fiber.

A high-fiber diet will require motivation on your part, however. To get results, you'll have to eat between 20 and 30 grams of fiber a day.

When you increase the fiber in your diet, drink lots of water, at least six glasses a day, to avoid constipation. It's also a good idea to increase your fiber intake gradually, to avoid cramping or bloating.

Work the following suggestions into your diet plan one at a time.

◆ Eat at least five servings of fruits and vegetables every day.
◆ Switch to whole-grain breads and cereals, and eat brown rice.
◆ Rediscover oatmeal, bran muffins, and popcorn.
◆ Eat a very high-fiber bran cereal for breakfast.

◆ Add 1/4 cup wheat bran to foods like applesauce or meatloaf.

◆ Give beans such as lentils, black beans, lima beans, pinto beans, and baked beans a permanent spot on your weekly menu.

**Eat four to six small meals instead of three square meals.** Participants in a recent study lowered their blood sugar levels and insulin requirements by grazing instead of eating three square meals a day. This doesn't mean you get to eat more — just eat smaller quantities more frequently.

If you're taking insulin, remember that you must eat at regular times, according to the time and amount of your injection.

**Stop smoking and stay away from alcohol.** Alcohol can cause hypoglycemia, interact with medication, and lead to liver damage. Smoking cigarettes doubles the risk of diabetes. It also damages the pancreas, which produces the insulin your body needs.

While many of the nutrition rules have changed, the game remains the same: Your diet is important. Counting calories and eating healthy can prevent complications and, for Type II diabetics, reduce your need for insulin.

*Sources:*
*American Family Physician* (51,2:419)
*Journal of the American Dietetic Association* (94,5:504)
*Medical Tribune for the Internist and Cardiologist* (36,7:18)
*Nutrition Today* (29,1:6)
*The American Journal of Clinical Nutrition* (55,2:461)
*The Journal of the American Medical Association* (271,18:1421)

# Zinc: the sight-saving mineral?

Losing your sight is one of the scariest complications of diabetes. Surprisingly, the solution to this common problem may be as simple as swallowing some extra zinc.

Many diabetics have low blood levels of zinc. A recent study of 50 diabetics revealed that only three of those people were getting their recommended daily allowance (RDA) of zinc.

Now, an even more recent study shows that diabetics with the lowest zinc levels have the highest risk of retina damage, the most common cause of blindness in diabetics.

Researchers speculate that low levels of zinc contribute to the breakdown of the retina by not protecting the eyes from damaging *free radicals* (unstable chemicals that injure cells).

The exciting news is that blood levels of zinc rose when researchers gave study participants 30 milligrams (mg) of zinc a day (twice the RDA). At the same time, signs of free radical damage decreased. It appears that the extra zinc protected the participants' eyes from further damage by the free radicals.

Even though the results of this early study look promising, don't start taking extra zinc supplements yet. Researchers can't guarantee the long-term safety of 30 mg of zinc taken daily. However, you may want to consider taking a daily multivitamin that contains the RDA for zinc (15 mg) just to make sure you're getting enough.

Also, consider making your meals a little zippier with zinc. Good natural sources of zinc include blackstrap molasses, crab, lamb, lean beef, lentils, lima beans, lobster, maple syrup, milk, oysters, pork, sesame seeds, soybeans, sunflower seeds, turkey, wheat bran and wheat germ, whole-grain foods, and yeast.

Other ways you can help protect your vision include keeping your blood sugar level as close to normal as possible and having a yearly eye exam. During this exam, your doctor should dilate your pupils so he can see the backs of your eyes to determine if you have any damage there.

If you do have some damage, your doctor may be able to use laser surgery to treat that damage or to at least prevent further complications.

In addition to this yearly exam, you should contact your eye doctor immediately if you have any problems with your eyes, such as blurry vision or if you start seeing dark spots, flashing lights, or rings around lights.

*Sources:*
*Complete Guide to Vitamins, Minerals, and Supplements,* Fisher Books, Tucson, Ariz., 1988
*Do Your Level Best: Start Controlling Your Blood Sugar Today,* National Institute of Diabetes and Digestive and Kidney Diseases, National Institutes of Health, NIH Publication No. 95-4016, Bethesda, Md., 1995
*Don't Lose Sight of Diabetic Eye Disease,* National Eye Institute
*European Journal of Clinical Nutrition* (49,5:282)

# CARING for diabetes the exercise way

If you think having diabetes gives you the perfect excuse not to exercise, think again. A diagnosis of diabetes means you need exercise more than ever.

Not only will regular exercise make you feel better and help you cope more easily with the disease, it also significantly reduces your risk of serious complications.

**CARING** for your body through exercise is one of the best ways to deal with diabetes. Here's how it works:

Controls blood sugar by helping your body use insulin more efficiently.

Aids in lowering blood pressure and cholesterol levels.

Reduces stress.

Improves appearance and increases self-esteem.

Nibbles away at excess weight.

Gives you a sense of "being in control" of a disease many diabetics consider uncontrollable.

The actual act of exercise uses some of the extra sugar diabetics often have in their blood, helping to lower blood sugar.

By keeping blood sugar as normal as possible, you reduce your risk of many of diabetes most serious complications, such as eye, nerve, and kidney damage. This is because normal blood sugar helps keep small blood vessels healthy. Studies consistently show that regular exercise helps prevent heart disease, the number one killer of people with diabetes.

Exercise may even help Type I (insulin-dependent) diabetics use less insulin and may eliminate Type II (noninsulin-dependent) diabetics' need for insulin completely.

Exercise is also one of the best ways to control stress. Controlling stress is important for diabetics because too much stress can send blood sugar soaring.

Regular exercise will also improve your appearance and self-esteem. While this benefit doesn't necessarily affect the course of diabetes, many people enjoy this extra bonus.

In addition, regular exercise is the secret to success in maintaining a healthy weight, which is another trick you can use to keep your blood sugar under control.

Be sure you talk to your doctor before beginning an exercise program. Since people with diabetes are often at risk of heart disease or circulation problems which may affect the eyes, hands, and feet, your doctor may need to help you establish some specific exercise guidelines to make sure you exercise safely.

Once you get your doctor's OK, get started. Make your exercise program a priority and be consistent. That's the only way you'll reap the long-term benefits of exercise. Finding one or more physical activities you enjoy will make sticking to an exercise program easier.

However, remember that as important as it is to exercise, it's also important not to overexercise. You should feel pleasantly tired after your exercise routine, not utterly exhausted.

A good book that will give you additional guidance on exercising safely and effectively is the American Diabetes Association's *The Fitness Book for People with Diabetes*. It's available in many bookstores. If you have trouble locating a copy of the book, you can order directly from the American Diabetes Association by calling 1–800–232–6733.

Although some people feel damage caused by diabetes is uncontrollable, that's not the case. How you choose to live your life often determines the course of the disease. Caring for your body through exercise can make all the difference.

*Source:*
The Fitness Book for People with Diabetes, American Diabetes Association, Alexandria, Va., 1994

## Aspirin heads off heart disease

Although diabetics are often warned against aspirin because large doses may cause blood sugar levels to drop too low, recent research reveals that moderate doses of aspirin can head off one of the common complications of diabetes — heart disease.

Heart disease can be deadly for anyone, but it often presents a greater danger to diabetics because it can be more difficult to recognize and treat. Both insulin-dependent and noninsulin-dependent diabetics have higher risks of heart disease than people who don't have diabetes.

Researchers stumbled across aspirin's apparent benefit for diabetics by accident. A study designed to test the effects of aspirin on *diabetic retinopathy* (damage to blood vessels in your eyes that can cause blindness) revealed some unexpected results. Apparently, aspirin didn't have any effect on retinopathy in the 3,700 insulin-dependent and noninsulin-dependent diabetics tested.

However, the experiment did show that the people who took two aspirin a day had a 17 percent lower risk of heart attack in the following five years than people who didn't take aspirin.

A more recent study found aspirin to reduce the risk of heart attack by one-third and the risk of stroke by one-fourth. Unfortunately, the study also found that aspirin doubled the risk of bleeding in the brain. However, researchers concluded that the protective benefits to the heart outweighed the risks of bleeding in the brain.

Since several studies look positive, consider discussing aspirin therapy with your doctor. Ask him to explain how the benefits and risks of aspirin therapy would affect you. Often, each person will be affected differently according to age, family history, and type and degree of diabetes.

Never practice preventive medicine on yourself at home by regularly taking aspirin. It may cause your blood sugar level to drop dangerously low or cause bleeding in your brain. Regular aspirin use must be monitored by your doctor.

*Sources:*
British Medical Journal (311,7006:641)
*Mayo Clinic Heart Book,* William Morrow and Company, New York, 1993
*The Diabetic's Book: All Your Questions Answered,* G.P. Putnam's Sons, New York, 1994

# Heart-smart surgery for diabetics

Not only does having diabetes increase your risk of developing heart and artery disease, it also makes these conditions trickier to treat. One common heart condition diabetics often face is blocked arteries. For two or more blocked arteries that a heart-healthy diet and exercise aren't helping, doctors often suggest surgery.

If your doctor has recommended heart surgery for blocked arteries, be sure you choose the heart-smart option. According to a recently released recommendation from The National Institutes of Health, *coronary artery bypass graft* (CABG) surgery is the safest surgery option for diabetics who take insulin or pills to control their condition.

Normally, doctors operating on people with blocked arteries have two surgery options to choose from. In the first type, coronary artery bypass graft surgery, the surgeon removes a piece of vein from your chest or leg and then sews it to your heart and artery to create a detour around the clogged area.

The second type of treatment is called *percutaneous transluminal coronary angioplasty* (PTCA). In this procedure, the doctor inserts a balloon into the blocked artery, then inflates the balloon near the blockage. This stretches the artery and gives blood room to flow around the blockage.

A recent study of 1,829 people revealed that CABG surgery is twice as safe for diabetics who take pills or insulin as PTCA surgery. In fact, researchers found that five years after surgery, death rates were twice as high among diabetics who underwent PTCA instead of CABG. For people with diabetes who did not take any drugs to control their conditions, the two surgeries appeared to be equally safe.

*Source:*
The Diabetes Advisor (4,1:1)

## Kudos for caffeine

Recognizing the sometimes subtle signs of low blood sugar (also called hypoglycemia) is not always easy. It often gets even harder once you've had insulin-dependent diabetes for a while. However, it's vitally important for diabetics to catch and treat hypoglycemia quickly, since it can cause a loss of consciousness, coma, and even death.

For this reason, researchers developed several different tactics to help diabetics recognize the signs of falling blood sugar before levels go too low. Unfortunately, none of those methods were particularly convenient or easy for people to use. Then, results from a previous study led scientists to suggest that the solution might be as simple as drinking several cups of coffee.

Scientists have known for a while that caffeine often intensifies the symptoms of low blood sugar in people who don't have diabetes. Therefore, they reasoned, caffeine would probably have the same effect on diabetics.

Two small, separate studies support this theory. In lab tests, caffeine actually intensifies diabetics' symptoms of low blood sugar, making them more noticeable and easier to recognize. Common symptoms of hypoglycemia include anxiety, blurred vision, difficulty thinking, feeling faint, hunger, irritability, rapid heartbeat, tingling, trembling, and sweating.

So, it seems that caffeine offers an added advantage for diabetics who use it to kick start the day. Not only will you feel pepped up, your system will be revved up and ready to warn you before your blood sugar level drops dangerously low.

Even if you've always stayed away from caffeine for fear of how it could affect your body's already delicate balance, you may want to consider having a little caffeine every day. It may be just what you need to help you stop a hypoglycemic attack before it gets out of hand. Two to three cups of coffee is plenty for most diabetics. You may even need less if you're sensitive to caffeine.

However, if you're at risk of heart disease or you've had a stroke, you should limit your caffeine consumption to one or two cups a day. In fact, whether you're at risk of heart disease or stroke or not, you should clear the use of caffeine with your doctor before you use it to help head off hypoglycemia.

*Sources:*
Medical Tribune for the Internist and Cardiologist (37,3:4)
The Lancet (347,8993:19)

## Handling hypoglycemia

The best way to handle *hypoglycemia* (low blood sugar) is to eat or drink something that contains sugar as soon as you recognize the symptoms. Some good choices include hard candy, orange juice, sugar-sweetened soda, or a glass of milk. Glucose tablets, sold over-the-counter in most pharmacies, also work well.

If your next meal is scheduled for more than 30 minutes after your low blood sugar reaction, you should eat a small snack, such as some crackers, half a sandwich, or a glass of milk.

*Source:*
*Do Your Level Best: Start Controlling Your Blood Sugar Today,* National Institute of Diabetes and Digestive and Kidney Diseases, National Institutes of Health, NIH Publication No. 95-4016, Bethesda, Md., 1995

## Teeth care tips for diabetics

As a diabetic, it's especially important to take care of your teeth and gums and protect them from possible infections, which can be hard to heal and send your blood sugar levels soaring. Here are some helpful tips:

◆ Brush your teeth with a soft nylon toothbrush and fluoride toothpaste every morning and every evening. Use a circular scrubbing motion to gently clean your teeth. Don't forget to give your tongue a gentle brushing as well. If possible, brush after every meal. If this is not convenient, at least make sure you rinse out your mouth after every meal or snack.

◆ Floss your teeth each evening before bed. Start with a piece of floss about 18 inches long. Use a gentle sawing motion to maneuver the floss between tightly spaced teeth. Curve the floss around each individual tooth and move it from the bottom of your gum line to the top of your teeth several times. Remember to rinse your mouth out after flossing.

◆ See your dentist for a checkup at least every six months, or more often if he recommends it. Let him know you have diabetes. Schedule your dental appointments after breakfast, so you won't develop low blood sugar during your visit. Carry some glucose tablets to use in case your blood sugar level starts to drop.

*Sources:*
*Diabetes & Periodontal Disease: A Guide for Patients,* National Institute of Dental Research, NIH Publication No. 95-2946, Bethesda, Md., 1995
*Do Your Level Best: Start Controlling Your Blood Sugar Today,* National Institute of Diabetes and Digestive and Kidney Diseases, National Institutes of Health, NIH Publication No. 95-4016, Bethesda, Md., 1995
*The Diabetes Sourcebook,* Lowell House, Los Angeles, 1990

## Diabetics, don't forget your feet

Resting your aching feet at the end of a long day is all the foot care most people need. But for adults with diabetes, your feet need a lot more attention to prevent some very serious problems.

Adults suffering from diabetes frequently develop sores on their feet. These foot ulcers are caused by dry, cracked skin; poor circulation; hardening of the arteries; loss of nerve sensitivity; and a weakened immune system. If not cared for properly, foot ulcers can lead to *gangrene* (an infection in dead tissue) and, eventually, amputation.

**Prevent or repent.** The only sure method for preventing foot problems is to protect your feet from injury, practice careful foot hygiene, and have frequent foot checkups by your doctor or podiatrist.

Ask the doctor who normally treats your diabetes to regularly test your ankle reflexes and examine your feet to determine how sensitive they are to touch. This can help determine if you have any nerve damage in your feet.

The two tests most commonly used are called *vibratory testing* and *monofilament testing*. These tests also help your doctor gauge your risk of developing diabetic nerve damage.

Call your doctor immediately if you notice any redness, swelling, soreness, tingling, numbness, or infection in either of your feet.

**Pass on that barefoot stroll.** As a diabetic, you should never walk barefoot or in sandals. Shoes protect your feet from injury.

**Search for shoes that fit.** A good fit is extremely important since nerve damage can prevent you from feeling the ill effects of improperly fitted shoes. You may want to have your shoes fitted by a professional familiar with your special needs as a diabetic.

Shop for shoes near the end of the day when your feet are a little swollen. This will help you avoid buying shoes that seem to turn too tight overnight.

Another way to help get a better fit is to stand on a piece of paper and draw an outline of your foot. Take your foot cutout to the shoe store and put it under shoes you've picked out to buy. If the shoe doesn't fit the outline, keep looking.

Shoes should be sturdy with ample toe room, good support, and soft leather uppers. Running or walking shoes are generally a good choice, but you may require specially designed orthopedic shoes, especially if your feet have an unusual shape.

You may need shoes with custom-made insoles so that they will fit your feet properly. Never use inserts or pads without consulting your doctor.

You want whatever shoe you choose to provide cushioning for your entire foot. Don't wear any shoe that is uncomfortable or causes blisters, and never walk around in wet shoes. Dry your feet as soon as possible.

Break in new shoes gradually to prevent blisters. Wear them for short periods of time at first and check your feet afterwards.

**Soften the blow.** Good socks protect your feet from the friction your shoes create as you walk, so never go without them. Buy thick socks made of acrylic fibers that shield your skin from moisture. Cotton socks hold moisture against your skin.

Make sure your socks fit your feet properly without bunching up. Be sure there are no seams that may irritate your feet. Select socks that are 1/2 inch longer than your longest toe. Avoid stretch socks as well as socks with elastic or garter tops.

**Change your shoes at least twice a day.** Different shoes have different pressure points. By changing your shoes twice a day, you can help protect your feet from blisters that could develop into sores later on. If you find this practice too troublesome, you should switch out your shoes every other day.

**Keep shoes clear of clutter.** Shoes tend to attract little annoyances like pebbles and other small prickly things. Remove this sort of stuff from your shoes every day to prevent possible injury to your feet. Also, look for torn linings and either have them repaired or replace the shoes.

**Take notice of their temperature.** If one foot feels warmer than the other, you may have an infection in the warmer foot. If one or both feet are cold, it may mean that your circulation isn't working well. In either case, contact your doctor.

**Treat your feet well.** Keep your feet clean and dry at all times. Daily foot care should include careful inspection of your feet, toes, and spaces between your toes; washing in lukewarm water with a soft washcloth and mild soap; drying thoroughly by blotting (don't rub, and don't forget to dry the spaces between your toes); and moisturizing with lotion, especially the heels.

If your feet tend to be sweaty, keep them dry with a daily dusting of a non-medicated powder before you put on socks and shoes.

Don't soak your feet in hot or cold water and never expose them to extreme temperatures, such as heating pads or very cold or hot outdoor weather. You also should not use adhesive tape, chemicals, or any type of massaging device on your feet.

Keep the bedsheets and blankets at the bottom of the bed loose so they won't press on your toes or heels. Nails should be trimmed straight across, not rounded. Corns, calluses, and plantar warts should only be removed by your doctor or podiatrist.

**Toss out all tobacco products.** Using any type of tobacco increases your risk of developing diabetes-related foot problems.

**Eat a diet fit for your feet.** Diabetic foot problems can also be prevented by controlling the underlying causes. Tight control of your blood sugar levels can reduce damage to your nerves and circulatory system.

If you spot a foot sore, see your doctor immediately. You may need treatment with antibiotics, new footwear, or whatever your doctor suggests to make sure your foot heals completely.

*Sources:*
*American Family Physician* (53,2:615)
*Diabetes Forecast* (46,5:42)
*Diabetes in the News* (13,6:46)
*Geriatrics* (50,2:48)
*Postgraduate Medicine* (96,5:177 and 99,3:147)

## Self-care guide for people with insulin-dependent diabetes

◆ Take an insulin shot before you eat.

◆ Avoid skipping meals, especially if you've just given yourself an insulin shot.

◆ Attempt to eat about the same amount of food at the same time every day.

◆ Exercise after you've eaten, but several hours before bedtime. Otherwise, your blood sugar may drop too low during the night. Remember to always test your blood sugar before, during, and after exercising. Don't exercise if your blood sugar is over 240.

Carry a snack with you while you exercise in case of low blood sugar. You should also carry an identification tag that states you have Type I diabetes and lists what medicines you take as well as whom to call in an emergency.

◆ Test your blood sugar daily, according to your doctor's recommendations. Some people need to check their blood sugar four or more times a day, others only once. Remember to test your blood sugar before beginning a difficult activity or stressful task since stress can affect your blood sugar levels.

◆ Keep careful records of when, how much, and what kind of insulin you give yourself. You should also note if you ate more or less food than usual, if your blood sugar was unusually low, if you felt tired or sick, and how long and what kind of exercise you did. Share your records with your doctor. They can help him prepare the most effective treatment plan for you.

You should also record your findings when you test your urine for *ketones* (acids produced by the body when you don't have enough insulin in your blood). You need to test for ketones if your blood sugar is over 240 before a meal. If a urine test reveals the presence of ketones, you should call your doctor immediately. You may have a condition called *ketoacidosis*, which can be fatal if not treated immediately.

◆ Let your doctor know if you have frequent low blood sugar reactions (feel shaky, sweaty, hungry, irritable, confused, tired, or sleepy). Be sure to let your doctor know if these reactions typically occur at a certain time of day or night.

You should also let your doctor know if low blood sugar has ever caused you to faint or to require a friend or family member's assistance. Ask him about *glucagon*, an emergency injection someone can give you if you faint. This medicine can help keep your blood sugar stable until emergency help arrives.

◆ Keep extra insulin in the refrigerator. Don't store it in the freezer or leave it in hot places like your car's glove compartment. You should also try to keep your insulin away from bright light. Both extreme temperatures and bright lights can damage insulin. Consider purchasing specially insulated bags designed to carry insulin and keep it from freezing or getting too hot.

*Source:*
*Do Your Level Best: Start Controlling Your Blood Sugar Today,* National Institute of Diabetes and Digestive and Kidney Diseases, National Institutes of Health, NIH Publication No. 95-4016, Bethesda, Md., 1995

## Tips for people with noninsulin-dependent diabetes

◆ Follow the meal plan recommended by your doctor or dietitian.

◆ Avoid skipping meals to prevent your blood sugar from falling too low or rising too high. This is especially important if you take diabetes pills. Consider eating several mini-meals throughout the day instead of three regular-sized meals.

◆ Consult your doctor before beginning an exercise program. If you haven't eaten in over an hour, have a small snack, such as an apple or a glass of milk, before you begin exercising.

Take a snack with you just in case you start to develop low blood sugar symptoms (feel shaky, sweaty, hungry, irritable, confused, tired, or sleepy). Always carry an identification card with you which states that you have Type II diabetes and whom to contact in an emergency.

◆ Be sure to test your blood sugar before and after exercise if you take diabetes pills.

◆ Always inform your doctor about any medicines you're taking.

◆ Let your doctor know if you experience low blood sugar reactions. This is especially important if you take medicine to control your diabetes. Your doctor may need to change your diet or your medicine.

◆ Test your blood sugar daily, according to your doctor's recommendations. Some people need to check blood sugar four or more times a day, others only once.

◆ Keep careful records of your blood sugar tests, including the time you tested. You should also note if you ate more or less food than usual, if your blood sugar was unusually low, if you felt tired or sick, and how long and what kind of exercise you did. Share your records with your doctor. They can help him prepare the most effective treatment plan for you.

**Source:**
*Do Your Level Best: Start Controlling Your Blood Sugar Today*, National Institute of Diabetes and Digestive and Kidney Diseases, National Institutes of Health, NIH Publication No. 95-4016, Bethesda, Md., 1995

# Caring for Your Kids

## Heading off soccer injuries

It's part of the uniform in football, baseball, hockey, boxing, and rollerblading, among other sports. Maybe protective headgear should be part of the game in soccer, too.

Soccer has become popular in the United States in the past several years. It's thought of as a safe, healthy game and a good cardiovascular workout. But soccer is the only popular sport where "heading," or hitting the ball with your head, is part of the game. Recent studies have shown that this is having more of an impact than people realize.

Researchers at the Medical College of Virginia found that players who "head" the ball frequently (more than 10 times per game) are risking brain damage. When tested in a study, these players had slightly lower IQs than nonheading players. They also scored lower on tests to measure attention, facial recognition, visual searching, and mental flexibility.

Part of the problem can be improper technique. Players should hit the ball at the flat part of the forehead at the hairline, with the head and neck rigid. Coaches should teach their players the correct way to head the ball to lessen the chance of injury or brain damage. Using lighter soccer balls might help, too.

If your child is playing soccer, make sure that he has a knowledgeable coach who will teach him proper technique to ensure his safety.

*Source:*
*American Family Physician* (52,8:2156)

## Shopping carts unsafe at any speed

Shopping carts are perfect for transporting groceries around a supermarket, but less than perfect for safely transporting children. In the period between 1990 and 1992, over 75,000 children under the age of 15 were injured in serious cart-related accidents. Most of the injuries affected children under the age of 5, and most involved falling out of the carts or the carts tipping over. Some of the injuries were even fatal.

If you are caring for a child and must put him in a shopping cart, don't take your eyes off him for a second. And be sure to use the seat belt provided in the cart to strap him in safely.

*Source:*
*Medical Abstracts Newsletter* (16,1:3)

## Surprising cause of infant ear infections

When your screaming baby latches on to his pacifier and stops crying, the quiet can be blissful, not just for you, but for everyone around you. But that peace and quiet may come at a price — the increased risk of ear infection.

For children under 3 years old, using a pacifier may cause more ear infections than not using one, according to a study in Finland. About one-third of children who used pacifiers got ear infections, compared to about one-fifth of children who didn't use them. The risk of ear infections for children was greatest at 2 to 3 years old.

During the first 10 months of your baby's life, using a pacifier doesn't promote ear infections. That's when his need for sucking is strongest, and ear infections are unlikely.

*Source:*
*Medical Abstracts Newsletter* (16,2:5)

## Number one cause of choking death in children

The bright yellow balloon bobbing in the breeze may be exactly what your grandchild wants, but it's just what she doesn't need. It seems like such an innocent toy, but that shiny balloon is the most frequent cause of choking death in children. It is the culprit in 29 percent of such deaths.

This is true for young children (under age 3), but the incidence is even higher for children between 3 and 14 years of age. If a balloon is swallowed or inhaled, it can block the flow of air to the lungs. The result is choking or suffocation. A broken piece of balloon can be as lethal an object as an intact one, and so can a latex glove. Let your grandchild admire that bright balloon from afar, but don't take it home with you.

*Source:*
*The Journal of the American Medical Association* (274,22:1763)

## Reducing children's risk of skin cancer

The lifetime risk of developing *malignant melanoma* (skin cancer) has risen from one in 1,500 people in 1930 to a projected one in 90 people in the year 2000. Children are as much at risk as adults, and they need adult guidance to help them fend off danger to their skin.

In a recent study, researchers concluded that the best way to control malignant melanoma is to educate doctors and parents to help children avoid behavior that makes their risk higher. The risk of a child developing skin cancer is increased by several factors. Only the last two can be controlled, but you need to be aware of all of them.

Some of the risk factors are:

◆ Many freckles and moles, especially large ones.
◆ A family history of skin cancer.
◆ Large moles present at birth.

◆ An immune system suppressed by illness or medication.
◆ Light skin and light-colored eyes.
◆ Many blistering sunburns before the age of 12 years.
◆ Frequent exposure to the sun without sunscreen, especially in the last 10 years.

If your child or grandchild has any of these risk factors, you need to be especially careful about his exposure to the sun. Avoid direct sunlight between 11:00 a.m. and 3:00 p.m., and apply a good sunscreen rated at least 15 SPF, or "sun protection factor," if he will be outdoors.

*Sources:*
*Alternative Medicine,* Future Medicine Publishing, Puyallup, Wash., 1993
*American Family Physician* (49,1:237)

## The fuss about fluoride

In the United States today, 121 million people drink artificially fluoridated water daily. The policy of adding fluoride to drinking water began in many large cities in the United States in 1950. The theory was that it would help prevent tooth decay, especially in children.

However, controversy surrounds the use of fluoride today, and many people question whether it has any benefits at all. Medical studies have implicated fluoride in a higher incidence of cancer and a higher incidence of hip fractures in older people. Fluoride is toxic, and even fatal, in large doses. It has already been banned in several countries in Europe.

To realize how much fluoride you consume, consider that fluoride occurs naturally in certain foods, including organ meats, eggs, apples, cod, canned salmon and sardines, and tea. The amounts of fluoride in these foods are influenced by the soil and water around them and can vary greatly. You probably get fluoride in the toothpaste and mouthwash that you use. Add to that the fluoride in your drinking water, if the city in which you live has fluoridated water. Include everything you cook or prepare with water, as well as bottled drinks and foods prepared in other cities with fluoridated water. So, you're probably getting more than your daily dose of fluoride, and so are your kids.

A safe amount of fluoride for daily adult consumption is 1.4 to 4 mg (milligrams). Children under a year old should consume less than 1 mg daily, and children under 6 months old should consume less than one-half mg. In addition to being dangerous in large doses, fluoride in small doses can cause a mottled discoloration of the teeth, called *fluorosis*, in children.

The American Academy of Pediatrics and the American Dental Association have changed their guidelines for fluoride supplements for children. They no longer recommend fluoride supplements for babies under 6 months old. And they have lowered the recommended doses of fluoride supplements for children 6 months to 16 years old.

Children younger than 6 years old should brush with only a small amount of toothpaste that contains fluoride, so they won't get too much fluoride if they swallow it. Consult your doctor before giving your child any kind of fluoride supplement for his teeth. If you are concerned about your child consuming high levels of fluoride, you might want to give him nonfluoridated bottled water to drink instead of tap water. You could also look for toothpaste and mouthwash that don't contain fluoride.

**Sources:**
*Alternative Medicine*, Future Medicine Publishing, Puyallup, Wash., 1993
*Medical Abstracts* (15,7:3)
*PDR Family Guide to Nutrition and Health*, Medical Economics Company, Montvale, N.J., 1995

## Save your child from SIDS

Sudden Infant Death Syndrome kills between 5,000 and 6,000 infants each year, and usually strikes between 2 and 4 months of age. The tragedy is often made worse by not knowing the cause. Researchers still have not pinpointed a cause or a cure, but they have discovered some simple actions that may reduce the risk of SIDS.

Babies who are put to bed in a face-down position seem to be at higher risk of SIDS than those who are placed on their backs or on their sides. In a study in Tasmania, the rate of SIDS deaths decreased 46 percent when most of the babies were switched from sleeping on their stomachs to sleeping on their backs or sides.

Never place soft pillows, blankets, quilts, or coverlets underneath a baby when he is sleeping. These increase the risk of suffocation or SIDS.

Also, don't expose a baby to passive smoke. It increases his risk of SIDS and of various childhood diseases.

**Source:**
*The Journal of the American Medical Association* (273,10:818)

## Removing foreign objects

Children are curious about their bodies and about everything in their surroundings. Sometimes in the rush to experience life first-hand, young children put small items, such as beads, seeds, crayons, or food, into their noses.

A doctor visit is usually necessary to remove the offending object. It can be a difficult experience, with the child restrained and the doctor using probes and forceps. But a new technique performed by a parent can be effective and much less difficult for everyone involved.

In a doctor's office, the child lies down on his back and opens his mouth wide. His parent holds the empty nostril closed, covers the child's mouth with hers and blows a puff of air into the child's mouth, as if doing CPR. The object should pop out of the child's nose. If it doesn't, a second or third breath will usually dislodge it.

**Source:**
*Medical Abstracts Newsletter* (15,10:3)

## Is this 'bug' bugging your child?

If your child frequently complains of stomach pain, there may be more to it than just too much candy or a virus that's going around. The *H. pylori* bacteria, which is a major cause of ulcers in adults, may also be a cause of *gastritis* (inflammation of the stomach) in children.

Researchers from the Indiana University School of Medicine studied 218 children with recurrent abdominal pain. They identified 38 children who had been exposed to the *H. pylori* bacteria, and 12 of these children tested positive for *H. pylori* infection.

The children were given a two-week treatment with bismuth (the chalky substance in antacids) and two antibiotics. The levels of the bacteria in their bodies decreased, and continued to decrease for six months after treatment. Even more important, their stomach pain was less frequent.

Children are not usually tested or treated for recurrent abdominal pain because of the assumption that it will eventually go away by itself. But for children with severe pain or blood in their stools, a test for *H. pylori* may be useful. Although *H. pylori* bacteria may not be a major cause of ulcers in children, it can sometimes be the cause of stomach pain and inflammation.

***Source:***
*Medical Tribune for the Internist and Cardiologist* (36,17:18)

## Facing a febrile seizure

You're answering your sick child's whimper in the middle of the night. She's had a runny nose, cough, and fever for the last 24 hours. As you reach her doorway, you see something you're totally unprepared for — she's having a seizure. What should you do?

First of all, don't panic. Febrile seizures may be frightening to watch, but they're not as dangerous as they seem. Febrile seizures are brought on by fever, last only a few minutes, and don't cause any brain damage. Most occur when a child is between the ages of 6 months and 3 years. They seldom occur after the age of 8.

If your child is having a febrile seizure, here's what you can do:

◆ Don't try to keep your child from moving during the seizure.
◆ Gently roll your child onto her side so that she won't get choked on saliva.
◆ Don't put anything in her mouth.
◆ When you see the seizure begin, check the time. If a seizure lasts more than 10 minutes, call 911.

Once the seizure has stopped, call your doctor so that he can help you find the cause of the fever.

***Source:***
*American Family Physician* (52,5:1409)

## How to stop the spread of strep throat

Strep throat, caused by *Streptococcal* bacteria, is a common illness among children. Once the extreme sore throat, fever, headache, and illness are diagnosed by your doctor as strep throat, it's a simple matter to give your child her prescribed antibiotic. But when should you send her back to school?

Many children return to school the next day after they start taking their medicine. But a recent study showed that children should not go back to school for at least 24 hours after they start taking their antibiotics.

Some experts even advise waiting five days after medication is begun. Although your child may be over her fever, and she may feel much better, she could still infect her classmates with strep throat if the medicine hasn't had a chance to work.

Be sure your child takes all of her medicine, even if she already seems well. It's important to take the entire dosage of medicine so that the infection doesn't come back and the bacteria doesn't change itself into a new strain.

**Sources:**
*Complete Guide to Symptoms and Surgery,* The Berkley Publishing Group, New York, 1995
*Medical Update* (17,6:6)

## Eating disorders prevent growth

If your adolescent daughter is not growing as much as she should, the problem may be an eating disorder. Among adolescent girls, eating disorders, including *anorexia nervosa* and *bulimia*, are the third most common chronic illness.

A young girl with anorexia nervosa thinks she is fat, no matter what her body weight. She refuses to eat normally, eventually refuses to eat at all, and gradually starves herself. A girl with bulimia will eat heartily and go on binges of stuffing herself with food. Then she'll induce vomiting, fast, or take laxatives to eliminate the food from her body.

People with eating disorders can be very good at keeping them secret, even from their families. The pre-teen and teen-age years are the time when a young person should be growing and developing rapidly. Sometimes the only sign of an eating disorder may be that your adolescent simply isn't growing.

The problem will not get better or go away. If you suspect that your young person may have an eating disorder, seek help from your doctor immediately. She can help you set up a program of psychiatric care, family therapy, and nutrition counseling to get your daughter back on the road to health and normal growth.

**Source:**
*Medical Tribune for the Internist and Cardiologist* (36,14:19)

## Controlling kids' cholesterol levels

French fries, chili cheese dogs, hamburgers, sausage pizza ... The world is full of high-fat foods just waiting to tempt adults and children alike. In the United States, about one-fourth of children have high or borderline-high cholesterol levels.

Most of those children grow up to be adults with high cholesterol, and all the health risks that go along with it. If your child has been diagnosed as having high cholesterol, a simple addition to his diet may make a healthy difference in his cholesterol level.

In a recent U.S. study of children with high cholesterol, half ate cereal fortified with the soluble fiber psyllium, and half did not. The fiber was given in two one-ounce boxes of cereal a day, each containing 3.2 grams of added psyllium. Those who ate the cereal with psyllium had lower cholesterol at the end of 12 weeks. The only negative side effects reported were a mild upset stomach and gas.

The authors of the study were encouraged by the fact that children's cholesterol levels could be affected by such a simple method. They recommend, however, that children only be given psyllium in food, not as a supplement that might replace essential calories.

Another study followed more than 650 children with high cholesterol over a period of three years. Some of the children were put on a low-fat diet and counseled frequently. At the end of three years, those who followed the diet had lowered their cholesterol levels.

The authors of this study suggest that lowering cholesterol levels in childhood may give you a better chance in the battle against high cholesterol and heart disease. Everyone, including children, should eat a healthy, low-fat, balanced diet.

**Source:**
*Medical Tribune for the Internist and Cardiologist* (36,14:18 and 36,11:11)

## Three cheers for chocolate milk

If your child never wants to drink his milk unless it's chocolate, don't worry. Flavored milk can be just as nutritious as plain milk. All types of milk are full of calcium and other nutrients, but the low-fat versions are the healthiest. Flavored milks contain two to four teaspoons more sugar per serving than plain milk, but they have all the same nutrients.

Here are some more points in favor of flavored milk:

◆ Calcium is absorbed just as well from flavored milk as from plain milk.

◆ Sugar can cause cavities, but the sugar in flavored milk is not sticky, so it doesn't adhere to the surface of teeth. The calcium and phosphorus in the milk help protect against cavities.

◆ The small amount of caffeine in chocolate milk doesn't have a negative effect on behavior or health.

◆ People with lactose intolerance may be better able to drink chocolate and other flavored milks without getting gastrointestinal symptoms.

For a healthy dose of calcium, vitamin A, potassium, phosphorus, and magnesium, let your child drink any flavor milk he wants — just as long as he drinks it.

**Sources:**
*Dairy Council Digest* (66,3:13)
*Food Values of Portions Commonly Used,* HarperCollins Publishers, New York, 1989

## Building bones for the future

Osteoporosis, a weakening of the bones, is a widespread problem for women as they age. It's the cause of hip fractures, backache, and stooped posture in older women. But it is a preventable disease, and the younger you start, the better chance you have of preventing it.

Most young girls don't get enough calcium, and calcium helps prevent osteoporosis. Supplementing the diets of young girls with calcium may prevent the onset of osteoporosis in later years.

In a Pennsylvania study, girls 12 to 14 years old took calcium supplements of 500 mg a day. By the time they reached the age of 16, they had increased their bone mass by 4 percent more than girls who didn't take the supplements. If the girls maintain their increased bone mass until the age of 21, they may reduce their risk of osteoporosis by as much as 50 percent.

Combined with the amount in their food, the calcium intake of the girls in the study was raised to about 1,300 mg per day. Most American females get no more than 800 mg daily.

The National Institutes of Health recommend a daily calcium intake of 1,200 to 1,500 mg for people ages 11 to 24. Young people can get sufficient calcium by adding some of the high-calcium foods listed below to their daily diets.

| FOOD | QUANTITY | MILLIGRAMS OF CALCIUM |
| --- | --- | --- |
| Skim milk | 1 cup | 316 |
| Plain yogurt | 1 cup | 413 |
| Swiss cheese | 1-1/2 ounces | 408 |
| Parmesan cheese | 1 ounce | 390 |
| Cheddar cheese | 1-1/2 ounces | 306 |
| Great northern beans | 1 cup | 120 |
| Navy beans (from dried) | 1 cup | 127 |
| Black-eyed peas (fresh) | 1 cup | 212 |
| Cooked spinach: | | |
|     Fresh | 1/2 cup | 122 |
|     Frozen | 1/2 cup | 139 |
|     Canned | 1/2 cup | 136 |
| Cooked turnip greens: | | |
|     Fresh | 1 cup | 197 |
|     Frozen | 1 cup | 248 |
| Canned salmon (with bones) | 4 ounces | 242 |
| Sardines | 4 ounces | 433 |

*Sources:*
*Medical Tribune for the Internist and Cardiologist* (36,19:4)
*Hamilton and Whitney's Nutrition Concepts and Controversies,* West Publishing Company, New York, 1994

## Good news for kids: sweet news about sugar

The thought of giving candy to a baby is not such a sweet idea if you've ever witnessed your two-year-old become a screeching, hyperactive terror after downing a cup of sugar-laden lemonade and a cookie. Some doctors and parents used to think that consuming food or drinks high in sugar would make most children wildly energetic, noisy, and irritable. Now the tide of opinion is turning against this theory.

A new look at past medical studies concludes that sugar is not a cause of hyperactivity in children. Researchers looked at 16 previous studies that tested children's reactions to consuming refined sugar. There was no hard evidence to prove that sugar affected the behavior of the children.

So, why do many parents believe that it does? Researchers have a couple of explanations. First, sugar is often consumed in settings such as birthday parties and holidays where there is already a lot of noise, activity, and excitement. The behavior of children consuming sugary foods at the party will reflect that.

The other possible explanation is that parents may automatically assume sugar causes their kids to be hyper, even when it doesn't. In one study, parents thought their children had been given a sugary drink and reported that it made them hyperactive. In fact, the drinks were artificially sweetened and didn't contain sugar.

Researchers haven't ruled out the possibility that some children, under certain circumstances, may have reactions to sugar. For most kids, however, this isn't the case. A little sugar, when it's part of a healthy, balanced diet, won't turn your little darling into a little devil.

*Sources:*
*Medical Abstracts Newsletter* (16,1:3)
*The Journal of the American Medical Association* (274,20:1617)

## Cut the caffeine for a calmer child

When you consider caffeine intake, you have to keep in mind that a child is putting caffeine into a much smaller body. For a 30-pound child, one 12-ounce cola drink contains the equivalent of five cups of instant coffee for a 150-pound adult. An energetic young child doesn't need the stimulating effects of caffeine. Try to keep caffeine at a minimum in your child's diet.

*Source:*
*Food and Mood,* Henry Holt and Company, New York, 1995

## A sweet remedy

It may indeed be true that "a spoonful of sugar helps the medicine go down." In a recent study of newborn babies, sugar was used as a pain reliever for little ones. The babies were given a small amount of sugar and water solutions on their tongues one minute before a heel stick, the method used to draw blood for testing from a baby's heel.

The babies who were given the solution with the greatest amount of sugar (50 percent) cried the least. Those given weaker concentrations of sugar, or just plain water, cried more. The sugar water proved to be a safe and effective pain reliever.

Sugar can also play a part in helping babies take unpleasant-tasting medicine. Dr. Rhonda E. Damschen of La Crosse, Wis., has an effective method of giving liquid medicine to bottle-fed babies. She fills a bottle with fruit juice and lets the baby drink until it is almost gone. Then she puts the medicine in the nipple and the baby swallows it down without even realizing it. He's then rewarded with a little more juice. This method might work for your baby, too.

*Sources:*
*Emergency Medicine* (27,3:64)
*Journal Watch* (15,15:119)

## Beware of baby bottle bacteria

Your baby drinks only part of her formula, and you put the bottle away in the refrigerator for later. It seems like a sensible thing to do, but you're actually putting your baby at unnecessary risk of illness. Even if you cool it quickly and reheat it properly before giving it to your child, the bottle may be breeding harmful bacteria.

When your baby drinks from a bottle, bacteria from her mouth can move from the nipple into the formula. There they can multiply quickly as your baby drinks, and those busy bacteria can contaminate the leftover formula or milk. So, toss out the remaining contents and start fresh again at the next feeding.

*Source:*
*Medical Update* (17,6:6)

## Lend a helping hand to kids too young to brush

If your young grandchild doesn't do a good job brushing his teeth, it may not be because he isn't trying. A child under the age of 10 may not have the physical skill and coordination to be really effective at toothbrushing.

In a study of 122 children ages 6 to 11, a pumice and dye mixture was painted on the children's upper teeth, and they were given instruction in toothbrushing. The 6 year olds left as much as 29 percent of their tooth surfaces unbrushed. The older children did much better.

Researchers concluded that parents or grandparents should help their younger children brush their teeth. If a child younger than 10 is wearing braces, he especially needs your help. You may also want to take him for professional dental cleanings more than the usual twice a year.

*Source:*
*Medical Abstracts Newsletter* (16,1:3)

## Take a shot at childhood diseases

You know that your child needs certain immunizations against childhood diseases. But did you know that in January 1995 the guidelines changed? The new immunization schedule was a cooperative effort among three groups: the Centers for Disease Control, the American Academy of Pediatrics, and the American Academy of Family Practice.

Here are some of the new recommendations of the immunization schedule:

◆ For children ages 11 to 12 who have not had three doses of the Hepatitis B vaccine, a series of three doses is recommended.

◆ At ages 4 to 6 or 11 to 12, a second dose of the measles, mumps, and rubella vaccine is recommended. This should be given at least one month after the first dose.

◆ Children who have weak immune systems, or who live in a home with someone else who has a weak immune system, should receive an inactive polio vaccine, instead of the live oral vaccine.

◆ At 12 to 18 months, children should routinely receive a vaccination for varicella-zoster (chickenpox). Children who haven't been vaccinated, and who have not had a documented case of chickenpox by age 11 or 12, should receive a vaccination.

Ask your child's doctor for a copy of the new immunization schedule, so that you can be sure your child is up-to-date on his disease-preventing shots.

*Source:*
*Journal Watch* (16,3:28)

## Fever: How hot is too hot?

The average body temperature of 98.6 degrees Fahrenheit was determined over 100 years ago. Recent research has shown, however, that there's much more variation in body temperature than scientists had realized. Normal adult temperatures can range from 96 degrees to 100.8 degrees.

For a baby, temperature can also vary according to his age and the season. Your baby's temperature is higher during the hot summer months. So, how can you know what's normal for your child, and when he has a fever?

For babies less than a month old, fever is defined as a rectal temperature of 100.4 degrees. For babies 1 month old, it's 100.6 degrees, and for babies 3 months old and older, fever is 100.8 degrees.

The way you measure your child's temperature can make a difference. Rectal temperature is considered to be the most accurate. It's recommended for children under 5 years old, but it can be awkward and uncomfortable for children older than 5.

Forehead-strip thermometers seem to give unreliable results. Oral thermometers work well, but many children don't like them. A good alternative is to place a thermometer in your child's armpit and hold his arm close to his body. The reading from this is called an axillary temperature.

A recent study showed axillary temperatures to be very accurate. By adding 1 degree Celsius or 1.8 degrees Fahrenheit, the axillary temperature can be made to equal rectal temperature. This way, you can measure your child's temperature without causing him any discomfort or anxiety.

**Sources:**
*Emergency Medicine* (25,2:125)
*Journal Watch* (16,4:34)
*The Journal of the American Medical Association* (270,22:2680)

# Preparing your child for a hospital visit

Every year, hundreds of thousands of children need surgery of some kind. Years ago, children were shuttled off to the hospital with little or no information about what to expect from their stay, but today the approach is different. Doctors realize that the more a child is prepared for his visit to the hospital, the less upsetting the experience will be for everyone.

Here are some helpful things you can do to make a hospital visit easier for your child:

◆ Keep a positive attitude. It's normal, as parents, to feel some anxiety, but don't communicate your worries to your child.

◆ Stress that the operation is going to make him feel better, and that's why he's having it. Let him know that your family will all feel better when it's over.

◆ Don't discuss pain that might go along with the operation. He'll be given a sedative or some kind of anesthesia to keep him from having pain.

◆ Don't talk about the risks of the operation or treatment. That could cause your child to worry.

◆ Never tell him he's going to be "put to sleep." He has probably only heard that phrase in connection with the death of a dog or cat.

◆ Visit your local library or bookstore and find entertaining children's books or videos about going to the hospital. Read or watch them with your child.

◆ Take your child's favorite stuffed animal, toy, doll, or blanket to the hospital to provide an extra measure of comfort.

◆ Take your child on a pre-surgery tour, if available, so that the hospital won't be a completely unfamiliar place.

**Source:**
*The Atlanta Journal/Constitution* (March 20, 1996, D1)

# Nutrition
# Know-How

## Eat like the Greeks to live longer

The Greeks really know how to live it up. They eat crusty whole-grain breads, fresh fish, and lush salads drenched with olive oil, and they drink wine in moderation. This all adds up to a long, healthy life.

Years ago, researchers discovered that Greeks lived longer than people in other parts of the world. In 1960, for example, Greek men had a 90 percent lower risk of death from heart disease than men in the United States. Greek women had less than one-half the risk of breast cancer that American women had. These statistics spurred researchers to take a close look at the Mediterranean diet.

**Plant foods.** Plant foods rather than animal foods make up the main part of the Mediterranean diet. Greeks consume lots of fresh fruits and vegetables, as well as pastas and breads.

**Olive oil.** Though most of the world avoids fat like the plague, the Greeks consume large amounts of olive oil. Olive oil contains monounsaturated fats, which may lower cholesterol, as well as the antioxidant vitamin E. It contains very little saturated fat, which is associated with a high risk of heart disease.

**Wine.** Moderate amounts of wine are a normal part of a Greek meal. For men this means two glasses of wine a day, and one glass a day for women. This amount seems to reduce the risk of heart disease. The Greeks eat dairy products, red meats, and sweets sparingly.

In a recent study of Greek men and women over age 70, those who ate a traditional Greek diet were more likely to live longer than those who ate more red meat and saturated fat.

Eat like the Greeks and live the good life ... longer.

*Sources:*
*Medical Tribune for the Internist and Cardiologist* (36,24:2)
*Nutrition Today* (30,2:59)
*The American Journal of Clinical Nutrition* (61,6S:1402S)

## Confucius say, 'Eat more rice'

The familiar food pyramid has a new twist. A new pyramid using the plant-based diets of Asian countries contains the latest eating plan for good health.

People in Asian countries have long been known for their low rates of heart disease, obesity, and many cancers. Following the eating patterns of these healthy people may be your path to greater health.

According to the new pyramid, most of your diet should consist of rice, noodles, bread, millet, corn, and other grains. The next level of the pyramid contains fruits, vegetables, nuts, legumes, and seeds. These items should all be eaten daily. Small amounts of vegetable oil, fish, shellfish, and dairy products may also be eaten daily. Sweets, eggs, and poultry should be eaten only weekly, and red meat should only be eaten about once a month.

The Asian diet has won the approval of many nutrition experts because it emphasizes plant-based, rather than animal-based foods.

*Source:*
*Medical Tribune for the Internist and Cardiologist* (37,4:5)

## Stay super healthy with 50 top nutrition tips

We all want to eat healthy, nutritious foods. Sometimes, however, that isn't as simple as it seems. For easy ways to eat more fruits and vegetables and prepare healthier meals, try these top 50 nutrition tips from the American Institute for Cancer Research:

1. Add more vegetables and less meat than called for in stir-fries, casseroles, soups, and other recipes.
2. If time is a problem, purchase prepackaged salads in the grocery store.
3. When possible, choose dark green salad leaves — the darker, the more nutritious.
4. Experiment with unfamiliar vegetables and fruits. Try collards, kale, red leaf lettuce, broccoflower, dandelion greens, jicama, mango, kiwi, starfruit, and lots more!
5. Instead of fruited yogurt, try plain nonfat or low-fat yogurt mixed with chopped apples and cinnamon, crushed pineapple with a drop of coconut extract, or raisins and your favorite cereal. Be creative!
6. Prepare your own "fruit-sicles" easily. Combine fruit juice and small chunks of fruit, pour into a paper cup, add a popsicle stick, and freeze until firm.
7. Make a refreshing, lower-calorie beverage by mixing fruit juice with seltzer water and crushed ice.
8. Add more vegetables to sandwiches. Lettuce and tomato are fine, but so are cucumber rounds, diced carrots, sprouts, green and red pepper strips, and broccoli.
9. Supplement store-bought pasta sauce or dishes like meatloaf with finely chopped veggies: fresh onions, green and red peppers, spinach, celery, or mushrooms.
10. Add more beans to soups, stews, and salads, or use them in burritos instead of beef.
11. Give tofu and other soy products a try. They are a good source of vegetable protein and contain phytochemicals which may reduce cancer risk.
12. Supplement a reduced-fat frozen meal with a tossed salad, skim milk, and fruit for dessert to ensure nutritional adequacy.
13. Take a break from rice with kasha, couscous, bulgur, barley, wild rice, millet, and other less familiar grains. Check out cookbooks for ideas — like couscous with chopped raisins, dried apricots, and a few toasted almonds.

14. Boost the fiber in your favorite breakfast cereal by sprinkling on a teaspoon or two of unprocessed bran or adding some 100 percent bran cereal. Be sure to drink plenty of fluids when increasing the fiber in your diet.

15. Turn baked potatoes into a main dish by topping with reduced-fat cheese and a generous helping of steamed fresh broccoli. Or top with a mixture of black beans, browned ground turkey breast, corn, and salsa.

16. Poach fish with reduced-sodium bouillon or wine and fresh herbs. Or bake fish in foil with thinly-sliced fresh vegetables, a small amount of olive oil, and some fresh basil.

17. Experiment with a variety of flavored vinegars on salads or in other dishes — a splash of raspberry vinegar on greens, or some balsamic vinegar on a brown rice salad with chopped fresh tomatoes and basil leaves.

18. Sauté foods in broth, water, or wine instead of oil or butter.

19. Try using only half the fat called for in a recipe.

20. Substitute evaporated skim milk for whipping cream in many recipes.

21. Try unsweetened applesauce for a portion of the fat in baking, usually up to one-half. Use prune purée for part of the fat in recipes with chocolate, as it is more compatible with the stronger flavor.

22. In many recipes, you can replace each ounce of unsweetened chocolate with three tablespoons unsweetened cocoa powder for the same flavor without the fat.

23. Much of the fat in cake comes from the frosting. Top instead with slices of fresh fruit, fruit sauce, or a sprinkle of powdered sugar.

24. Those innocent looking muffins and scones may be just as high in fat as Danish and donuts. Choose bagels instead and smear with just a light layer of reduced-fat cream cheese or jelly.

25. In recipes which call for fat-free cream cheese or sour cream, consider using reduced-fat versions instead. You are likely to get more taste and a more acceptable texture for just a few more grams of fat.

26. Replace mayonnaise on sandwiches with mustard or salsa for a fat-free taste sensation.

27. Try broth-based soups — they are far lower in fat than cream-based alternatives.

28. At salad bars, skip over the mayonnaise-laden salads and oily marinated beans. Emphasize fresh greens and vegetables with fat-free or reduced-fat dressing.

29. When eating pizza, blot the surface with a paper napkin. Order vegetable toppings instead of extra cheese, pepperoni, or ground beef.

30. Enjoy a fat-free cookie or two, but remember that "no fat" doesn't mean zero calories.

31. Keep healthy, low-fat snacks on hand: flavored rice cakes, sliced fruit, fat-free caramel popcorn, vegetable sticks with salsa, baked tortilla chips, unsalted pretzels with mustard, fruit bars, or dried cereal.

32. To prepare guacamole that's lower in fat, try using canned asparagus or

cooked peas instead of avocado. The result will be surprisingly similar to the real thing.

33. Try powdered butter substitute as a low-fat alternative to butter or margarine. It's wonderful on pasta, potatoes, hot cereal, rice, and in recipes where a buttery flavor is desired.

34. You can substitute two egg whites or one-fourth cup egg substitute for each whole egg in most recipes.

35. It's okay to alter cooking directions on the back of processed foods to control fat or salt. Use two-thirds of the seasoning packet in a rice mix, or make macaroni and cheese mix without the butter or margarine.

36. Always eat a variety of foods for good health. Cancer-fighting nutrients and phytochemicals, natural disease fighters that come from plants, vary from food to food.

37. Too busy to cook during the week? Set aside some time on the weekend to prepare a low-fat vegetable lasagna or vegetable bean stew that can be refrigerated for a quick meal on busy days.

38. When dining out, ask questions about ingredients and preparation methods. Most restaurants will go out of their way to make you happy.

39. If you eat at fast food restaurants often, choose meals carefully to control fat and calories: consider the grilled chicken breast with mustard (no special sauce!), a single hamburger, skim milk, a fat-free muffin, a low-fat milkshake, or fat-free frozen yogurt.

40. Prepare a pot of turkey chili, hearty minestrone soup, or a vegetable casserole, store in individual-size containers, and freeze. Defrost in the microwave for a quick supper or a nutritious lunch at work.

41. Roast a turkey breast, slice and separate the meat into portions of two to three ounces. Place portions in their own plastic zipper bags and freeze for later use in stir-fries, casseroles, and sandwiches.

42. When traveling by air, call ahead to request a low-fat or low-calorie meal.

43. Avoid charring or overcooking grilled foods. Remove any visible fat before grilling to help eliminate flare-ups and the formation of potential carcinogens, substances that cause cancer.

44. To avoid food-borne illness, always cook poultry and other meats thoroughly. Never cut fruits and vegetables with the same knife or on the same cutting board used for raw meat.

45. When reading food labels, always look at the serving size first. This way you'll know the amount of food the nutrient analysis refers to.

46. If you're trying to manage your weight, don't deprive yourself. Just eat high-fat favorites less often and in smaller portions. Fill up on fresh fruits, vegetables, and whole grains to feel more satisfied.

47. At times, people eat for reasons other than physical hunger: for social reasons; for psychological reasons; and in response to the smell, taste, and appearance of food. Listen to your body and try to eat only when you're truly, physically hungry.

48. Try ordering a salad and a low-fat appetizer (or two appetizers) in a

restaurant instead of an entrée. This strategy can accommodate a smaller appetite, satisfy the desire to try more than one item, and cost less as well.

49. Experiment with herbs and spices as a substitute for fat — and the salt shaker. Try rosemary with peas, dill with green beans, oregano with zucchini, or basil with tomatoes.

50. Above all, remember to enjoy food — for its wonderful variety of flavors, textures, colors, and nutritional qualities.

*Source:*
Adapted with permission from the *American Institute for Cancer Research Newsletter* (50:1)

## Meat that makes the grade

If you've always been a meat and potatoes kind of person but decided to sacrifice meat for the sake of your low-fat diet, there's reason to rejoice. As long as you exercise a little control, it's OK to eat meat.

Be a fat detective. Fat likes to hide in innocent-looking foods, so read labels carefully. Many people think that meat is their main source of fat, but meat only accounts for about one-fourth of their fat consumption. For example, did you know that one glazed doughnut contains more fat than three ounces of top sirloin? Try to choose low-fat foods from each food group rather than eliminating meat from your diet.

Though 70 percent of our dietary cholesterol comes from the meat group, over half of that amount comes from eggs. Also, studies have shown that substituting chicken or fish for beef and pork does not result in lower cholesterol.

If you give up on meat, you may be depriving yourself of more than a food that you love to eat. Lean meat is an important source of protein, vitamins, and minerals. Meat supplies lots of iron, which is particularly important to women, and elderly people sometimes need the extra zinc that meat provides.

Instead of cutting meat out of your diet, choose your cuts of meat carefully. Select beef cuts with the words "loin" or "round" in the name. Pick "choice" instead of "prime" and choose those cuts graded "USDA Select." When buying pork, pick cuts with the word "loin" or "leg" in the name.

Once you've chosen your meat carefully, trim away the excess fat. You should also practice low-fat cooking methods like broiling, steaming, baking, roasting, or grilling. If you're careful, you can maintain your low-fat diet and still enjoy a good steak now and then.

*Source:*
*Postgraduate Medicine* (98,4:113)

## How does your breakfast cereal stack up?

When Toucan Sam or Tony the Tiger tells you to make cereal part of your complete breakfast, you should listen. Those animated animals know that nutrition experts recommend doing just that.

You can whip up a nutritious breakfast of cold cereal with milk, fruit, and juice in no time. It's quick and easy, but which cereal should you choose?

Try to pick high-fiber cereals. Fiber helps reduce your risk of colon cancer, regulates bowel function, lowers cholesterol, and may help with weight control. You should get 25 to 30 grams of fiber a day, and high-fiber cereal gives you a good start on your daily requirement.

Cereals like puffed wheat may be considered a "diet" breakfast, but that may be because they're mostly air. Since a stomach full of air isn't very satisfying, you may end up grabbing a not-so-nutritious candy bar or other snack mid-morning.

If you're an active person, you need to eat about a 300-calorie bowl of cereal (check the nutrition information on the side of the box), with another 200 to 300 calories in the form of milk, fruit, and juice. This should give you plenty of energy to last until lunch, without any of those naughty trips to the candy machine.

If you take vitamin supplements, you could just eat a bowl of cereal every morning instead. A large bowl of fortified cereal may provide as much as 75 percent of several important vitamins and minerals. Check labels carefully for the exact amounts.

Stock your cupboard with several different kinds of cereal for variety in taste and nutrition. Your mornings may become a little less hectic with the convenience of lots of nutritious breakfast cereal at your fingertips.

**Source:**
*The Physician and Sportsmedicine* (22,12:21)

## The killer green vegetable

You should eat lots of green vegetables. However, eating one vegetable when it's green could make you a little green around the gills yourself.

Potatoes weigh in right behind wheat as the second largest food crop in the world. Since potatoes make up such a large part of our diets, we should be aware of the problems this seemingly innocent vegetable can cause.

Potatoes contain several chemical compounds which could be toxic. Green or damaged potatoes can have higher levels of these compounds. Eating these potatoes may cause nausea, vomiting, diarrhea, and damage to the intestinal tract. Rare cases of death have been reported, but not definitely confirmed, due to eating green potatoes.

The effect of these compounds on pregnant women hasn't been established yet, but if you're pregnant, perhaps you should be especially careful about the potatoes you eat.

If you love your potatoes, don't panic. They are an important and safe part of our diets. Just watch out for the green, and you can still enjoy your spuds.

**Source:**
*The Lawrence Review of Natural Products,* Facts and Comparisons, St. Louis, Mo., 1995

## Is butter better?

Slathering your bread with butter has long been a nutritional no-no. Experts recommended that you use margarine instead. Although margarine contains the same amount of fat and calories as butter, butter contains mostly saturated fat, the kind you've been warned to avoid. However, margarine contains trans-fatty acids which are formed during the process of turning liquid fats into solids.

Trans-fatty acids, like saturated fat, increase the level of LDL or "bad" cholesterol in your blood. Unlike saturated fat, however, trans-fatty acids also lower the level of HDL or "good" cholesterol.

So, which should you use, butter or margarine? Since a diet low in total fat improves your health, cutting out butter and margarine would be best. However, if you must have your bread and butter, the best alternative is the soft "tub" type margarine.

***Sources:***
*American Institute for Cancer Research Newsletter* (47:9)
*The Journal of the American Medical Association* (273,21:1699)

## Quicker picker upper

Do you run out of steam halfway through your workout? Maybe you need a little pick-me-up before you begin.

Many people think that you shouldn't eat before you exercise, because the food doesn't get digested until afterward. However, as long as you exercise at a moderate intensity, your body is able to digest food and send it to your muscles for energy. People who rush off to the gym without eating breakfast tend to struggle through their workouts rather than getting the most from their exercise.

This need for energy during exercise inspired the creation of the sports bar (a convenient snack food, not a place in which to watch football and drink beer). These bars have become increasingly popular for athletes. They provide a convenient source of calories, mainly in the form of carbohydrates.

However, you can get the same calorie boost from a banana or a bowl of cereal. Sports bars cost more per calorie than many other energy-boosting foods. Though some sports bars are fortified with vitamins, they shouldn't be considered an important part of your nutritional plan. They simply provide convenience and quick energy. If you choose to use sports bars for your pre-exercise snack, always drink eight to 16 ounces of water to help digestion.

Whether you choose sports bars or raisins for your workout energy, fuel up and go full steam ahead.

***Source:***
*The Physician and Sportsmedicine* (23,9:7)

## Give peas a chance

Once upon a time, a boy named Jack traded the family cow for a handful of beans. Jack's mother thought he was crazy. But by the end of the story, those beans brought them untold wealth. In the real world, beans may not be a magical key to greater wealth, but they can definitely be your key to greater health.

Beans are generally either canned, dried, or fresh. Right now we'll deal with dried beans — so called because they've been picked, allowed to dry, and then packaged for long-term storage.

Dried beans are also called *legumes* (leg-OOMS), which are vegetables that have seed-bearing pods such as peas, beans, and lentils. There are two different types of legumes: grain legumes, which are grown mostly for protein, and oilseeds, which are grown for their protein and oil content. The most common grain legumes include pinto, navy, Great Northern, lima, and garbanzo beans, as well as lentils, cowpeas, and common peas. The most common oilseeds are peanuts and soybeans.

**Fat and calories.** Beans are a surprisingly low-fat, low-calorie food. Most grain legumes contain between 110 and 140 calories per half-cup serving, with a fat content of less than one gram of fat per serving. Oilseed beans have a higher fat content, with 7.5 grams of fat per half-cup serving for boiled soybeans and 14 grams per ounce for dried peanuts.

**Fiber.** The high fiber content of legumes helps to reduce blood sugar levels, which helps control diabetes. Their soluble fiber has been shown to lower cholesterol. They also contain insoluble fiber, which improves digestion and aids in weight control by moving food more quickly through the intestines. Eating high fiber foods also tends to make you feel full sooner — good news to anyone trying to lose weight. A sudden increase in fiber can cause stomach discomfort, so add fiber to your diet gradually, so that your body has time to adjust.

**Protein.** Although animal protein is a complete source of all the amino acids (important building blocks of protein), it's high in fat and calories. Legumes provide a low-calorie, low-fat alternative to animal protein, but they are missing two types of those valuable amino acids. The trick is to mix your beans with other foods containing grains or flour so you'll get the other two amino acids you need. Such complementary pairs include pasta and bean soup, refried beans with corn tortillas, and red beans and rice.

**Vitamins and minerals.** Legumes contain generous helpings of important minerals such as iron, calcium, phosphorus, zinc, potassium, and magnesium. They also supply several water-soluble vitamins such as thiamin, niacin, and riboflavin. Since your body only stores water-soluble vitamins for a short time, you need to take in these vitamins daily.

**Carbohydrates.** Legumes are loaded with carbohydrates, mostly in the form of starch. Some of these carbohydrates contain sugars which are hard to digest. This can cause gas or a bloated feeling, especially in people who aren't used to eating legumes.

One way to lessen the gas effect is by soaking your beans for 4 to 5 hours before cooking (some people even soak them overnight). Then discard the water and start cooking the beans in a fresh pot of water. Replace the used cooking water with fresh water every half hour of cooking time.

If all else fails, a product called Beano, which you can buy at any drugstore, provides an enzyme to help digest those pesky sugars.

So, it looks like Jack's beans are a wealth of good nutrition.

*Sources:*
*The Journal of the American College of Nutrition* (13,6:549)

*The Journal of the American Diabetic Association* (93,12:1446)
*The Physician and Sportsmedicine* (23,6:13)

## Smooth and creamy health protection

Remember those old television commercials with people who said they lived to be over 100 years old by eating yogurt? Maybe those advertisements were more true than we thought at the time. Research shows that yogurt provides a variety of health benefits.

**Provides calcium.** Yogurt, like most dairy products, provides lots of calcium, which helps to maintain strong bones. Many people who are lactose intolerant and can't eat most dairy products may be able to eat yogurt.

**Fights infections and diarrhea.** Yogurt kills many types of bacteria in the body, including the common *E. coli* germ that causes diarrhea. Women have long eaten yogurt to help fight yeast infections. Now some women even apply it directly, mixed with water as a douche, or full strength. Yogurt also battles potentially dangerous bacteria such as *Salmonella enteritidis* and *Staphylococcus aureus.*

**Lowers cholesterol.** Yogurt helps lower cholesterol, which helps reduce the dangers of heart disease and high blood pressure. One study found that people who supplemented their regular diets with three cups of yogurt daily lowered their cholesterol by almost 10 percent in a week.

**Cancer preventive.** Men who eat yogurt on a regular basis have a decreased risk of developing colorectal cancer. Yogurt also reduces the incidence of breast cancer in women.

**Stomach soothing.** Yogurt contains a natural substance called *Prostaglandin E* which coats the lining of the stomach and protects it from irritating substances like cigarette smoke and alcohol. Prostaglandin E is also a prescription ulcer medication which can be obtained naturally from yogurt.

How many different kinds of food would you expect to pile on your plate to get all these health benefits? Now you can get it all in one smooth and creamy bite.

*Sources:*
*The Food Pharmacy,* Bantam Books, New York, 1988
*The Lawrence Review of Natural Products,* Facts and Comparisons, St. Louis, Mo., 1995

## This little fruit packs a powerful nutrition punch

The avocado is the talented, unknown starlet of the fruit world. This humble little fruit packs a powerful nutrition punch.

**Fiber.** The avocado has more dietary fiber than any other fruit. Fiber helps control diabetes, reduces cholesterol, and may help prevent certain types of cancer.

**Folate.** Folate, a B vitamin, reduces the tendency of the blood to clot, which may lead to heart disease. Pregnant women and children need folate because it is essential for proper cell division. Avocados contain lots of folate, as well as other B vitamins. Folate shows up in other foods as well, such as liver, pinto beans, and asparagus. However, much of it is destroyed in cooking. Because avocados are usually eaten raw, the folate isn't destroyed.

**Fatty acids.** Though the avocado contains more fat than most fruits, 60 percent of its fat is monounsaturated, which may reduce cholesterol levels, and only 17 percent is the less desirable saturated fat. Avocados can replace some of the high-fat butter and cheese in your diet. If you substitute avocado for cheese in a salad, you can reduce the fat content by one-third. Avocados harvested early in the season, between November and March, also contain about a third less fat than those harvested in September and October.

**Antioxidants.** Avocados contain lots of vitamins C and E, which are both well-known for their antioxidant prowess. Antioxidants protect your body's cells from the damaging effects of free radicals (unstable oxygen molecules) in the blood and guard against many diseases, including cancer and heart disease.

**Minerals.** Avocados contain 13 essential minerals, including potassium, magnesium, and iron. Potassium protects against high blood pressure and stroke, while iron and magnesium work together to build healthy blood.

The avocado, a well-rounded fruit, contributes to moist, healthy skin as well as great nutrition. You can make a moisturizing mask by crushing up avocados and mixing the mash with a little oatmeal, or you can simply rub the inside of the avocado skin over your skin.

Stir up some guacamole, toss some on your salad, or smear some on your face. Whatever you choose to do with your avocado, put its talent to work for you.

*Sources:*
*Nutrition Today* (29,3:23)
*Super Healing Foods,* Parker Publishing, West Nyack, N.Y., 1995

# Natural healing nectar

Honey is being hailed as the new wonder drug. However, this news isn't really new. Ancient Egyptians mentioned honey as an ingredient in numerous remedies. Almost all ancient civilizations used honey as a treatment for wounds, sores, and skin ulcers. Modern cultures are beginning to discover what the Egyptians knew thousands of years ago. Honey can help many common ailments.

**Wounds.** Many studies have confirmed honey's healing powers on wounds, sores, and skin ulcers. Honey has been found to be very effective in the treatment of burns, and some doctors routinely apply honey to surgical wounds.

**Diarrhea.** Honey kills many of the bacteria which can cause diarrhea. Drinking a solution containing honey often relieves traveler's diarrhea.

**Asthma.** Some doctors once scoffed at the idea that honey could prevent asthma. However, a theory arose that perhaps the pollen in honey could desensitize you to allergies the same way allergy shots do. Then a study found that allergy-prone children who drank a pollen solution had fewer allergic symptoms than they did before. This lent weight to the argument that honey can indeed prevent asthma.

**Cancer.** One of the most dreaded diseases may be sweetened by honey. Honey has been used to stop the growth and spread of tumors.

**Cataracts.** Honey has been effective in the treatment of cataracts and other eye disorders.

**Coughs.** Many cough and cold preparations contain honey. It soothes itchy sore throats and calms coughs.

**Insomnia.** Eating honey increases a chemical in the brain that calms you down and helps you sleep.

One caution about using honey: don't ever give it to an infant under a year old. It contains a bacteria which could cause deadly botulism in infants.

Ancient civilizations knew the sweet secret of honey. You, too, can benefit from the healing power of honey ... even if you're not ancient.

*Sources:*
*The Food Pharmacy,* Bantam Books, New York, 1988
*The Lawrence Review of Natural Products,* Facts and Comparisons, St. Louis, Mo., 1995

# Special cell rejuvenator

What the wine leaves behind may help your health. Red grape seeds, obtained as a by-product of wine-making, can be ground up to make grape seed oil. This oil contains essential fatty acids and vitamin E compounds. It helps prevent cancer, triggers cells to renew themselves, and helps fight tooth decay. If you don't drink red wine, you can still partake of the benefits it leaves behind.

*Source:*
*The Lawrence Review of Natural Products,* Facts and Comparisons, St. Louis, Mo., 1995

# 'KO' cholesterol and cancer with this seed

What would you say if a friend offered you a muffin that would lower your cholesterol, give you a good dose of vitamin D and healthy fatty acids, relieve your constipation, *and* help you fight cancer? You'd ask for the recipe, of course! Then you'd share your health secret with all your family and friends.

Research on flaxseed has generated an impressive list of important benefits:

◆ It's high in heart-healthy omega-3 oils like those in fish.
◆ It contains as much fiber as oat bran and acts as a natural laxative.
◆ It reduces total cholesterol and LDL ("bad") cholesterol.
◆ It helps fight malaria and cancers of the breast, prostate, and colon.
◆ It may help diabetics maintain control of their blood sugar.
◆ It works like an anti-inflammatory on arthritis and psoriasis.
◆ It's high in vitamin D, which is important in preventing osteoporosis.

The oil extracted from flaxseed contributes to the beneficial effects of a high-fiber diet. When used in moderation, it helps reduce cholesterol and lowers your risk for cardiovascular disease, heart attack, and stroke.

Flaxseed is easy to add to your normal diet. Stir some into your orange juice or sprinkle it on hot or cold cereal. You can even sprinkle some on salads or soups. It has a pleasant, nutty flavor. You can add flaxseed flour to any baked goods, like muffins, breads, or pancakes.

If you want to sample this nutritional powerhouse, start slowly. Eat only small amounts at first, because it may cause gas until your body adapts to it. Three teaspoons is all the average adult needs. People with diabetes or hemophilia, a blood clotting disorder, should consult their doctors before adding flaxseed to their diets because it can change certain blood properties that affect the management of these diseases.

Flaxseed and flaxseed oil may be purchased at most health food stores and some supermarkets. You can make your own flaxseed flour by grinding the seeds in a blender or coffee grinder.

*Sources:*
*Cereal Foods World* (38,10:753)
*Information Bulletin*, Flax Institute of the United States, Fargo, N.D., 1995
*Journal of Endocrinology and Metabolism* (77,5:1215)
*Journal of the National Cancer Institute* (87,7:484)
*The American Journal of Clinical Nutrition* (59,6:1304; 61,1:62; and 86,23:1746)
*The Lawrence Review of Natural Products*, Facts and Comparisons, St. Louis, Mo., 1995

# The healthy new way to cook

You buy healthy foods for your family, and you want to cook them so they will retain all their nutritious value. Why not try poaching for a change of pace?

Poaching basically involves cooking food in a covered pan of simmering liquid. The liquid usually consists of broths and juices. You can use vegetable juice, broth, or water flavored with wine or lemon juice, and seasoned with herbs and spices. Keep the poaching liquid at a slow simmer instead of a full boil. This method makes wonderfully flavored, moist, and tender fish and poultry.

You can also poach fruits in sweetened juices. Select firm fruits that aren't overripe. Brush all fruits, except plums, with lemon juice to prevent browning.

You can create healthy, tasty main dishes as well as sweet, fruity desserts with poaching. It isn't just for eggs anymore.

*Source:*
*American Institute for Cancer Research Newsletter* (47:12)

# Cooking up good health

Stocking your kitchen for good health doesn't just mean buying fresh, nutritious foods. You need the right tools to prepare the food properly.

**Microwave.** This little miracle of modern technology is an important tool for good nutrition. Vitamins in foods disappear rapidly when exposed to heat, water, and air. Your microwave provides a quick way to cook food with a minimum of nutrition loss.

**Vegetable steamer.** Steamed vegetables retain more nutrients than those boiled for a long time. You can buy steamer baskets which fit into a saucepan. Cover tightly and steam for just a few minutes.

**Nonstick cookware.** Loading the old cast-iron skillet with lard will soon load your hips with the same. Nonstick cookware can reduce your fat intake by making it possible to use less oil, or even just a vegetable spray. Nonstick cookware also makes cleanup a breeze, which might encourage you to use it more often.

**Pressure cooker.** The comeback kid of cookery, the pressure cooker, can help you prepare a moist, tasty meal in minutes. If you've ever had a pressure cooker splatter beans all over your kitchen, you'll be relieved to know that the improved, modern version of this 1950s relic provides safety as well as speedy cooking.

Supply your kitchen with the right tools for healthy food preparation, and soon you'll be cooking up a nutritious storm.

*Source:*
*The Physician and Sportsmedicine* (24,2:45)

# Required reading: food labels

Do you spend hours in the grocery store trying to figure out the information on food labels? You want to buy healthy food for your family, but sometimes you need an interpreter to explain the meanings behind those confusing numbers.

**Percent daily value.** The most important number on a food label, percent daily value, is based on a 2,000 calorie a day diet. Of course, if you're watching your weight, you may not take in this much, and if you're an athlete in training or a growing teenager, you may take in more. However, you can still use the percent daily value to give you an idea of how a particular food fits into your nutritional plan. You should try to eat 100 percent of the daily value for each nutrient every day. If the percent daily value listed on the label is 5 percent or less, the food doesn't contribute much of that nutrient to your diet.

**What do those terms mean exactly?** The government has set definitions for certain terms to meet before they can be used on a food label. Some of the terms:

♦ High-protein: at least 10 grams of high-quality protein.
♦ Fat-free: less than 0.5 grams of fat per serving.
♦ Low-fat: less than 3 grams of fat per serving.
♦ Good source of calcium: at least 100 mg per serving.
♦ Sugar-free: less than 0.5 grams per serving
♦ Reduced or fewer calories: at least 25 percent fewer calories per serving than the regular food
♦ Light: one-third fewer calories or half the fat of the regular food, or a "low-calorie," "low-fat" food with half the sodium content of the regular food

**American Heart Association symbol.** If all the numbers still confuse you, just look for the American Heart Association symbol of a heart with a check in it. This certifies certain foods as being heart-healthy. In order to earn the AHA symbol on its package, the product must meet the definitions for low fat, low saturated fat, and low cholesterol. Meat products must be extra lean. All products must be low in sodium and contain at least 10 percent of at least one of the following nutrients: protein, vitamin A, vitamin C, calcium, iron, or fiber. You can find the symbol on many of your favorites, like pork and beans and Cheerios. It's an easy way to ensure that the food you buy contributes to your family's improved health.

Sources:
American Heart Association news release (February 1996)
FDA Consumer (29,7:19)

## Bad to the brain

Could two common food additives be deadly brain-cell destroyers? At least one expert thinks so. Dr. Russell Blaylock, author of *Excitotoxins: The Taste that Kills* believes that MSG (monosodium glutamate) and aspartame (also known as Nutrasweet) excite nerve cells to a point of hyperactivity that severely damages your brain.

He calls the substances *excitotoxins* and says that they may cause brain cancer, Parkinson's disease, Huntington's disease, Alzheimer's disease, and symptoms similar to multiple sclerosis. Dr. Blaylock says that MSG also causes many learning disorders, such as attention deficit disorder. MSG causes brain lesions in laboratory animals, but whether it has that effect in humans has not been determined. Aspartame has been shown to cause a high incidence of brain tumors, as well as uterine and ovarian cancer, in laboratory animals.

It's the substance that is formed when aspartame breaks down that actually causes the damage, says Dr. Blaylock. Aspartame breaks down into more and more of this toxic substance as time goes on, and it breaks down much faster when heated. He theorizes that aspartame may be behind the Gulf War Syndrome. A soft-drink company donated cases of diet soda containing aspartame to the military personnel during the war. These soft drinks may have become toxic while sitting on loading docks in the desert heat.

Since aspartame breaks down when it is heated, Dr. Blaylock is particularly concerned about manufacturers' attempts to develop similar sweeteners for cooking.

Of course, not everyone agrees with Dr. Blaylock, including the U.S. government. The Food and Drug Administration says that these substances are safe for human consumption. They believe MSG causes allergic reactions in some people and breathing problems in asthmatics, but otherwise it's harmless.

According to Dr. Blaylock, avoiding excitotoxins seems to be a wise choice, especially since they don't provide any essential nutritional value.

Dr. Blaylock suggests using saccharine instead, or at least cutting back on aspartame. That may not be easy, since he also thinks that aspartame may be addictive. That's why it's particularly dangerous for children. He says, "A couple of diet sodas can be very dangerous for a child. The smaller the child, the more dangerous."

"As for me, I wouldn't touch the stuff, period." Dr. Blaylock says. If he's right, many people need to be seriously concerned about their brain cells.

Sources:
Dr. Russell Blaylock, M.D., Neurosurgeon, private practice, Jackson, Miss
FDA Consumer (29,9:2)
Healthy and Natural Journal (3,1:22)

## Vitamin supplements: help or hype?

Most of us sink a large chunk of our incomes into insurance — car insurance, life insurance, health insurance, and homeowner's insurance. Taking a multivitamin a day could be inexpensive insurance against disease.

Vitamin A, vitamin C, and beta carotene all provide significant antioxidant protection. One recent study suggested that smokers who took beta carotene supplements actually had a higher risk of developing lung cancer and dying from it. However, the study was done on people who had already been smoking for 30 years, so the damage had probably already been done.

Many other studies have demonstrated the beneficial effects of vitamins in fighting heart disease, cancer, and infections. One study found that men who had the highest intakes of vitamin C and beta carotene were 37 percent less likely to die of cancer, and 30 percent less likely to die of heart disease. Vitamins also give your immune system a little extra boost, and vitamin C helps prevent cataracts.

Eating fruits and vegetables every day provides you with the best source of vitamin and mineral protection. They also provide many other healthy benefits, such as fiber. However, since multivitamin supplements in recommended doses usually don't cause any harmful side effects, a little extra insurance couldn't hurt.

*Sources:*
*Journal of the American College of Nutrition* (14,2:124)
*Medical Tribune for the Internist and Cardiologist* (37,2:2 and 37,3:1)
*The Journal of the American Medical Association* (273,14:1077)

## The best source of bone-building calcium

As you get older, your need for calcium increases. However, older people only get about half of the calcium they need from their diets, so a calcium supplement may be necessary. Which supplement provides the best source of calcium?

Calcium from supplements containing calcium carbonate, like Tums or Rolaids, may not be absorbed by the body very well. Supplements containing calcium citrate are more easily absorbed and cause less bloating, gas, cramping, and constipation than calcium carbonate. Steer clear of natural calcium supplements, such as bone meal or oyster shell, which may contain lead.

Lots of protein in your diet can deplete your calcium supply. Many other foods and medicines can interfere with calcium absorption, so it's best to take your calcium pills between meals.

You need about 1,500 mg of calcium daily, so read labels carefully to make sure you get the right amount and the right kind of calcium

*Source:*
*Consumer Reports* (60,8:510)

## Iron irony

Balancing iron can be a weighty problem. You may be tempted to take iron supplements, just to be sure you get enough. However, too much iron can be toxic, so supplements may not be a good idea.

People with *hemochromatosis* absorb twice as much iron from their food as other people. Hemochromatosis occurs more often than any other genetic illness among whites. The liver, pancreas, heart, and brain store all that extra iron. This extra iron usually causes no problems at first, but after about age 50, it begins to damage organs, especially in men. How do you know if you have an excess of iron in your blood? The symptoms include fatigue, impotence, persistent thirst, and frequent urination. However, if you want to know for sure, get tested. Your doctor can give you a simple blood test to determine your *ferritin* (the form iron takes in the blood) level. A ferritin level above 200 could indicate excessive iron storage. Treatment consists of removing extra iron by giving blood.

Now you may be tempted to avoid all iron, but iron also accounts for the most common nutritional deficiency — anemia. Symptoms include fatigue, irritability, difficulty swallowing, and paleness. Menstruating women are victims of anemia more often than any other group. Iron deficiency not severe enough to cause anemia can still cause attention disorders and chronic fatigue.

Since too much iron can hurt you and not enough iron can hurt you, what should you do? First, you should get tested so that you know your ferritin level. Consider donating blood regularly. It's a great public service as well as the only way to safely lower ferritin levels in your blood. Don't take iron supplements unless a health care professional recommends them. Instead, try to get your iron from your diet. Good sources of iron include liver, red meat, shellfish, greens, and soybeans.

Current recommendations for iron intake:

◆ Children, men over 18, and women over 50: 10 mg a day
◆ Males ages 11 to 18: 12 mg a day
◆ Females ages 11 to 50 and lactating women: 15 mg a day
◆ Pregnant women: 30 mg a day

*Sources:*
*Nutrition Action Healthletter* (23,1:8)
*The Real Vitamin and Mineral Book,* Avery Publishing, Garden City Park, N.Y., 1990

## Zap the zinc

When choosing a multivitamin, perhaps you should pick one without zinc. Zinc can interfere with your body's copper levels, which can alter your cholesterol unfavorably. A recent study found that you need no more than 9 mg of zinc daily, which should be easily obtained from your diet. Meats, shellfish, and poultry are good sources of zinc.

*Source:*
*The American Journal of Clinical Nutrition* (61,3S:621S)

# Fun and Fitness

## The best prevention against disease

Exercise may be the most perfect medicine. Doctors often prescribe exercise to treat the following diseases·

- ◆ Heart disease. The number one killer today is coronary artery disease. This disease claims about 2,000 lives a *day* in the United States alone. Exercise can reverse the effects of heart disease and reduce many risk factors, such as high blood pressure, high cholesterol, and obesity.
- ◆ Stroke. Vigorous exercise provides protection against stroke and helps to restore function following a stroke.
- ◆ High blood pressure. Regular aerobic exercise may enable many people to reduce their blood pressures without taking medication. Those with severe cases may be helped by using exercise therapy as a supplement to their drug therapy.
- ◆ Diabetes. Diabetes is often responsible for damage to the brain, heart, kidneys, eyes, and legs. Exercise can prevent or delay many of these complications, as well as helping to reduce insulin requirements.
- ◆ Arthritis. Exercise strengthens muscles, improves flexibility, and increases range of motion.
- ◆ Osteoporosis. Osteoporosis causes bones to become porous and weak, resulting in loss of height and increased risk of bone fractures. Exercise can prevent or reverse bone loss, reducing the chances of fractures.
- ◆ Obesity. Excess body fat contributes to a number of serious diseases, including heart disease, diabetes, high blood pressure, and some types of cancer. Exercise helps maintain a healthy level of body fat.
- ◆ Depression. Depression is the most common type of mental illness, affecting about one in 20 people. Exercise therapy can improve self-image, reduce stress, and increase feelings of well-being. Exercise also triggers the release of endorphins, which can give people an attitude boost. Some therapists even walk or run with their depressed patients rather than just talking to them in an office.
- ◆ Cancer. Exercise has been shown to be effective in the treatment of colon cancer and breast cancer.
- ◆ Chronic obstructive pulmonary disease. Recent studies suggest that exercise can be beneficial even to people with severe air flow obstruction.

If your doctor prescribes exercise for your condition, follow his advice. Remember, though, exercise doesn't require a prescription. It's available to everyone and best of all ... it's free.

*Source:*
*The Physician and Sportsmedicine* (24,2:72)

## Increase your life span

Have you been a couch potato all your life and think that starting an exercise program now would be a waste of time? Think again. Studies have shown that increasing your level of fitness can reduce your mortality risk significantly. In fact, the reduction in risk is about the same as for people who quit smoking.

It's never too late to add years to your life. Just get off the couch and get moving!

*Source:*
*The Journal of the American Medical Association* (273,14:1093)

## Maximize your exercise

That leisurely stroll you take every day is good for you. However, if you are really serious about increasing your life span, you may need to step up the pace. Though many experts say that 30 minutes of moderate exercise is enough to improve your health, studies show that more vigorous exercise can help you live longer.

One study found that the level of HDL or "good" cholesterol in the blood rose with the number of miles run per week. The most changes in cholesterol levels were found in those who ran 7 to 14 miles per week at a mild to moderate intensity.

Another study followed 17,000 men for 20 years. There were significantly fewer deaths among those who engaged in vigorous activities, such as brisk walking, running, swimming, or playing tennis, than among those who were less active.

If you want to get the most out of your exercise program, follow these recommendations. Exercise intensely enough to produce light sweating or hard breathing for 20 minutes at least three times a week. Keep in mind that moderate exercise is better than no exercise, so don't stop strolling unless you start running instead.

*Sources:*
*Archives of Internal Medicine* (155,4:415)
*The Journal of the American Medical Association* (273,15:1179)

## Ageless fitness

Face facts. Everyone ages. Our bodies are not the same ones we had 20 years ago. Beginning about age 40, you tend to lose over six pounds of lean body mass every 10 years. Your metabolism slows, body fat increases, glucose tolerance (your body's ability to regulate the level of sugar in your blood) decreases, and blood pressure rises. The question is, are you going to take this sitting down, or are you going to do something about it?

People have been searching for a fountain of youth for centuries, to no avail. However, you may have an untapped fountain at your disposal — exercise. One study found that older people who exercised vigorously lived longer and developed fewer disabilities than others their age. A separate study found that people over age 50 who participated in a running program on a regular basis had fewer medical problems and took fewer medications than nonrunners.

You can also increase your aerobic capacity by 20 to 25 percent by beginning a program of vigorous exercise. This translates into about a 20-year rejuvenation in cardiovascular fitness. Wouldn't you take 20 years off your heart if you knew you could?

Being physically fit becomes more important the older you get. Many older people think they can't exercise like they should. However, in most cases, that just isn't true. First, you have to believe that you can do it, and then just do it.

*Sources:*
*The Physician and Sportsmedicine* (23,11:109)
*The Saturday Evening Post* (267,2:14)

## 8 simple tips recharge your exercise program

Regular exercise provides numerous benefits, including prevention of many serious diseases. Yet only 22 percent of the people in the United States exercise at the recommended levels. If exercise reaps such great rewards (and what greater reward than longer life and improved health), then why aren't more people taking advantage of these benefits?

Some people think that vigorous, continuous exercise is the only kind that will do them any good. However, experts say that activity which is only moderately vigorous, such as brisk walking, is enough to reduce your risk of heart disease. Thirty minutes a day is recommended, and this can be broken up into 10 minute sessions throughout the day.

Making time for exercise is easier than you think. You just have to be creative and persistent. Here are some ways to get you started.

**Don't drive when you can walk.** Running errands nearby, visiting friends in the neighborhood, or going to church are good excuses for making your exercise pull double duty.

**Take the stairs.** Walking up or down stairs is good exercise, and it's usually just as quick as waiting on an elevator.

**Make exercise a family affair.** Evening walks with your family will give you an opportunity to talk about the day's events. You'll become a closer family and more physically fit.

**Early to rise.** Some people find that getting up earlier in the morning to exercise starts the day off right.

**Turn work into an exercise opportunity.** Yard work and housework can both be excellent ways to exercise while accomplishing something useful.

**Keep weights and exercise clothes in your car or office.** Then, if you have some unexpected free time, you'll be prepared to take advantage of it.

**Buddy up.** Find an exercise buddy, at work or at home. You'll help keep each other motivated, as well as keep each other company.

**Make it a priority.** Find time to exercise by adjusting your daily schedule. In other words, just make exercise fit, and it will make you fit.

*Sources:*
*Medical Tribune for the Internist and Cardiologist* (37,2:3)
*Scientific American Medical Bulletin* (18,10:3)
*The Physician and Sportsmedicine* (24,2:83)

## Fitness guidelines for people over 40

These guidelines can give you an idea of exactly how fit you are in comparison to others your age. In order to judge aerobic capacity (your body's ability to use oxygen), you should see how long it takes you to walk one mile, and then compare your time with the ones listed below.

| AGES | MEN'S TIME | WOMEN'S TIME |
|------|-----------|--------------|
| 40-49: | 15:00 to 16:00 min. | 14:00 to 14:42 min. |
| 50-59: | 15:36 to 17:00 min. | 14:24 to 15:12 min. |
| 60-69: | 16:18 to 17:30 min. | 15:12 to 16:18 min. |
| 70-79: | 20:00 to 21:48 min. | 15:48 to 18:48 min. |

Upper body endurance can also be measured by how many repetitions of bicep curls with a five-pound weight you can do in 30 seconds.

| AGES | MEN | WOMEN |
|------|-----|-------|
| 40-49: | 30 to 34 repetitions | 21 to 27 repetitions |
| 50-59: | 29 to 33 repetitions | 20 to 25 repetitions |
| 60-69: | 26 to 31 repetitions | 19 to 22 repetitions |
| 70-79: | 24 to 28 repetitions | 18 to 21 repetitions |

*Source:*
*Medical Tribune for the Internist and Cardiologist* (37,3:9)

## Warm-up to exercise

You probably know instinctively that warming up before exercise is a good idea. People have long believed that warming up helps prevent injuries and improves performance. Warming up can also decrease stress on your heart. If you jump right into a strenuous exercise, your heart will probably not get enough blood flow and oxygen. However, warming up slowly increases blood flow to the heart, which could reduce your risk of a heart attack.

**Correct warming.** Many people think that stretching before exercise is a good way to warm up. However, stretching cold muscles could actually cause an injury. The best way to warm up is to start gradually whatever activity you plan to be doing. If you run, begin by walking. If you swim, begin with leisurely laps, slowly getting faster. This gradual increase warms up the specific muscles you will be using during your exercise. You will need to warm up more in cold weather and less in hot weather. If you plan to exercise outdoors in cold weather, try warming up inside so you won't have to remove extra clothing as you get warmer.

**Too cool.** Cooling down is just as important as warming up, but most of us neglect this. We want to hit the couch immediately after exercise, but this is really *not* cool. Cooling down helps to remove some chemical by-products of exercise from your muscles. It also helps lower levels of adrenaline in your bloodstream which increase during exercise. If this extra adrenaline remains in your bloodstream during rest, it can place extra stress on your heart. Sudden inactivity after vigorous exercise can cause blood to pool, especially in your legs. This could lead to lightheadedness and decreased blood flow to your heart.

**Stretch it out.** Okay, now you can stretch. Bring down the pace of your workout slowly, and then stretch those muscles. This will help prevent some of the stiffness you may experience after exercise. In cold weather, cool down indoors to help prevent chills by slowing the loss of body heat.

Get the most out of your exercise program by making warming up and cooling down a routine practice.

*Source:*
*The Physician and Sportsmedicine* (23,9:97)

# Exercise: out with the old, in with the new

Ah ... the good old days, when sit-ups were a breeze, push-ups were for show, and running was just as easy as walking. Now, as you get older, you find it takes a little more effort to do the exercise and much more time to recuperate. However, that nagging pain you feel after working out may not be entirely due to age — it may be the way you're exercising.

As you age and your body changes, your choice of exercise may need to change also. Over time, muscle mass decreases and bones weaken, making bodies weaker and less flexible. This allows your body to become more easily injured. Therefore, the exercises of your youth may do you more harm than good at this point.

Many common exercises, such as sit-ups and toe touches, place tremendous stress on the lower back and neck. Young people can bounce back from the tension, but an older adult may not be able to endure the added pressure. Fortunately, there are safe alternatives to these and other classic exercises. Try these alternatives for the same healthy benefits without the pain.

♦ To stretch the back of your thighs, try the one-legged stretch instead of the standing toe-touch. Sit on the side of a bed or couch with one leg extended in front of you. Bend at your hips and grasp lower leg. Extend your chin toward your knee until you feel a comfortable stretch through your back and shoulders and hold. Repeat with other leg.

♦ Full sit-ups are stressful to the lower back. Try crunches instead. Lie on your back, knees bent, and feet flat on the floor. Cross your arms over your chest. Raise your chest, shoulders, and head a few inches and hold, then lie flat again. Repeat.

◆ Donkey kicks are dangerous to the neck and lower back. Try rear thigh lifts instead. Get on all fours, with your knees bent to 90 degrees. Keep your neck in a neutral position. With your neck and lower back straight, slowly raise one leg until the thigh is parallel to the floor. Hold for a second and then let your leg down. Repeat with other leg. You can also do this exercise lying on your stomach, with a pillow under your stomach.

◆ Rolling your head in a complete circle puts stress on the upper spine. To stretch your neck muscles safely, gently tilt your head to the side, then the front, then the opposite side, and then to the back.

◆ Yoga "plows" risk injury to your neck. The fold-up stretch safely stretches your back muscles and is much easier to do. Kneel down and sit on your heels, bow forward with your arms extended until your forehead nearly reaches the floor. Keep your buttocks resting on your heels. Stretch from your fingertips through your back as far as you can comfortably hold. This exercise may also be done by sitting in a chair and reaching down between your legs to touch the floor.

◆ Full "squats" strengthen the upper thighs, but they can be damaging to your knees, so instead try partial squats. Start in a standing position, then bend your knees, keeping your back straight and your knees parallel over your feet, until you can just see the ends of your toes. Straighten back up slowly and repeat.

*Source:*
*The Physician and Sportsmedicine* (23,6:87 and 23,8:7)

## Pain-free workouts

Proper technique is vital to your health no matter what your age. Here are some common rules that everyone should follow.

◆ Don't alter an exercise. If you can't do the exercise as directed, don't do it.

◆ Stop when you get tired. You're more likely to injure yourself when your body is weak.

◆ Never bounce. Use slow, controlled movements.

◆ It's better to hold a stretched position longer than to repeat it for shorter periods. Start out holding your stretches for six seconds. Slowly build up to two-minute stretches.

◆ If you are in pain, stop immediately. Your body is trying to tell you something is wrong. Whatever is wrong cannot be fixed by continuing the exercise.

◆ Don't do twisting exercises, like "windmills." They are very stressful on the back.

◆ Avoid "jumping jacks." They can be damaging to your knees. If you land on your toes, the tendons in the back of your heel could tear if you aren't in good shape.

By doing exercises with caution and the proper techniques, you can take the pain out of working out and start enjoying your gains.

*Source:*
*The Physician and Sportsmedicine* (23,6:87 and 23,8:7)

## Easy ways to soothe side stitches

During exercise, you suddenly feel a stabbing pain in your side. Although side stitches are quite common, no one is sure what causes them although theories abound. Some people believe that muscles starved for oxygen during exercise spasm, causing the pain. Others think that the body produces too much *lactic acid* (excess glucose particles in the muscles) during exercise, causing the same effect as the rubbery legs you get after a hard run. A shortage of potassium or water may also trigger side stitches. However it happens, if you get a side stitch, you can try one of these methods for relief.

♦ Bend forward while tightening your abdomen.
♦ Breathe deeply and exhale slowly.
♦ Hold the painful area tightly with your fingers.
♦ Try stretching your arms up above your head. This may help stretch out the muscles in the affected area.

Preventing side stitches is also a bit of a mystery, but you can use some commonsense suggestions.

♦ Wait 30 to 90 minutes after eating to begin your exercise.
♦ Warm up before exercise.
♦ Make sure you get enough potassium. Fruit juice is one good source.
♦ Drink plenty of water before beginning your exercise, instead of trying to quench your thirst in the middle of a workout.
♦ If you have a problem with side stitches, try slowing down your workout and build up intensity gradually.
♦ Keep it up. As your fitness level increases, the chances of getting a side stitch decrease.

The more fit you are, the less likely you are to experience side stitches. Don't let stitches drive you away from exercise. Instead, exercise to drive away the stitches.

*Source:*
*In Health* (4,4:84)

## Wrap and don't worry

You've sprained your wrist or twisted your knee. One of the things you are most likely to do for your injury is to wrap it with an elastic bandage, such as an

Ace bandage. Does this really help? Many people feel that it provides extra support and stability for the injured joint during exercise, but most experts say an elastic bandage is not strong enough to provide support for a joint. The bandage's advantage may simply be that it makes the wearer more aware of the joint's movement; therefore, they are more careful during exercise. You are then less likely to aggravate the injury by placing too much stress on it. The rule seems to be that it can't hurt, and it may help, so if it makes you feel better, wrap it up.

*Source:*
*The American Journal of Sports Medicine* (23,2:251)

## Natural way to beat muscle aches

A vigorous workout or a day spent gardening can leave you sore and tender. You vow not to push your body so hard again, but next time, you just can't resist.

British researchers say that vitamin C may prevent those achy muscles. Exercisers who take 400 mg of vitamin C before doing one hour of step aerobics wake up feeling less sore than usual, the researchers report.

Try vitamin C before you spring-clean or plow up your garden patch. It won't make the work easier, but tomorrow will be a better day.

*Source:*
*Medical Update* (19,4:6)

## Vitamin fends off muscle damage

Vitamin E supplementation may be essential to older people who exercise on a regular basis. Though exercise provides great health benefits to older people, it can cause muscle damage. Some muscle damage during exercise is normal and occurs even in young people. Our bodies have a built-in immune response to this and repairs the damage. However, older people's bodies don't seem to repair the damage as easily. Vitamin E helps to boost this immune response.

Exercise also may increase the body's production of free radicals. Radicals are unstable oxygen molecules which can damage muscle tissue and cell membranes. Because you take in more oxygen when you exercise, more of that oxygen may be converted into radicals. Vitamin E is an effective antioxidant, and it may help control those damaging radicals.

*Sources:*
*American Journal of Physiology* (264:R992,1993)
*Cancer Weekly* (March 22, 1993)
*The Journal of Nutrition* (122,3S:796)

## Walking: the wonder drug

The excuses range from, "I can't find enough time in the day" to "I'm already overweight, so why bother?" to "I can't afford to go to a health club." Although the excuses may sound reasonable, they can't hide one plain fact: If you want to feel better, look better, and live longer, you need to start exercising.

If you are making too many excuses to avoid exercising, it may be that you've chosen the wrong exercise program. Find something you like to do — something simple and easy to do wherever you are, with very little expensive clothing or equipment.

We've got the answer for you: Try the one exercise human beings are perfectly designed to do. Walk!

Research has proven that just plain walking for 30 minutes a day provides long-lasting health benefits. And there are no fancy outfits, no weights, no classes to attend.

Not only does walking get you out in the sunshine, or at least the mall, it also enriches your health, both physically and mentally. Look what walking can do for you:

- ◆ Burns calories at the rate of approximately 100 calories per mile.
- ◆ Improves digestion. Heartburn, gas, constipation — whatever you're troubled with, exercise is sure to help.
- ◆ Improves your mood. People who exercise regularly are less likely to be depressed. Several studies reveal that exercise helps lift depression as much as regular counseling does.
- ◆ Reduces your risk of high blood pressure, heart disease, diabetes, osteoporosis, and colon cancer.
- ◆ Improves your circulation.
- ◆ Helps relieve stress.

**Find the time.** Studies show that a lack of time is the number one reason most adults don't exercise. If time is a major concern to you, break up your 30 minute walking routine into three 10-minute intervals. You'll receive the same health benefits as walking the 30 minutes all at one time.

**Don't worry about speed.** If you're an overweight beginner, don't worry about how hard or fast you walk. The important thing is to get up and get moving. To achieve the best results, adults should build up to a moderate-intensity workout, which translates to a walking speed of 3 to 4 miles per hour. Walking 30 minutes at this pace is equal to walking about two miles.

A higher intensity workout such as speed walking will naturally help burn fat and build muscle, and it may help suppress your appetite. But studies show that fat loss is more related to the amount of energy you use during exercise rather than the intensity of the exercise itself. So, a low-intensity workout that lasts a long time can dramatically change the composition of your body.

**Lose fat without dieting.** Walking programs that gradually increase the length of time that you walk and the pace are great for many overweight people. Although your body weight may not change a lot at first, the composition of your weight will. Many people lose a noticeable amount of fat and gain lean body mass without even dieting. Imagine what a walking program coupled with a low-fat diet will do for your profile!

**Start with a stroll; finish with a power stride.** In an organized walking program you'll gradually move through the three stages of walking. The first style, strolling, is for beginners. This involves walking at a slower pace for 20 minutes, four days a week.

After two weeks, move up to the second stage known as striding. Striding is faster-paced and requires longer steps. Your heart rate will increase, and you'll really begin to reap the health benefits of your efforts. Although breathing will be harder, you should still be able to carry on a conversation with your walking partner without getting short of breath.

After three to four weeks of striding and the approval of your doctor, you can graduate to the third stage of walking known as power striding. This stage involves holding hand weights and vigorously swinging your arms. Swinging the weights builds up your shoulder and arm muscles. Legs, heart, lungs, arms, and shoulders — they all benefit from power striding.

**Set your pace with music.** To help you keep up a good pace, check out the cassette tape section at your local music store. You can buy tapes of music chosen specifically for walking. Music with 108 beats per minute keeps you walking at 3 mph. For all of you "power walkers," you can even get tapes that go up to 175 beats per minute, which will keep you striding along at a brisk 5 mph.

**Before hitting the open road, think about your feet.** Choose safe and comfortable walking shoes. Running shoes are not the same as walking shoes. Because your feet have more contact with the ground during walking, you need the greater flexibility and smaller tread of walking shoes. Don't forget to replace your walking shoes every four to six months. Worn-out shoes can lead to injury.

One final tip to help jump-start your exercise program: Turn off the television. Instead of heading for the couch to watch a movie on a sunny afternoon, go outside and take a brisk walk.

If you can't get motivated, recruit a friend to help you out. The more the merrier applies to exercise. Instead of meeting your friend at a restaurant, meet at the park for a walk. A friend provides encouragement and motivation. Besides, it's safer to walk with a partner.

Once you start a walking program, you'll probably want to keep it up forever. It's that easy. When you realize how much better you look and feel, you'll ask yourself why you didn't start sooner.

*Sources:*
*The Journal of the American Dietetic Association* (95,6:661)
*The Journal of the American Medical Association* (273,5:402)

## Safe ways to walk with weights

Weights can turn walking into a vigorous workout, but only if you know what you're doing. You don't want to strain your body or injure your bones and joints. To safely build fitness and upper body strength with weights, follow these precautions:

◆ Start out with one-pound weights.

- If possible, use hand weights one day, ankle weights the next, then vest weights, then no weights. When you finish the cycle, start over with hand weights. (A weighted vest works like a well-packed backpack. Either a vest or a backpack is a good option because they won't stress your joints like hand or ankle weights can. Depending on your size, it may take as much as 50 pounds worn close to the chest to increase the intensity of your workout.)
- If you have trouble with wrist pain, you may not be comfortable holding hand weights. Consider buying wrist weights.
- Don't lengthen your stride when you use weights, especially ankle weights. If you want to work harder, walk faster.
- Never let your arms swing freely when you hold weights. Use controlled movements so that you won't stress your shoulders and elbows.
- Carry a shoelace so that you can let go of your weights if your joints begin aching. Tie one weight to each end of the string. Loop the lace over your shoulders and behind your neck.
- Don't let the weights just hang at your side. That won't contribute to your workout. Bend your elbows and pump the weights from thigh level to eye level.
- To take stress off your shoulder and elbow joints, alternate pumping with some other motions — shrug, raise your arms out to the sides, or punch at a pretend opponent.

*Source:*
*The Physician and Sportsmedicine* (23,10:81)

## Top-ranking exercise machine

If you prefer to exercise in the privacy and comfort of your own home, a treadmill may be your best bet.

When different exercise machines were rated according to how much energy was actually expended at various levels of difficulty, the treadmill came out on top. For example, at a difficulty level of "somewhat hard," the average person expends about 700 calories an hour on a treadmill. At the same level of difficulty, the same person would only expend about 500 calories an hour using a cycle ergometer (a stationary bike which measures energy output). Therefore, you get a better workout on the treadmill, even though it seems just as easy.

Since an exercise machine won't do you any good if you don't use it, try to find a machine that you enjoy using. If you prefer cycling to walking or running, a stationary bike might be a better choice for you than a treadmill.

Price is always a consideration. Exercise machines come in a wide variety of price ranges. Try buying a used machine at first, at least until you find one you like. Shop around for a machine that's right for you. Most importantly, once you find the right machine, don't just put it in the closet. Instead, put it to good use.

*Source:*
*The Journal of the American Medical Association* (275,8:1424)

## Better bones for women

When you hear about weightlifting, you generally think about muscle-bound young men "pumping iron" in a gym. However, recent studies conducted on women ages 50 to 70 show that weightlifting isn't just for the young. These studies found that women who engaged in weight training gained bone density and muscle mass, improved their balance, and adopted a more active lifestyle. Weight training strengthens bones and helps protect them from osteoporosis, a disease that makes bones brittle.

*Source:*
*Nutrition Today* (30,2:52)

## Location motivation

Business people know that one of the most important ingredients for the success of a business is location. Turns out, that may be true for exercise, too. Though you can get the same physical benefits running on a treadmill as you can running outdoors, the psychological benefits may not be as great.

Psychologists have found that running outdoors increases your "feel-good" hormones and invigorates you. Running on a treadmill indoors, however, may make you depressed and tired. Your heart may not care where you exercise, but your head does. And if exercise makes you feel good, you're much more likely to stick with it.

*Source:*
*American Family Physician* (52,4:1091)

## Garden your way to fitness

Do you enjoy gardening but also want to find time to exercise? Don't leave your garden to dash off to the gym just yet. Gardening can provide you with a great exercise program as well as beautiful flowers and tasty vegetables.

Gardening can burn as many calories as an aerobics class. It's all in how you go about it. Different gardening activities require different levels of energy. The toughest gardening feats include mowing the lawn (with a push mower), chopping wood, shoveling, and tilling. More moderate tasks include digging, raking, and planting.

Make the most of your gardening workout by following a few simple tips:

- ◆ Begin your gardening session by warming up, and make sure you cool down slowly afterward.
- ◆ Bend at your knees, not at your waist.
- ◆ Try switching your grip occasionally from your dominant hand when raking, hoeing, or digging.
- ◆ Garden in two to three hour spurts, rather than those all day long weekend sessions.

◆ Add stretching exercises to your gardening activities, such as the "lunge and weed."

Gardening is an excellent way to reap the rewards of your labor, and not just by growing an immaculate lawn or luscious tomatoes. You can enjoy yourself and watch your fitness blossom.

*Source:*
*The Saturday Evening Post* (267,5:14)

## Golfers beware

All golfers heed the warning when they hear "Fore," but there is another warning they should also heed. Golfers increase their risk of exposure to tick-borne infections when they chase balls into the woods. To reduce your risk:

◆ Use insect repellent.
◆ Wear long sleeves.
◆ Check for ticks upon leaving wooded areas.
◆ Consider taking an extra stroke instead of chasing that ball into the woods.

*Source:*
*The New England Journal of Medicine* (333,7:420)

## Get a grip on golf

If golf is your game, you can improve your grip using an old phone book. Open the phone book and moisten your fingertips. Using one hand, press down with your fingertips, and rip, crumple, and discard one page. Continue doing this until fatigued, alternating hands. You should be able to do more pages with your dominant hand. This exercise will improve grip strength, endurance, and flexibility.

*Source:*
*The Physician and Sportsmedicine* (24,1:22)

## The headache you shouldn't shrug off

Sore muscles after strenuous exercise are usually a good sign that your exercise program is working. A headache after intense exercise or movement of the neck, however, may warn of a serious injury.

On rare occasions, the violent motion from a roller-coaster can damage the tissues and blood vessels in the neck. This can lead to a stroke in a perfectly fit person, as one 31-year-old woman found out. After a trip to an amusement park, she suddenly developed neck pain and a severe headache.

After several days, she also developed dizziness and nausea. She then went to the hospital, where it was discovered that she had suffered a stroke, caused by damage to arteries in her neck. The same type of stroke can occur following an automobile accident (whiplash), hair washing by a beautician, chiropractic manipulation, certain yoga or gymnastic exercises, and prolonged overhead painting or upward gazing.

This type of headache may be caused by blood leaking out of a blood vessel in the brain. If you experience a severe headache for the first time after riding a roller-coaster or after strenuous exercise, go to the emergency room immediately.

*Source:*
*The New England Journal of Medicine* (332,23:1585)

# The Thin Within

## Forever free from weight worries

The mere mention of the word "diet" can take the joy out of life. You immediately envision a struggle against seemingly insurmountable odds. After all, millions of people are on a diet at any given time. Most of them will fail to lose weight, or fail to keep it off. The problem may be that diets just aren't any fun. You feel deprived and tired, and eventually give up. It doesn't have to be that way. A healthy lifestyle will naturally lead you to a healthy weight.

**Set realistic goals.** The first step to losing weight is to set a realistic goal. See "How to Calculate Your Healthy Weight" later in this chapter to determine your ideal weight, or ask your doctor to help you set a reasonable goal.

**Take your time.** Quick weight loss is usually temporary weight loss. If you want to lose weight and keep it off for years, you have to change your habits for good. Shortcuts and fad diets just don't work in the long run.

**Balance your diet.** You should eat a wide variety of foods and not deprive yourself of your favorites. Moderation is the key. There are no "good" or "bad" foods. You can enjoy the foods you love in reasonable amounts. In fact, depriving yourself of your favorite foods may result in craving and binge eating, which will make you *gain* weight. Balance your diet over several days, so that if you happen to have a special occasion, and want to eat cake, you can cut back a little on other days. What counts is the overall picture.

**Make exercise fun.** Exercise does not need to be a grueling two-hour workout every day. Moderate exercise totaling 30 minutes a day effectively helps control your weight. You can space the exercise out with a few minutes here and a few minutes there, so you don't tire yourself out. If exercise is fun, you're much more likely to continue it.

Losing weight does not have to be an agonizing process. Eat healthy foods, stay active, and let nature take its course.

*Sources:*
*FDA Consumer* (30,1:16)
*Nutrition Today* (30,3:108)

## Calculating your healthy weight

You may think you'd like to weigh 100 pounds, but would that really be healthy for you? In a society of willowy role models, it's tough to be an oak, but maybe that's best for you. How do you determine your healthy weight? Doctors usually use the body mass index (BMI) to determine what you should weigh. This method involves a little math, so have a calculator handy.

**Step 1.** Calculate your height in inches. For example, if you're 5 feet 8 inches tall, this number would be 68.

**Step 2.** Square your height in inches. Using the above example, 68 squared would be 4,624 (68x68).

**Step 3.** Divide your weight in pounds by your squared height. Let's say you weigh 159 pounds. You would divide 159 by 4,624, which equals .034.

**Step 4.** Multiply the number you calculated in step 3 by 705 to get your BMI. Using our example, you would multiply .034 by 705 to find the BMI, which in this case is 23.9.

A body mass of 19.1 to 25.8 is considered healthy for women. A BMI of 25.8 to 27.3 is considered slightly overweight and moderately risky. If you're a woman, the higher your BMI goes above 27.3, the greater the health risks you're likely to face.

Because men generally have more muscle mass than women, their average BMIs are slightly higher. Men with a BMI of 20.7 to 26.4 are considered healthy. A BMI of 27.8 to 31.1 is considered slightly overweight and moderately risky. If you're a man, the higher your BMI goes above 32.2, the greater your health risk.

Though BMI is the best method for calculating desirable body weight, it does not take into account the difference between lean muscle mass and fat. Therefore, if you are very muscular, your BMI might indicate that you are overweight. However, for most people, this method works well.

*Source:*
*Hamilton & Whitney's Nutrition Concepts and Controversies,* West Publishing, New York, 1994

# 10 ways to lose a pound a week

Did you ever wonder what it takes to lose a pound (or gain one)? 3,500 calories to be exact. That means to lose a pound, you must burn 3,500 calories more than you take in. Sound tough? It doesn't have to be. If you cut a few calories here and a few calories there, over the course of a week, those saved calories can quickly add up and take a pound off your frame.

◆ Drink water or fruit juice without added sugar instead of soda or other sweetened beverages.

◆ Substitute skim milk for whole milk and save 60 calories per cup.

◆ Choose meat cuts carefully. Those graded "select" tend to be the lowest in fat.

◆ Trim excess fat from meat and remove skin from chicken before cooking.

◆ Buy canned tuna packed in water instead of oil. You'll save 60 calories per three ounce serving.

◆ Make smart snack choices. Two chocolate chip cookies have about 90 calories, but 10 pretzel sticks only have about 10 calories. Read labels carefully.

◆ Consider reduced-calorie mayonnaise. It has only about 35 calories per tablespoon, while real mayonnaise has 100.

◆ Use low-fat cooking methods, such as broiling, poaching, grilling, and baking instead of frying.

- ◆ Eat a variety of healthy foods to get proper nutrition and avoid cravings.
- ◆ Cut the fat. All fats contain nine calories per gram. All carbohydrates contain four calories per gram. Cutting fats in favor of more carbohydrates will soon help eliminate those excess pounds.

*Sources:*
*Foods That Cause You to Lose Weight,* The Magni Group, McKinney, Texas, 1992
*Shopping for Food and Making Meals in Minutes Using Dietary Guidelines,* U.S, Department of Agriculture, Human Nutrition Information Service, Home and Garden Bulletin No. 232-10

# Control your food cravings

"Once a month, I crave chocolate candy bars."

Is this a compulsive overeater talking? Nope. It's food disorder expert Dr. Dina Zeckhausen.

"It's pretty normal to have a food craving. But I can have one chocolate bar and stop. Compulsive overeaters can't," she explains.

There's a big difference between simply overeating and *compulsively* overeating. "We all go a little overboard occasionally, particularly when food is abundant and we're in a celebratory mood," says Marietta, Georgia-based psychologist Dina Zeckhausen. "It's also normal to sometimes eat in response to stress — like getting ice cream as comfort food after a bad day at work. Normal eaters are aware they are doing this, and they quickly reestablish their normal eating patterns. This is not compulsive overeating."

On the other hand, if you think about food most of the time and find it difficult to stop eating once you start, you may be a compulsive overeater. It's not what compulsive eaters consume that's their biggest problem — it's the emotional problems behind their food obsession.

Any emotion can spark a compulsive eater's binge — sadness, happiness, or boredom. "Once they start eating, they find it difficult to stop. Many feel they're in a trance-like state," Dr. Zeckhausen comments.

**Food can be addictive.** It may literally have drug-like effects on some people. Researchers have discovered brain chemicals called endorphins (natural tranquilizers) that are boosted by eating. Neurobiologist Sara Leibowitz of Rockefeller University suspects compulsive overeaters may have an imbalance of endorphins.

Emotional stress can deplete your brain cells of another chemical, serotonin, resulting in depression and a loss of energy. Since eating sugars and starches hikes serotonin levels and perks up your mood, some researchers believe low levels of serotonin may also spur compulsive overeating.

According to Dr. Zeckhausen, compulsive overeaters' behavior — using food to alter mood, sneaking and lying about it, the resulting self-loathing — is similar to that of drug abusers. But while addicts and alcoholics can give up the substances wreaking havoc in their lives, compulsive overeaters can't live without food.

**You can develop a healthy relationship with food.** If you think you may be a compulsive overeater, here are some steps you can take to regain control of your eating:

◆ Learn to love and accept yourself. Make a list of your good qualities and read it often.

◆ Find a group of people, such as a network of friends, a church group, or a support group led by a person trained in eating disorders, where you will be accepted while you work on your eating problem.

◆ Don't try to be "cured" by a strict diet. Nerve chemicals and hormones go wildly out of whack during quick weight loss diets. The result is more cravings and binge eating. Have several small meals a day, balanced with carbohydrates, protein, and fat, instead of a couple of huge ones. You'll keep your blood sugar and brain chemicals stable, and you'll help curb your overeating.

◆ Learn to recognize your trigger foods. If potato chips are irresistible, don't buy them. Don't go grocery shopping on an empty stomach; compulsive eaters are likely to grab everything in sight. Rent a video instead of going to the movies if the smell of popcorn sets you on a binge.

◆ Get in touch with your feelings. Is your stomach hungry, or is it really your heart? What emotional traumas do you need to deal with? Get these issues out in the open and deal with them.

How long does it take to normalize your eating? "There's no quick fix, but you can change these problems if you are committed to it," answers Dr. Zeckhausen. "Sometimes it's very hard to look at the pain you have been trying to avoid. But it's worth it. You are getting back something precious — your ability to love yourself and make healthy choices for yourself."

*Sources:*
Dina Zeckhausen, Ph.D., clinical psychologist, private practice, Marietta, Ga.
*Food & Mood,* Henry Holt and Company, New York, 1995
*The Atlanta Journal/Constitution* (Oct. 18, 1995, E3)
*The Complete Life Encyclopedia,* Thomas Nelson Publishers, Nashville, Tenn., 1995

# Miracle mineral boosts metabolism

*Chromium picolinate.* Though it may sound like a shiny car part, or maybe a hot Mexican dish, don't let the funny name fool you. It may be the secret weapon you need to help you win the weight loss war.

If you've been to a health food store lately, you've probably seen chromium picolinate supplements advertised as "fat burners." It may look like just another weight loss fad. After all, people have been searching for years for an easy way to lose weight. "Miracle" products always attract a lot of attention before they fade away. But this time the research seems to show that chromium picolinate is more than just another weight loss gimmick.

Chromium appears to aid weight loss in two ways:

**Lowers body fat.** Because chromium helps your body burn up fat more quickly, it can lower your percentage of body fat and help you lose weight.

**Builds muscle.** Chromium was tested on athletes who used it along with an exercise program. The athletes who took chromium picolinate supplements increased their muscle mass significantly after only two weeks, and they lost weight, too.

It certainly seems that chromium can play a part in weight control. However, about 90 percent of Americans don't get enough chromium in their diets. Recent surgery, a severe burn, a chronic wasting disease, or alcohol or other drug abuse may increase your need for chromium.

In addition, manufacturing often removes chromium from foods. Most people tend to eat a lot of prepackaged, highly processed foods such as sugar and white flour. This could be the reason so many people don't get enough chromium. Heavy exercise, such as long-distance running, can cause your body to lose chromium faster than usual.

Also, sometimes your body doesn't absorb chromium very easily. Some scientists think that less than 1 percent of the chromium in foods you eat is actually absorbed by your body. Taking calcium carbonate supplements can also limit how much chromium your body can absorb. To make it easier to absorb, some manufacturers add picolinate acid to chromium. This results in chromium picolinate, which is more easily absorbed.

If you're curious about your chromium level, ask your doctor for a serum chromium test. Always talk to your doctor before taking chromium (or any other supplement), especially if you have diabetes or a lung, liver, or kidney disease.

One recent study also raised concerns about chromium's possible ability to cause chromosome damage that could lead to cancer. Researchers found a normal dose of chromium picolinate damaged chromosomes in the ovary cells in Chinese hamsters. Researchers noted that the type of chromosome damage they observed can eventually cause cancer. Chromium nicotinate, another popular form of chromium supplement, did not have this effect.

If you would rather get your chromium from the foods you eat, try some of these delicious natural sources of chromium:

- Apples with skins
- Asparagus
- Brewer's yeast
- Liver
- Mushrooms
- Nuts
- Oysters, fish, and other seafood
- Prunes

Even though chromium isn't a miracle cure for controlling your weight, it may help. Just remember that no supplement will ever take the place of a sensible diet and exercise program. More study is needed to determine chromium's full potential as well as possible side effects. In the meantime, chromium may offer hope for those who constantly fight the battle of the bulge.

**Sources:**
*FASEB Journal* (9:1643)
*Hamilton & Whitney's Nutrition Concepts and Controversies*, West Publishing, New York, 1994
*Medical Tribune for the Family Physician* (35,10:19)
*Nutrition Health Review* (53:14)
*The Complete Guide to Vitamins, Minerals, and Supplements*, Fisher Books, Tucson, Ariz., 1988
*The Doctor's Complete Guide to Vitamins and Minerals*, Dell Publishing, New York, 1994
*The Physician and Sportsmedicine* (22,8:30)
*The Real Vitamin and Mineral Book*, Avery Publishing Group, Garden City Park, New York, 1990

# Fill up with fiber

When you're trying to lose weight, that gnawing, empty feeling in your stomach can sabotage even the strongest will. To feel full longer and delay the onset of hunger, eat meals that are high in fiber.

Fiber fills you up because it absorbs water and swells, taking up more space. Fiber also slows movement of your food through your upper digestive tract, so that you don't get hungry again as quickly.

Foods that are high in fiber include:

◆  fruits
◆  vegetables
◆  legumes
◆  grains such as oats, barley, wheat, rice, and rye

**Source:**
*Hamilton and Whitney's Nutrition Concepts and Controversies*, West Publishing Company, New York, 1994

# Unmasking the insulin resistance myth

Bad news travels fast, good news travels slow. However, when weight loss is involved, any news travels like wildfire. The latest rumor on the weight-loss grapevine is that most overweight people are insulin-resistant and should eat high-fat, low-carbohydrate diets. Great news if you've always struggled with your weight because you love fatty, fried foods. But before you fill your shopping cart with lard for all those pork chop and gravy dinners you've already planned, make sure you've gotten the facts straight.

**What is insulin-resistance?** You probably know that insulin is a hormone associated with diabetes. The fact that many diabetics must have insulin shots may have led you to believe that they have less insulin than the rest of us. That's not always true. While Type I diabetics (insulin-dependent) don't produce enough insulin, most diabetics (Type II noninsulin-dependent) have plenty of insulin. Their insulin just doesn't do its job properly, which is letting sugar pass from the blood into the body's cells to be used for energy. Having ineffective insulin, or insulin-resistance, causes your body to produce more and more insulin to try to get the job done. While many diabetics are insulin-resistant, some nondiabetics may also be insulin-resistant, which can lead to too much insulin in the body.

**How can insulin hurt you?** Too much insulin in your body raises your risk of heart disease, diabetes, and high blood pressure. Experts estimate that perhaps as many as one-fourth of the population (besides diabetics) may be insulin-resistant. While excess insulin does occur more often in overweight people, it may be the result of the weight problem and not the cause. When people who are insulin-resistant lose weight, their insulin levels usually return to normal.

**How should insulin-resistant people eat?** Although a high-carbohydrate, low-fat diet will raise insulin levels in insulin-resistant people, if that diet helps you lose weight, your insulin will then drop. The bottom line seems to be that you need to maintain a healthy weight whether or not you are insulin-resistant. What's the best way to do that? Any diet that cuts calories will help you lose weight. Regular exercise will help you lose weight. So, what's the word on the high-carbohydrate, low-fat diet as opposed to the high-fat, low-carbohydrate diet? Studies find that people lose the same amount of weight on either diet as long as the calorie intake is equal. However, studies also prove that high-fat diets increase your risk of heart disease and cancer, and evidence indicates that low-fat diets are easier to maintain.

**How do you know if you're insulin-resistant?** If you want to know if you're insulin-resistant, have your doctor give you a blood test. If your triglyceride level is over 200 and your HDL cholesterol is below 35, you're probably insulin-resistant.

Now that you know the facts, you can make an informed decision about your diet. Your best bet will probably be to cut the fat in favor of a sensible diet and exercise.

*Source:*
*Nutrition Action Healthletter* (22,4:4)

# Fight flab with breakfast

If you wish to prevent unwanted weight gain, then eat a hearty breakfast, suggest researchers from the Department of Nutrition at Complutense University in Madrid, Spain.

The secret of how to prevent unwanted weight gain really is that simple, according to their recent study of 122 people between the ages of 65 and 95. Their findings support several earlier studies which indicated that going without breakfast or eating a skimpy breakfast sabotages other attempts to eat healthy for the rest of the day. People with poor breakfast habits are more likely to choose fattier or higher calorie foods throughout the day. They're also more likely to snack impulsively.

The researchers found that normal weight people who ate breakfast generally had healthier eating habits than their fatter friends. For example, normal weight people preferred fruit, juices, and bread for breakfast while the heavier people preferred fried, fattier foods.

Normal weight people also included more variety in their breakfasts, eating many different foods from several different food groups, with a focus on their favorite food, fruit. Normal weight people got more fiber, iron, and vitamin E from their breakfasts, too.

They also spent more time eating breakfast and consumed more calories at breakfast than the heavier people. Some nutrition specialists recommend that 20 to 25 percent of your daily calories come from breakfast.

Take time for breakfast. It helps make sure you eat healthy for the rest of the day, which goes a long way toward helping you maintain a healthy weight.

**Source:**
*Journal of the American College of Nutrition* (15,1:65)

## Nighttime eating: a no-no or not?

Have you heard that everything you eat after five p.m. turns straight into fat — that you might as well take that late-night snack and apply it directly to your hips? Well, now hear this. According to a recent study of women's eating habits, that old belief doesn't add up to extra pounds after all.

The study found that a calorie has the same effect no matter what time of day it is consumed. However, according to the study, women who ate most of their calories at night got less vitamin C, vitamin B6, folate, and carbohydrates from their diet than women who spread their calories out more over the day. Nighttime eaters were also more likely to get more calories from fat, protein, and alcohol. This could be because they were so hungry by the time they ate, they made poor nutritional choices.

If you choose to eat more after the sun goes down, just make sure you're eating a balanced diet. That cheesecake has the same amount of calories at 10 p.m. as it did at 10 a.m.

**Source:**
*Medical Tribune for the Internist and Cardiologist* (36,18:8)

## Diet pills don't measure up

Do you pop a diet pill every day in the hopes that it will make your struggle to be slim easier?

Most over-the-counter (OTC) diet pills contain phenylpropanolamine (PPA) as their active ingredient. Products such as Dexatrim and Acutrim usually contain 75 mg of controlled release PPA. These products are meant to be used along with a diet and exercise program. However, according to the FDA's Office of OTC Drug Evaluation, using these diet pills probably won't help the pounds come off much faster. Even the best studies only show a half-pound a week greater weight loss with the pills than with diet and exercise alone.

Of course, a half-pound a week does add up. However, you should be careful not to exceed the recommended dosage of these drugs because of possible side effects, like high blood pressure and rapid heartbeat. Since some OTC cough and cold remedies also use PPA as a nasal decongestant, read labels carefully. You could easily get too much PPA by using it in two different products.

A study is currently underway to determine whether PPA may contribute to the risk of stroke. At the present time, the FDA says that they still consider PPA safe to use in the recommended dosage.

If you think you need the extra boost that OTC weight loss drugs may give, just be aware of the possible side effects, and don't get your expectations too high.

*Source:*
*FDA Consumer* (30,1:16)

# Anti-obesity drug promises relief from emotional eating

Do you drown your sorrows in ice cream or ease your stress with potato chips? Do you ever wonder why food has the power to make you feel better? Though you probably think there is a psychological reason for this, the answer may actually be physical.

A chemical in the brain called serotonin affects both eating and emotions. Certain foods trigger the body to make more serotonin, and set off the brain's stress-relieving system. When you are down or upset, you crave these foods because your body knows that eating them will make you feel better.

What kind of foods have this power? Carbohydrates, which come in two forms, sugars (simple carbohydrates) and starches (complex carbohydrates). That's why when you have the urge to binge, it's usually for sweet or starchy foods.

The FDA recently approved *dexfenfluramine* (Redux) for use as an anti-obesity drug. Dexfenfluramine releases serotonin in order to reduce your appetite. In one study by the FDA, six out of 10 people taking dexfenfluramine lost weight. Only three out of 10 who were not taking the drug lost weight.

The FDA does not say how long a person can take dexfenfluramine, but will require it to carry a warning label that says results have not been studied for more than one year. Though some doctors are concerned that it may cause brain or lung damage, the FDA says that the only side effects so far are diarrhea, dry mouth, sleep problems, and a general feeling of weakness.

*Sources:*
*Healthy Weight Journal* (10,4:65)
*The Serotonin Solution*, Fawcett Columbine, New York, 1996

# Eat more, weigh less

You've been counting calories for years, but did you know you should count fat grams, too?

A study from Indiana University found that overweight people ate about the same amount of calories as lean people. However, the plump people ate more fat and added sugar, while the lean people ate more fiber. This study seems to indicate that you can eat more food if you just change the form of the calories from fat and sugar to more fiber.

*Source:*
*Healthy Weight Journal* (10,3:45)

## The biggest source of saturated fat

Do you love cheesy lasagna, grilled cheese sandwiches, and macaroni and cheese? If so, you have lots of company. A recent study found that American women get most of their saturated fat from cheese. If you don't want to give up the food you love, try some of the modified-fat or fat-free varieties. While the modified-fat versions can lower cholesterol, they contain about the same amount of calories as regular cheese. Fat-free cheese, on the other hand, is lower in both calories and fat.

*Source:*
*Medical Update* (19,8:6)

## Good burgers without grease

If you love burgers, but hate the fat, try this cooking method. Microwave your patties for one to three minutes, pour off the liquid, and then fry, broil, or grill them. This method cuts the fat content by almost one-third, and has another benefit besides. Substances which may cause cancer are sometimes formed when cooking burgers at high temperatures. This method reduces those substances by as much as 90 percent.

You can also cut about half the fat out of the ground beef you use for spaghetti, chili, or other recipes that call for crumbled meat. Take the following steps:

◆ Brown the meat in a skillet.
◆ Place the meat on paper towels and blot it dry.
◆ Put the meat in a colander and rinse with water.
◆ Drain well.

*Source:*
*Food, Nutrition, and Health* (19,8:5)

## Nutritional flaws of fake fats

Isn't the genuine article always better than a fake? Maybe not. If you're an environmentalist, you probably wouldn't be caught dead wearing a mink ... unless it's fake fur. And if you're concerned about your weight, you may be considering using "fake fat."

A healthy diet means limiting the amount of fat you eat. However, you may find it difficult to sacrifice the taste and texture of fat for the sake of good health. Fat substitutes attempt to mimic the flavor and creaminess of fat without adding calories and clogging arteries like real fat.

Many of the numerous fat-free and reduced fat products on the market use some type of fat substitute. *Simplesse* has probably been around the longest. It has been in use since 1989. *Simplesse* is made from protein and can be found in many types of desserts, cheese, mayonnaise, and other refrigerated foods. It may not be listed by name on the product label, but may instead be described as a protein complex. *Simplesse* isn't available for cooking, and if you are on a protein-restricted diet, you may not be able to eat *Simplesse*.

The Food and Drug Administration (FDA) recently gave the thumbs up to the newest kid on the fat substitute block — olestra (*Olean*). Olestra is a compound of fatty acids and sugar. Your body does not absorb olestra, so it doesn't contribute any calories or fat to your diet. Olestra can be used for cooking. Some scientists have protested the FDA's approval of olestra for public sale. The FDA admits that olestra may cause loose stools and stomach cramps in some people, and may rob the body of certain fat-soluble vitamins like A, D, E, and K, as well as the antioxidant beta carotene. Before they approved this fat substitute, the FDA required the manufacturer to agree to add extra amounts of these vitamins to products containing olestra. These products must also carry a warning label about the possibility of stomach cramps.

Though fat substitutes obviously have their drawbacks, so does real fat. Fat-free products offer new variety, but there is still no substitute for foods that are naturally low in fat, like fruits and vegetables.

*Sources:*
Arthritis Today (10,3:48)
Science News (149,5:68)

## Still flabby after all those fat-free foods?

Fat-free products have flooded the market. Fat-free ice cream, cookies, and cakes line grocery store aisles, enticing you with their tantalizing guilt-free taste. With all these fat-free goodies at your fingertips, why are you still getting fat?

If a product is fat-free, you can eat as much of it as you want, right? Wrong. While eating low-fat helps control weight as well as protecting you from many serious diseases, you cannot take in an unlimited amount of calories without gaining weight.

Pay special attention to serving size on a food label because all other information listed is on a per-serving basis. Low-fat and even low-calorie foods can still cause you to gain weight if you eat multiple servings.

If you want to lose weight, you have to burn more calories than you take in. Limiting fat helps, but does not give you a gold card to carefree calorie consumption. You must watch your fat *and* your calories for a healthy lifestyle.

*Source:*
Nutrition Research Newsletter (14,6:71)

## The up side of yo-yo dieting

Have you experienced the ups and downs of weight cycling? If so, you may have heard that it's better to remain at a constant weight, even if that weight is roughly equivalent to that of a minivan. New studies, however, prove that weight cycling may not be so bad after all.

One reason that weight cycling has gotten such a bad rap is that it supposedly had a negative effect on metabolism. A review of 43 studies on weight cycling revealed no evidence that the losing and regaining merry-go-round permanently lowers metabolism The same review also found no connection between weight cycling and fat distribution or lean body mass. The main drawback to the ups and downs of weight loss could be the psychological effect — the harm to a dieter's self-esteem.

Another recent study on heart disease followed 153 overweight people for almost two and a half years. They were divided into groups who lost weight, gained weight, remained at a constant weight, or lost and regained. At the end of the study, those who lost weight had significantly reduced their risk factors for heart disease, while those who gained were at the greatest risk. The weight cyclers actually showed improvement in some risk factors when compared to those whose weight remained constant.

Of course, no one wants to keep losing the same ten pounds over and over. But evidence indicates that it's just as easy to lose it the tenth time as it was the first, and you may be giving your heart a little boost. In the "weighting" game, even temporary losses seem to help, so if you can't stop the diet roller coaster at the bottom of a hill, just hold on tight and try again the next time around.

*Sources:*
*Medical Tribune for the Internist and Cardiologist* (36,16:20)
*The Journal of the American Medical Association* (272,15:1196)

# Battling your body's resistance to change

Even the most adventurous person sometimes resists change. A new job, a new home, or a new school might sound exciting, but it also causes feelings of apprehension. There's comfort in familiarity. Your body feels the same way about weight loss. While a new, slim body may be healthier for you, your body tends to try to return to your "normal" weight.

A recent study measured energy use in overweight people who lost 10 to 20 percent of their body weight, and people who were not overweight who gained 10 percent of their body weight. In people who lost weight, metabolism slowed to conserve energy. In people who gained weight, metabolism sped up to try to get rid of the new pounds.

This explains why it is so difficult to keep those pounds off once you shed them. However, persistence will pay off when you've maintained your new weight level long enough for your body to consider it your "normal" weight.

*Source:*
*Nutrition Today* (30,2:53)

# Extra benefits of extra weight

The government's weight guidelines for healthy weight changed in 1995. This meant many people who were at a healthy weight were suddenly unhealthy. This main basis for this change was a study of women ages 30 to 55.

This study found that even small weight gains around middle age could result in a higher death rate. The old guidelines had a different set of healthy weights for people over 35. Because this study found that gaining weight as you age can be unhealthy, the new guidelines have one set of suggested weights for all adults

However, if you're over 65 and a little overweight, it may be better to stay that way.

An older person who is a little overweight by the new guidelines, but is otherwise healthy, probably should not attempt to lose weight. A little extra weight may provide extra energy during times of illness and helps preserve bone and muscle mass as well.

*Sources:*
*The Journal of the American Medical Association* (275,23:1828)
*The New England Journal of Medicine* (333,11:678)

## Two steps to permanent weight loss

Diet and exercise work hand in hand to help you lose weight and keep it off. The only way to lose weight is to burn more calories than you take in. You can do that simply by restricting your calorie intake. However, if you add regular physical activity to your diet plan, you can afford to indulge your appetite a little more, and not feel so deprived.

Exercise can help you eat a healthier diet. According to a recent survey, people who get little exercise eat more fat than those who are physically active. Another study found that women who exercise on a regular basis are less likely to fall off the diet wagon than women who are inactive. This could be because the exercising women are too busy to think about food, or they experience a greater boost in self-esteem which helps them exert more control over their food choices. Whatever the reason, it seems that exercise not only burns calories, it also helps in the diet department.

Many people say that they simply cannot find time to exercise. However, these same people always find time to eat. Of course, if you didn't eat, you'd soon drop dead. Maybe you should view exercise the same way — as essential to sustaining life as eating and drinking. A mere 30 minutes of moderate exercise a day expends an extra 200 calories for most people. That 30 minutes of exercise doesn't even have to be all at one time. You can spread your exercise out over the day, 10 minutes here and 10 minutes there.

Add physical activity to your diet, and you'll lose weight quicker, stick to your diet better, and achieve a feeling of accomplishment that will help you maintain your healthy weight.

*Source:*
*Nutrition Today* (30,3:108)

## Creative exercise

You know you need to exercise to lose weight, but you break into a cold sweat at the very thought of sweating in front of a roomful of leotard-clad women and muscle-bound men. Calm down and mop off your brow. Exercise doesn't necessarily mean aerobic classes with a bunch of skinny strangers or pumping iron in a gym. If you enjoy those activities, great! But if you don't, you can still use exercise to become lean and fit.

In order to ensure that you stick to it, exercise should be as pleasurable as eating. Find activities that you enjoy and be creative.

◆ Yard work and gardening can be great exercise as well as giving you the spiffiest lawn in the neighborhood.

◆ Shopping in the mall burns up some extra calories and enables you to take care of important errands at the same time.

◆ Volunteer to chaperone a Boy Scout outing. Keeping up with energetic boys will definitely burn some calories, and you'll contribute to your community at the same time.

◆ Learn to dance. Many ballet schools offer classes for beginning adults, so you won't have to squeeze into a tutu and plié with eight-year-olds. There are also many other types of dance lessons available. There are square dance clubs, line dancing organizations, jazz and modern dance, and ballroom dancing.

◆ Though perhaps not very creative, the most common physical activity by far is walking. It doesn't require any expensive equipment and you can do it almost anywhere, at any time. You can make it more interesting by walking with a partner, jamming to some tunes on headphones, or finding interesting new places to walk.

*Source:*
*Nutrition Today* (30,3:108)

# Best gut buster: no pain, all gain

If you're carrying a "spare tire" around your waist, you should know that the fat that gathers around and above the waist is the most deadly kind. It can cause an increased risk of high blood pressure, heart disease, diabetes, and some cancers.

An easy way to decide if you need to lose that paunch is to wrap a tape measure around your waist. If you're a man, your waist should be no bigger around than 37 inches. Women should have a waistline no bigger than 34.7 inches. If you failed to measure up to a healthy waistline, there's still hope. You can melt off that belly fat easier than you think.

You know that you should maintain a healthy diet and get regular exercise, but your exercise should work all your muscles, not just your stomach. So forget those gut-wrenching sit-ups, and go for a brisk walk.

You should also take time every day to relax. For some reason, chemicals that are released when you are under stress will cause your body to redistribute fat from other parts of your body to your waist. If you can successfully limit your stress, you'll have better luck losing that dangerous belly fat.

*Sources:*
*Medical Abstracts Newsletter* (15,9:4)
*Medical Update* (19,6:2)

# Natural Care for Nails, Skin, and Hair

## A little gray hair can break your back

Those gray hairs on your head may be telling more about you than your age. Researchers say there is a link between premature gray hair and osteoporosis. Premature gray hair is defined as more than one-half of your hair graying before age 40.

In a study of 63 people being treated for osteoporosis, a strong link was discovered between early graying and low bone density. Researchers have two theories on the gray matter. One is that the genes responsible for early graying may also be responsible for bone mass. Others believe that bone weakening and hair pigmentation are related.

To prevent osteoporosis, exercise regularly and eat foods high in calcium. Milk and milk products, broccoli, and sardines are good sources of calcium.

*Source:*
*American Family Physician* (50,6:1193)

## Getting to the root of excess hair

From the time they're old enough to shave their legs, women fight the battle of excess hair in the interest of looking feminine. It's a tough enough battle with a normal amount of hair, but if you suddenly have lots of thick, dark hair on your face, chest, stomach, and back, it's a nightmare. This condition is called hirsutism, and it affects both men and women. In many cultures, it's only a problem for women.

A hormone imbalance can cause hirsutism. When your body produces too many male hormones, called androgens, an excess of hair grows. This can also happen when your hair follicles are overly sensitive to the androgens. If you're overweight, the best self-help method for dealing with hirsutism is to lose weight. This reduces the amount of hormones in your body that caused the excessive hair growth.

Hirsutism can be triggered by taking birth control pills or anabolic steroids, hormone replacement therapy, or developing tumors. You should see your doctor if you develop hirsutism.

*Source:*
*American Family Physician* (52,6:1845)

## Hair loss culprits

Having too little hair can be just as upsetting as having too much. If hair loss is hereditary, there isn't much you can do about it. But some things you might not suspect can cause hair loss, and you might be able to avoid or eliminate them if you know what they are. Some possible causes include illness, nutritional deficiency, fungal infection, problems with your thyroid or parathyroid glands, extreme stress, rapid weight loss, high fever, childbirth, exposure to pesticides or toxins, beta-blocker drugs, and anticoagulant drugs.

If you are bothered by hair loss, check with your doctor. It might be caused by something within your control.

**Source:**
*The Journal of the American Medical Association* (273,11:897)

## Turn up the power of your dandruff shampoo

If you have embarrassing flakes of dandruff, you're probably using a dandruff shampoo and wishing the results were better. Well, they can be.

To get the most benefit from your dandruff shampoo, leave the shampooing for last when you take a shower. Lather up with the shampoo, wrap your head in a towel, and wait 30 minutes before rinsing. This should dramatically increase the effectiveness of your dandruff shampoo.

Dandruff shampoos don't usually cure the problem the first couple of times you use them. It may take six weeks or more for you to get the maximum benefit.

**Source:**
*American Family Physician* (52,7:2017)

## Hair today, green tomorrow

If you're the lead singer in a rock band you might want green hair. But if you live in a more conservative environment and your lovely blond locks are suddenly ghastly green, you might not be so pleased.

Green hair can result from exposure to copper in the water you bathe or swim in. When tap water is fluoridated, the water becomes more acidic, and this can cause household pipes to release copper into the water. When electrical grounds connect to copper water pipes, the current can dissolve copper into the water. And if water stands in copper pipes for more than 48 hours, or even flows through corroded copper plumbing, it can have a high copper concentration. Swimming pools may have copper-based chemicals added to the water to kill algae.

Not everyone with blond, white, or gray hair will acquire the green hue, even when they're exposed to copper in their water. If you have really healthy hair, and the *cuticle* (outer surface) of your hair is not damaged, you probably won't get the odd color. If your hair is damaged from bleaching, perming, sun exposure, or overuse of blow dryers and curling irons, it has a much better chance of turning green. Coming in contact with alkaline shampoo, which changes the acidity of hair, or chlorinated water, such as in a swimming pool, can complete the unwanted tinting process.

Some home treatments for your green hair problem are shampooing regularly, soaking your hair in a 3 percent hydrogen peroxide solution, treating your hair with warm vegetable oil, and using a special shampoo to remove the copper deposits. See your doctor if your green hair persists, unless you're considering a career in rock music

**Source:**
*Cutis* (56,1:37)

## Stop skin cancer before it starts

Although skin cancer can be fatal, being informed can help protect you from this deadly disease. Here are some general, common-sense rules to follow:

◆ Avoid outside activities in the midday sun (between 10 a.m. and 2 p.m.).
◆ Wear a wide-brimmed hat.
◆ Wear sunglasses that block ultraviolet (UV) rays.
◆ Protect as much of your skin as possible by wearing clothing made of tightly woven fabric, such as broadcloth or denim.
◆ Use a sunscreen with a sun protection factor (SPF) of at least 15 whenever you're planning to be in the sun longer than 15 minutes.
◆ Eat a healthy diet including lots of fresh fruits and vegetables.

**Source:**
*FDA Consumer* (29,6:10)

## ABCs of skin moles

The incidence of skin cancer has increased rapidly in the last 50 years, and today it's the most common form of cancer. The good news is that skin cancer is usually curable, if diagnosed early enough. That's why it is important to examine yourself for early signs of the disease.

Counting the number of moles you have is a fairly reliable indicator of how likely you are to develop skin cancer. By adulthood, the average person has 15 to 20 moles. People with mole counts higher than average have a greater risk of developing skin cancer.

When you are counting your moles, it is important to recognize the difference between moles and freckles or age spots. The best time to count your moles is in midwinter, when freckling is at a minimum. Liver spots or age spots are also sometimes mistaken for moles. They are flat, brown spots which usually appear after age 55, especially on the face and hands. Moles first appear as flat, dark-brown spots, but they eventually rise and become rounded, sometimes turning light brown or pink.

Although most moles are harmless, melanoma, the deadliest form of skin cancer, sometimes arises from them. Because early diagnosis is critical in curing melanoma, you should examine your skin once a month. Note any changes in your moles, and check for any new growths. Report this information to your doctor.

The kind of mole most likely to develop into melanoma is called *dysplastic nevi*. It has varied shades of brown, pink, and tan, and it has blurred edges.

However, these moles are rare, and most melanomas appear as new growth on normal skin.

Melanomas can be identified using the "A-B-C-D" method of diagnosis.

**Asymmetry**: If you drew a line down the middle of a melanoma, the two halves would not match.

**Border:** The border of a melanoma is not smooth; it is usually notched or blurred.

**Color:** Unlike most moles, a melanoma is a mixture of colors, including blue, black, brown, tan, red, and white.

**Diameter:** A melanoma usually grows to at least a quarter of an inch in diameter.

Also look for these other signs of trouble when you are checking your moles:

◆ Sudden or continuous growth
◆ Rising above the skin
◆ Bleeding, crusting, or oozing
◆ Pain or itching
◆ Change in consistency (hardening or softening)
◆ Redness or swelling

Melanomas most often occur on the back, calves of legs, upper arms, ears, and the back of the neck, so examine those areas frequently.

*Sources:*
*British Medical Journal* (310,6984:912)
*FDA Consumer* (29,6:10)
*Medical Update* (14,10:1)
*Public Health Reports* (108,2:176)

# Best skin-saving sunscreen

Slapping on a little sunscreen before you go to the beach isn't enough to protect you from the sun's damaging effects. You need to protect yourself from the ultraviolet (UV) rays of the sun every day, even if you're only outside for a few minutes. Sunscreens with a high sun protection factor (SPF) are helpful, but they don't screen out the longer UVA-I rays that cause your skin to age. These rays strike deeper into your skin and change the underlying structure. UVB rays, which cause sunburn and skin cancer, are either reflected or absorbed by surface skin.

Broad spectrum sunscreens protect against UVB rays and the shorter UVA-II rays but not against UVA-I. The only chemical that can successfully screen these out is *Parsol 1789*, a new ingredient that isn't in most sunscreens yet. However, one sunscreen, Shade UVAGUARD, does contain it. Even if you think you are seldom exposed to the sun, you need to wear sunscreen daily, especially on your face. At the beach, use a water-resistant sunscreen with an SPF of at least 30, and apply it liberally.

Alternatives for screening out harmful rays are wearing a sunscreen containing titanium dioxide or wearing clothing made of tightly woven fabric, such as cotton broadcloth or denim, which can screen out UVA light.

*Source:*
*Medical Tribune for the Internist and Cardiologist* (36,5:19)

## No such thing as a safe tan

You're going to a tanning salon because you want to build up a "starter tan" before your trip to the beach, or you just think that the tan you get from a tanning salon is safer. Sorry, you've been misled. It's true that indoor tanning beds don't emit the harmful UVB rays that can cause skin cancer. But the UVA rays they do emit can be just as damaging.

A tanning lamp gives you two to three times the dose of UVA that you get from sunlight in the same amount of time. UVA light penetrates deeply into the layers of your skin, destroying supportive fibers and damaging your skin's elasticity. This causes premature aging and wrinkling, but it can also contribute to skin cancer.

If you choose to use a tanning salon anyway, be sure to wear the protective goggles that are provided with each tanning bed. Not using goggles can cause severe damage to your eyes. Read the instructions for proper use, and stay in the tanning bed for the shortest recommended time. Don't let an attendant or anyone else mislead you into thinking that you can use a tanning salon as much as you like and still be safe.

*Source:*
*Medical Tribune for the Internist and Cardiologist* (36,16:10)

## Effective, drug-free treatment for eczema

Eczema is a common problem that causes inflammation, blisters, and severe itching of your skin. An allergic reaction to a food or any substance that comes in contact with your skin, chemicals, or even microorganisms can cause eczema. When you have it, all you want to do is scratch. You may scratch so much that your skin bleeds, and that just makes the eczema worse. Usually doctors prescribe antihistamines or cortisone cream for the condition. But a recent study found an effective way to treat eczema without drugs.

A group of 113 people learned relaxation techniques to reduce their stress, along with behavior training to control scratching. Three months of this training led to more improvement than medication.

*Sources:*
*Complete Guide to Symptoms, Illness, and Surgery,* The Berkley Publishing Group, New York, 1995
*Medical Abstracts Newsletter* (15,11:8)

## Success secrets for stopping psoriasis

If you have psoriasis, your skin cells grow faster than they should. Your skin can't shed old cells fast enough, so patches of thick, raised skin form. Your knees, elbows, scalp, and trunk are most often affected, but it can occur even under your nails, which become ridged and pitted. Psoriasis seems to run in families, but it isn't contagious. So, what can you do if you have it?

There isn't a cure for psoriasis yet, but it tends to come and go, with the most recurrence in the winter when your skin gets dry. Try these methods when you have an attack:

**Remove the excess scaly skin** every day with soap and water, and apply a soothing skin cream.

**Apply a lotion or cream** containing coal tar, a traditional treatment, or a corticosteroid cream. You may need to ask your doctor for a prescription.

**Sunbathe or sit under a sun lamp**, but do so very carefully. Ultraviolet light can help psoriasis, but sunburn will only irritate it.

**Try PUVA therapy** if psoriasis covers a large area of your body. This involves taking a medicine that makes your skin very sensitive to sunlight, then sunbathing or sitting under a sun lamp for short periods of time. The treatment requires a doctor's care.

If these methods don't work, your dermatologist may prescribe *methotrexate*. This drug is usually used to treat cancer, but it may also help severe cases of psoriasis.

*Source:*
Postgraduate Medicine (98,6:206)

# Rebound against rosacea

It doesn't indicate a drinking problem, but it can make you look a little like W.C. Fields. Rosacea most often shows up on people between the ages of 30 and 50. Those people of Northern European ancestry who are fair-skinned and who blush easily are most at risk. Women are three times as likely to be affected as men.

Rosacea begins as a flushing of your nose and cheeks, sometimes extending to your chin and forehead. As it progresses, the flushing becomes permanent, bumps and nodules resembling acne appear, and the bumps may abscess and cause scarring.

In advanced stages of rosacea, your nose may become red, bulbous, and pockmarked, known as *rhinophyma* (this most often happens to men over 40). It can involve your eyes, with symptoms such as inflamed lids, redness, swelling, and a burning or stinging sensation.

Rosacea can't be cured, but there are some things you can do to control it. Your best bet is to avoid the substances and situations that you know can cause or worsen it. Anything that makes your face flush should be avoided. Here are some of the most common triggers of a rosacea attack and how to avoid them:

**Eating or drinking hot foods or liquids**. Try food and drinks at room temperature. Sometimes they taste even better when they're not boiling hot.

**Eating spicy foods**. Develop a taste for milder, more delicate flavors.

**Strenuous physical exertion**. Ask someone else to move those heavy boxes for you. Don't give up exercising, but try longer or more frequent sessions with less exertion.

**Exposure to sun, wind, and temperature extremes**. Avoid staying outside in the hottest part of the day, and bundle up well in cold weather, including a scarf to cover your face.

**Facial massages, saunas, hot baths, and showers**. It's easy to avoid saunas and massages, and your skin will be healthier overall if you take more temperate baths and showers.

**Emotional stress.** Try relaxation techniques or biofeedback to help you stay calm in the face of daily pressures.

**Smoking or being in a smoke-filled environment.** Avoid both of these for your health's sake, as well as to avoid rosacea outbreaks.

**Hot flashes caused by menopause.** Hold ice chips in your mouth to cool down your body temperature.

In addition to avoiding the triggers that can bring on an attack of rosacea, see your doctor. She can give you medicine to treat the symptoms, either in pill form or in cream form to apply to the affected areas of your face.

To find a dermatologist in your area who specializes in treating rosacea, you can write to the National Rosacea Society, 800 S. Northwest Highway, Suite 200, Barrington, Ill. 60010, or call (708) 382-8971 for their physician referral service. You can also ask for their free newsletter, *Rosacea Review*.

*Sources:*
*Taber's Cyclopedic Medical Dictionary*, F.A. Davis Company, Philadelphia, 1989
*U.S. Pharmacist* (20,4:41)

# Skin care secrets for people with rosacea

When you have rosacea, caring for your skin is more challenging, but it can make a real difference in your condition. Washing your face is an important part of treating rosacea. Wash your face twice a day with a mild, water-soluble cleanser, either liquid or a bar. The cleanser should not contain alcohol, fragrance, granules, or witch hazel. Don't use a rough washcloth or scrub your face vigorously. Instead, use your fingers, a natural sponge, or a very soft shaving brush to apply the cleanser. Splash your face with tepid or cool water to remove all traces of the cleanser. After washing your face, allow it to dry completely for about 30 minutes before applying any medication or makeup.

The National Rosacea Association recommends the nonsoap cleansers Cetaphil, Ponds Foaming Face Wash, and Dove for washing your face. For moisturizers, they recommend L'Oreal Moisturizer with SPF 12, Eucerin Dry Skin Care, and NutraDerm.

Don't use toners, astringents, or any products that could irritate your skin. Avoid using anything that contains alcohol, witch hazel, menthol, eucalyptus oil, clove oil, peppermint oil, or salicylic acid. If anything you put on your skin causes redness or stinging, stop using it immediately.

Use a sunscreen as part of your daily routine. Exposing your skin to the sun can cause flare-ups of rosacea, even during winter months.

When you use cosmetics, be sure they are water-based and fragrance-free. Avoid heavy formulas that can clog pores and highlight imperfections. The National Rosacea Association recommends Clinique Sensitive Skin Foundation with SPF 15 and MAC Foundation as makeup bases. To mask the ruddiness of your condition, use a color corrector in shades of yellow or green. Use a base makeup with neutral or yellow tones instead of pink or orange ones. And be sure to use makeup to enhance your best features and draw attention away from areas of your face most affected by rosacea.

*Source:*
*U.S. Pharmacist* (20,4:41)

## New treatments stop shingles faster

It begins with a vague feeling of illness and stomach upset and breaks out a few days later with searing pain and a line of blisters down one side of your body. It's shingles, and it's caused by the *herpes zoster* virus. This virus lodges in a nerve in your body where it may wait for years until extreme stress or a weakening of your immune system allows it to burst out.

A Florida doctor tried a successful new method of treatment on a 72-year-old man with shingles. The man was suffering from an extremely painful case of shingles when he went to the doctor. Five days later, he felt "100 percent better." The doctor prescribed *acyclovir*, an antiviral drug, to be taken in 800-milligram (mg) doses five times a day for seven days, along with a daily 250-mg dose of *zinc* and a twice-daily dose of 400 mg of *cimetidine*, a drug that decreases the amount of acid your stomach produces.

For the blisters, the doctor made a solution of aspirin and chloroform for the man to apply to his skin with a cotton ball. Each dose contained 10 grains of aspirin dissolved in 15 milliliters (ml) of chloroform. The solution dried into a white powder and began to relieve the pain in two to three minutes, providing pain relief for three to four hours.

If you are suffering with shingles, ask your doctor if this treatment might work for you.

*Source:*
*American Family Physician* (51,8:1861)

## Win the war on warts

When you hear the word "warts," you may have a vision of frogs, witches, and burying something in the backyard under a full moon. People have been trying all sorts of methods to get rid of these pesky growths. Warts probably don't seem like a major health concern if you don't have them, but if you do, they are a major annoyance. Here are two examples of people who took wart treatment into their own hands and won.

An Ohio dentist had tried conventional wart treatment for eight months with no success. The warts had begun to interfere with his work. His dermatologist at the Medical College of Ohio suggested a bold course of treatment. He prescribed massive doses of beta carotene. The dentist took eight 15-milligram (mg) capsules of beta carotene daily. By the end of the second month, the warts were smaller, and by the end of the fourth month, they were gone.

The dermatologist treated several other people with the same good results. The negative side effect of this treatment is that your skin temporarily looks yellow from all the beta carotene. But the effect goes away after you stop taking the megadoses of vitamins.

An elderly Florida man successfully used an old family remedy to get rid of a wart on the sole of his foot. Every night, he would smooth the wart with a pumice stone and then cut a very thin slice of raw potato slightly larger than the wart. He would tape the potato over the wart for the night. After six weeks of this treatment, the plantar wart was gone. This method hasn't been clinically proven, but it's certainly an easy and inexpensive wart treatment.

*Sources:*
*American Family Physician* (51,8:1861)
*Cutis* (55,6:332)

# A+ acne care

The days of fighting acne by denying young people their favorite foods and acting as if acne is some kind of punishment are over. If you are a teenager or adult with a not-too-severe case of acne, help is as close as your drugstore.

Benzoyl peroxide, which comes in a number of brands and formulations, is an effective acne treatment. If you use it twice a day for five days, it will kill 95 percent of the acne-causing bacteria on your skin. Even though 10 percent benzoyl peroxide is available, a solution of 5 percent delivers the most possible benefit, with fewer of the side effects of stinging, burning, redness, and scaling. In this case, more is not better.

Benzoyl peroxide shouldn't be mixed with any other acne medications. If you're going to use another product along with it, be sure that you wait several hours between applications.

*Source:*
*Cutis* (56,5:261)

## Super relief for cracked skin

Superglue is good for more than just mending broken dishes. If you have painful cracks in the skin of your fingers, especially around your fingernails, try superglue for a temporary fix. Use only a small amount, and try not to squeeze it down into the moist area of the crack. Let the glue dry thoroughly (about five minutes) before you touch anything. The glue should hold your skin together until it has a chance to heal.

*Source:*
*Postgraduate Medicine* (99,2:38)

## Selecting the best skin moisturizer for you

Itchy, flaky, irritated, dry skin can be very uncomfortable and put a damper on even the best day. Your dry skin may be caused by an allergic reaction, a genetic tendency, an occupation that requires harsh chemicals or frequent hand washing, too many hot showers, or the normal effects of aging. Whatever the cause, you just want some relief.

Don't waste money buying moisturizers that won't help your dry skin. Here are the five basic kinds of moisturizers. Choose one that's right for you.

**Ointments** are the heaviest and greasiest moisturizers, combining *petrolatum* (a grease derived from petroleum) and waxes or other ingredients, such as lanolin.

**Emollient creams** are good for dry, flaky skin on your hands and body. They are emulsions of water in oil.

**Creams** are made with a higher ratio of oil to water. They rub completely into your skin and are usually not greasy. They are often combined with *humectants*, such as glycerin, propylene glycol, or sorbitol, which attract moisture to your skin.

**Lotions** are liquid emulsions with a higher ratio of water to oil. They spread easily, but they aren't as effective as heavier moisturizers.

**Oils and bath oils** can be added to your bath water or applied to wet skin immediately after a bath or shower.

Urea, lactic acid, and other *alpha hydroxy acids* are sometimes added to over-the-counter moisturizers to improve their effectiveness. These particular ingredients work to change the texture of your skin instead of temporarily helping the dryness. Alpha hydroxy acids can cause skin irritation on sensitive skin, and they shouldn't be used on inflamed skin.

Other additives can cause you to have an allergic reaction to a moisturizer. Gums, synthetic polymers, sunscreens, preservatives, humectants, and fragrances can cause irritation for some people. If you have a history of allergies, you should avoid lanolin, a natural product derived from sheep's wool. Read labels carefully to watch out for these ingredients. If you still have questions about the type of moisturizer you should use, ask your pharmacist for help.

*Source:*
*Pharmacy Times* (62,2:24)

# Realistic wrinkle relief

Let's face it ... getting wrinkles is a fact of life. It happens slowly, so it's one of those things you may not notice until it's too late. But you can start right now to take better care of your skin so that wrinkles don't catch up with you too soon.

Here are some tips for skin care that will help keep you looking younger longer:

- ◆ After washing your face, apply a skin lotion or moisturizer. It helps flatten the skin cells and holds moisture in your skin, which makes wrinkles less visible.
- ◆ Avoid using rough washcloths, scrubbing pads, or brushes and products with grainy abrasives such as facial scrubs. They can increase the tendency of the top layers of skin to pull away from the deeper layers, which makes skin more prone to wrinkling.
- ◆ Wear a sunscreen and sunglasses whenever you go outside. In addition to

reducing your risk of skin cancer, you'll avoid squint lines around your eyes.

**Source:**
*U.S. Pharmacist* (20,4:17)

## Reversing wrinkle damage with natural nutrient

In order for your skin to form *collagen*, the fibrous support tissue that keeps your skin looking young, it must have the antioxidant vitamin C. The problem is, you can only get a certain amount of vitamin C in your diet or with supplements. A new 10-percent solution of vitamin C applied to your skin delivers 20 to 40 times as much.

This vitamin C lotion, called Cellex-C, gives your skin the signal to build new collagen, reducing wrinkles and other signs of aging and sun damage. In clinical trials, Cellex-C reduced wrinkling and sun spots on people's skin when they applied it daily for eight months. It also increases your skin's natural protection against ultraviolet rays by two to three times. Cellex-C is available at selected cosmetic boutiques.

Researchers are also investigating whether vitamin C applied to your skin can prevent the sun damage to your skin that causes skin cancer.

**Source:**
*Geriatrics* (50,11:23)

## Treat yourself to an in-home spa

A few simple ingredients from your kitchen pantry can make your bathtub seem like a spa. Fresh lemons or limes squeezed into your bath make it fragrant and cooling in hot weather. For a refreshing foot soak, use one-half lime, two teaspoons of sage, three teaspoons of parsley, one teaspoon of rosemary, and eight peppermint leaves. Raid your herb garden for fresh herbs, or use half the amounts of dried herbs plus a little bit of peppermint oil. Tie the herbs in a piece of cheesecloth and steep in hot water for five minutes. Let your feet soak for 10 minutes in the herbal citrus bath and follow with a foot massage with sweet almond oil.

For sloughing off dead, flaky skin, start with a bath scented with your favorite essential oil (oils scented with the aromatic substances of plants). After soaking for a few minutes, sit on the edge of the tub and slather yourself with sweet almond oil. Then take a handful of coarse salt and begin scrubbing your skin from toes to neck. Slip back into the tub for a relaxing 20-minute soak, follow with a body moisturizer, and slip into bed for a good night's sleep.

**Source:**
*The Joy of Healthy Skin,* Prentice Hall, Englewood Cliffs, N.J., 1996

## Nail salon nightmares

Believe it or not, your nails actually serve a purpose. They enhance your feeling of touch and your fine motor skills. They protect your delicate fingers and toes. They may also indicate when you have a health problem by the way they grow.

For most people, however, they're a handy area to decorate. If you want to get your nails done in the United States, you can choose from almost 35,000 free-standing nail salons, in addition to the hundreds of thousands of beauty salons that offer manicures.

Getting a manicure carries some risk. With the increased use of nail products and services in recent years, people have become more concerned about safety. It's possible to get infections from artificial nails or unclean tools and to have allergic reactions to chemicals in the nail products. Some nail products are poisonous if they're ingested, and many of them are flammable. However, there are precautions you can take to keep from experiencing the negative side of nail care.

You should choose your nail salon carefully. Use these guidelines to be sure a salon provides safe, sanitary service:

◆ Is the salon licensed? If you don't see a license posted, ask to see it.

◆ Are the nail technicians licensed? These are usually posted, too.

◆ How are the nail tools sanitized? Heat sterilization in an autoclave is the best treatment, but most states allow chemical sterilizing if the tools stay in the solution for at least 10 minutes between customers. Ask the technician which practice is followed. If they're using a chemical solution, check to see that the product's label says "germicidal" or contains other words that indicate it's antibacterial.

◆ Is there a pre-service hand washing? Both the technician and the customer should wash their hands with antibacterial soap before nail work begins.

◆ Does each customer get her own fresh bowl of soapy water to soak her nails? Does the technician use a new nail file for each customer?

◆ Is the facility neat and clean? Is there a strong smell of fumes? If so, it's a sign that the building is not well-ventilated. Inhaling fumes from nail products can make you sick.

If a nail salon doesn't pass the test when you evaluate it, look for another salon. If it makes you feel more comfortable, take your own tools to use on your nails. If you have a complaint about a salon providing nail services, contact your state board of cosmetology.

*Source:*
*FDA Consumer* (29,10:20)

# Healthy nail tips

If you love the look of long, luxurious fingernails but can't quite achieve it with your own two hands, artificial nails may be for you. Many people have great success with artificial nails. You simply need to be aware of a few precautions so that yours can be healthy as well as gorgeous. Here are some things to remember about artificial nails:

♦ If you're worried that you might be sensitive to something in the artificial nail materials, have just one nail done and wait a few days to see if you have a reaction.

♦ Don't apply an artificial nail if your own nail or the skin around it is infected or irritated. Let it heal first.

♦ If you're using do-it-yourself nails, be sure to read all instructions carefully before you apply them. Save the list of ingredients in case you have a reaction and need to tell your doctor about it.

♦ Don't use household glues for nail repairs. Use only products specified for nail use, and follow directions.

♦ If an artificial nail separates from your nail, dip your fingertip into rubbing alcohol to clean the space between the nails before reattaching them. This should help prevent infection.

♦ Keep nail glues and other nail products out of the reach of children. They can be harmful and even fatal if they are ingested or inhaled.

♦ Treat your artificial nails with care, and try not to bump or knock them against hard surfaces. They are strong, but they can still break or separate. Find new ways of doing tasks so you don't put stress on your nails.

♦ Don't wear your artificial nails for longer than three months at a time. Remove them for one month to give your natural nails a rest.

*Source:*
*FDA Consumer* (29,10:20)

# Outgrow your ingrown toenail

An ingrown toenail doesn't sound like a serious malady, but if you've ever had one, you know how painful it can be. It starts when a corner of your toenail grows into the flesh of your toe. This can be caused by a nail that curves too much, clipping your toenail too closely, wearing shoes that are too small, or an athletic activity that causes your toes to be jammed against the end of your shoe.

The result is pain, swelling, tenderness, redness, and heat in your toe. Once your toe becomes inflamed, infection can set in, and then you have to take an antibiotic to prevent the infection from spreading. You may even need surgery to remove the nail.

To avoid all this, it's better to prevent an ingrown toenail in the first place. Clipping your toenails carefully and wearing roomy shoes that fit your feet correctly should eliminate the problem. However, if you do get an ingrown nail, there's a much simpler treatment that should help you fix the problem yourself at home.

This method comes from Dr. Joseph E. Scherger of San Diego. Here's what to do:

♦ Each day, soak your ingrown nail in warm water for 20 to 30 minutes. Then massage the skin away from the ingrown nail.

◆ Use a butter knife, cotton swab, or some other small, blunt object to clean the skin in the area all around the ingrown nail.

If you use this soaking and cleaning routine daily, it should keep your nail from getting infected and eliminate the need for antibiotics and surgery. Your nail can grow back into a healthy position.

*Sources:*
*American Family Physician* (53,2:499)
*Complete Guide to Symptoms, Illness & Surgery,* The Berkley Publishing Group, New York, 1995

## Ingenious fix for ingrown toenail

You've tried soaking your feet, cutting a notch in the top of your toenail, and changing your shoes, but you're still plagued with ingrown toenails. Here's a new technique that's worth a try and may bring the relief you're looking for.

Apply a one-fourth-inch or one-half-inch wide strip of athletic adhesive tape to your toe, starting at the skin over the ingrown area. Using the tape, gently pull the skin away from the nail and wrap the tape snugly around and under your toe, back over your nail and over the beginning point of the tape.

The tape pulls the irritated skin away from the offending nail, giving it a chance to heal. Apply the tape twice a day, and monitor the healing process. If your toenail gets infected and looks red, swells, or oozes pus, it's time to let the doctor treat it.

*Source:*
*The Physician and Sportsmedicine* (23,7:22)

# Arthritis Advisor

## Outwit osteoarthritis

Osteoarthritis (OA) often takes a painful stand in your back, hips, and knees. By making some changes in your lifestyle, you can have more control over OA. The new guidelines for treating OA include a balanced diet, exercise, and pain-relief medication.

Obesity can cause OA to progress more quickly and cause more pain. So, if you're overweight, lose weight to take the stress off your knees and make joints less painful. Losing 11 or more pounds can lower your risk of developing osteoarthritis in your knees by 50 percent.

Following a balanced diet will help keep your body healthier overall. But certain foods may have a special impact on arthritis. Some studies have indicated that a vegetarian diet may be especially beneficial. If you don't want to make a radical change in your eating habits, eating more fruits and vegetables, cutting down on meat, and eating more deep-water fish, such as salmon, mackerel, and herring, could help relieve your arthritis.

You might want to try eliminating dairy products from your diet to see if there is an improvement in your symptoms. Some researchers think that certain foods, such as wheat, black walnuts, and dairy products, may trigger arthritis. If you do eliminate certain foods, be sure to find alternate ways of getting the nutrients that they provide.

If you exercise regularly, you will be better able to maintain a complete range of motion in your joints, and this will help strengthen the muscles surrounding them. The best approach is to balance periods of activity with rest. Exercises such as fitness walking, aerobics, exercising in water, and strengthening exercises are important to fight the pain and stiffness of OA. Swimming and cycling can be good exercise choices, too, especially if you have OA of the hip joints.

A few tools can make your exercise program easier. When you're resting, try using a straight-backed chair instead of a recliner. If your bed is soft, try switching to a firmer mattress. Shoes with good shock-absorbing properties help make walking more comfortable, and a walking stick can reduce the pressure on a painful hip by 20 to 30 percent. Be sure to choose a sturdy wooden or metal stick, with a comfortable handle, that comes to the top of your pelvis. Hold the walking stick on the side opposite your painful joint.

When you choose medication for OA, look for something that will relieve your pain, instead of something to reduce inflammation. According to the guidelines, an over-the-counter pain reliever, such as acetaminophen, should be your first choice. If that doesn't work, an over-the-counter nonsteroidal anti-inflammatory drug (NSAID), such as ibuprofen, may help. For stronger pain relief, you'll need a prescription from your doctor.

*Sources:*
*British Medical Journal* (311,7009:853)
*Environmental Nutrition* (16,9:2)
*Medical Tribune for the Internist and Cardiologist* (36,21:5)

## ACE arthritis with antioxidants

Antioxidants are those valuable vitamins that do battle with free radicals, forces in your body that can damage your cells and immune system. Now the little nutrients have another service to perform for people with arthritis.

In a Boston study, researchers found that antioxidants (vitamin C, vitamin E, and beta carotene) may help keep the osteoarthritis (OA) in your knees from getting worse.

People who consumed extra vitamin C, in foods or supplements, decreased the risk of their OA getting worse by 300 percent. They also reduced their risk of knee pain. Vitamin E and beta carotene also seemed to reduce the risk of OA getting worse, but the benefit was not as evident.

If you already have osteoarthritis, increasing your consumption of foods rich in antioxidants, such as fresh fruits, green and yellow vegetables, nuts, seeds, wheat germ, and soy products, may help you keep it at bay. These foods are a healthy addition to anyone's diet.

*Sources:*
Arthritis Today (10,1:51)
*Prescription for Nutritional Healing,* Avery Publishing Group, Garden City Park, N.Y., 1990
*Super Healing Foods,* Parker Publishing, West Nyack, N.Y., 1995

## Stop stomach pain before it starts

If you are taking medication for your arthritis, you are probably taking antacids to deal with the stomach discomfort that goes along with it. But don't be fooled into thinking that the antacid is protecting your stomach.

According to two new studies, antacids may be masking serious gastrointestinal problems caused by arthritis drugs, even simple nonsteroidal anti-inflammatory drugs (NSAIDs), such as ibuprofen. Older people and those with a history of peptic ulcers are particularly vulnerable to problems.

There is a new drug that can be taken along with your NSAIDs, and it will prevent them from causing ulcers. The drug is called *misoprostol*, and its brand name is *Cytotec*. Ask your doctor about it, so he can help you decide if it's a drug that you need.

If you are having stomach pain from your arthritis drug, talk to your doctor. Don't let a minor stomach problem become a serious one.

*Sources:*
AIMplus (23:24)
*The Newnan Times-Herald* (Jan. 17, 1996, 4B)

## Ease arthritis with exercise

For many years, doctors prescribed rest for people with arthritis. Today, the approach is much different. Doctors recommend regular exercise to maintain mobility in joints and strengthen the muscles surrounding them. Strength training and range-of-motion exercises are important, but now aerobic exercise is also being recognized as a valuable tool.

For some people who already have arthritis, light aerobic exercise may be better than the more vigorous kind. Nonweight-bearing exercises, such as bicycling, swimming, and water aerobics, are good choices.

But researchers are beginning to recognize that for some individuals, intense, vigorous, aerobic exercise is the therapy that can keep their arthritis under control. They prefer such exercises as running, walking, and aerobic dance to improve their arthritis, their overall physical conditions, their mental attitudes, and their quality of life. This can be true even for people with Rheumatoid Arthritis (RA).

Vigorous exercise can also help prevent weight gain, a problem for many people with arthritis. Added weight puts more stress on your joints and makes arthritis worse.

Older athletes who have exercised all their lives may be able to avoid most arthritis symptoms. But even if you're older and begin an exercise program for the first time, you may be able to keep arthritis symptoms at bay. And you may be able to lessen the symptoms you already have, if you commit to an exercise program at least three times a week for 30 minutes each time.

You must find your own best level of fitness, with advice from your doctor and physical therapist. Besides giving you greater strength and physical well-being, exercise can give you a feeling of control over your arthritis.

*Source:*
*Arthritis Today* (6,4:34)

## Tai chi takes ache out of arthritis

Centuries ago, long before running and aerobics dance classes became popular, people in China were exercising and staying healthy by practicing the art of tai chi. This involves a series of slow, concentrated movements, done over a period of 10 minutes to an hour, that take the body through a wide range of motions. Tai chi is excellent for people whose bones and joints can't take the jarring effects of more vigorous exercises.

Composed of a series of fluid, graceful postures, called *forms*, tai chi was first developed as a form of nonaggressive martial art. It was based on the Taoist religion and was intended to avoid force by turning an attacker's own energy against him. The forms are based on animal movements and have imaginative, poetic names.

Tai chi can be a very good exercise choice for people with arthritis. Motions are slow and deliberate, beginning with the feet, then rising up through the knees, torso, and shoulders and ending with the hands. The process continues through a smooth series of forms and postures. Tai chi not only improves balance and coordination, but also strengthens the muscles, an important aspect for people with arthritis.

Even though tai chi is very gentle, people with arthritis need to be careful. If a certain posture is painful, listen to your body and adjust the movements to accommodate the painful areas. You can bend your knees less, shorten steps, reduce the amount of hip twisting, pull swinging motions closer to your body, and limit the height of overhead motions. If you have pain in your feet, wear well-cushioned athletic shoes and try distributing your weight more evenly.

Any motions in tai chi can be changed to meet your needs. Just be sure that if you change a motion on one side, you also change it on the other. This way your body is exercised and developed evenly. If you are taking a tai chi class, your teacher should be able to help you do this.

If you want to learn tai chi, look for a good class. Most large cities in the United States and Canada have classes available today. Many fitness centers and some martial-arts centers offer tai chi, also. With more than 200 million people practicing it, tai chi is the most widely used physical training system in the world.

*Sources:*
*American Fitness* (10,5:46)
*Arthritis Today* (7,1:30)
*Women's Sports and Fitness* (17,1:45)

# Living well with arthritis

Much of life involves learning to cope with challenges, and finding out which strategies work for you and which don't. If you have arthritis, here are some ways you can adapt your surroundings to make your challenges easier to meet:

◆ To make a pen or pencil easier to grasp, have someone twist a large rubber band around it just below the area where your fingers rest. Or take the plastic center out of a foam roller and slide a pencil into the center of the foam. You can also get a pencil grip made of soft rubber where school supplies are sold. A ballpoint pen is easier to use than a felt-tip pen or pencil.

◆ Consider buying a speakerphone to replace your regular telephone so that you don't get a stiff or sore neck and shoulder from cradling the receiver for long periods of time.

◆ When you're reading, place the book on several pillows in your lap to raise it to a comfortable height. To turn the pages of a book, use the eraser end of a pencil or a rubber fingertip. Blow gently along the edges to separate the pages.

◆ To play a game of cards without aching hands, insert the cards into the side of a closed box of aluminum foil or waxed paper. You can also put the bottom of a shoe box into its lid and stand cards in the space between the box and the lid.

◆ In the kitchen, create a lower work space so that you can sit while working. Pull out a drawer and place a cookie sheet over the opening. Roll jars and bottles on the counter instead of shaking them. Open a bottle or jar more easily by having someone wind a rubber band around the lid.

◆ If you have trouble gripping your car door handle, especially when it's cold or wet, glue a piece of rubber (like the kind that opens jars) to the underside of the door handle. Make your steering wheel easier to grip by padding it with a foam cover (available in automotive stores). And add extra cushioning to the car seat to keep your back, hips, and legs more comfortable while driving.

◆ If you have trouble standing up for a shower, try putting a webbed lawn chair in the shower stall so you can sit while you bathe. It's easier to dry off after a shower by putting on a terry cloth bathrobe. And if you're bathing a baby in a sink or bathtub, wear a soft cotton glove on the supporting hand to keep him from slipping out of your grasp.

◆ When you're getting dressed, put the garment on your weaker limb first. When undressing, take the garment off the stronger limb first. Try knee-high or thigh-high hose to eliminate the hassle of putting on pantyhose.

*Source:*
*Arthritis Today* (10,1:12,22)

## Punch out pain

Here are a couple of quick tips to relieve arthritis pain at home while you're watching television or just relaxing:

◆ Place a plastic dish tub containing a little water on your lap. Dip a towel in the water, then wring it out. The action of twisting the towel, first one way and then the other, is a good exercise for strengthening and flexing the fingers, wrists, and arms.

◆ To soothe the discomfort of arthritis, fill a clean, dry, cotton sock with uncooked rice and tie the end closed. Heat in your microwave oven for three minutes, and you have a flexible heating pad that will conform to any aching part of your body. The sock will stay warm for up to an hour, and you don't have to worry about burns. Just don't get it wet, or you'll have a soggy mess!

*Sources:*
*Postgraduate Medicine* (98,2:34)
*The Physician and Sportsmedicine* (23,11:17)

## Fish oil fights arthritis

For people with arthritis, the sea may yield an important product. Recently, a study was conducted in Australia on the effect of fish oil supplements on people with arthritis.

A fatty acid called EPA has a beneficial effect on arthritis, as well as on heart disease and high blood pressure. The Australian study showed that taking fish-oil supplements raised the concentrations of EPA in the body.

Fish oil supplements may even be able to take the place of pain relievers for some people with arthritis. Another recent study replaced nonsteroidal anti-inflammatory drugs (NSAIDs) with fish oil supplements and tested the results. The fish oil relieved pain in tender joints and helped with morning stiffness.

However, there is some evidence that fish oil supplements may give you concentrations of vitamins A and D that are too high, and that ocean contaminants, concentrated in the supplements, may be harmful. Be sure to check with your doctor before adding fish oil supplements to your arthritis-fighting program.

Omega-3 fatty acids are the ingredients in fish oil that fight against inflammation in your joints. To consume enough of the omega-3 fatty acids to get results, you can make fish a main ingredient of your diet. Some of the best sources of omega-3 fatty acids are salmon, mackerel, sardines, anchovies, tuna, bluefish, and herring.

*Sources:*
*The American Journal of Clinical Nutrition* (61,2:320)
*Environmental Nutrition* (19,2:2)
*Medical Tribune for the Internist and Cardiologist* (36,18:1)
*Hamilton and Whitney's Nutrition Concepts and Controversies,* West Publishing Company, New York, 1994

# B vitamin banishes side effects of popular arthritis drug

In the last few years, the anti-cancer drug Methotrexate has become a common treatment for rheumatoid arthritis (RA). The treatment can be very effective, but nausea, anemia, liver problems, and hair loss can be some of the unpleasant side effects. Doctors at the University of Alabama at Birmingham have come up with a solution to the problem.

Methotrexate causes a deficiency of folic acid, one of the B vitamins. When people taking the drug for their arthritis also took a folic acid supplement, most of the side effects, especially the gastrointestinal ones, were reduced. And the drug was still effective against arthritis.

People in the study took high doses of folic acid. But the doctors say that a daily dose of 400 mcg (micrograms) of folic acid, the amount usually found in over-the-counter multivitamins, should be enough to prevent side effects. Check with your doctor before adding the supplements to your RA treatment.

*Source:*
*Arthritis Today* (9,4:9)

# Stress busters relieve RA

Doctors are still not sure how it works. But a recent study found that people with rheumatoid arthritis (RA) who learn techniques for coping with stress can reduce their pain and increase their mobility.

People in the study continued to take their medicine as usual, so the improvement wasn't based on any change in drug treatment. The 10-week program helped them cope with family problems, deal with depression, and learn biofeedback techniques to manage stress.

If you have RA, you know what it's like to live with stress every day. Since you never know when a flare-up may occur, you can't always make plans and follow through with them the way you'd like to. Many kinds of physical activities are out of the question, and this can cause problems in a marriage and family. It can also make you feel that you have no control over your life.

Surprisingly, learning to fight stress and regaining a feeling of control can actually *give* you that control. The pain in your joints is reduced, and you are able to move more easily. The process becomes a circle of improvement.

Ask your doctor to help you find a stress management program, or look for one at your local hospital.

*Source:*
*Medical Tribune for the Internist and Cardiologist (37,2:5)*

# Helping others helps relieve arthritis

Women with rheumatoid arthritis (RA) who work outside the home tend to be healthier than those who are homemakers. This finding was presented to the annual meeting of the American College of Rheumatology.

Of the women who were studied, those who worked outside the home for six or more years were healthiest. Doctors don't know the reason for this, but they think that it may have something to do with the satisfaction in life of the working women.

Perhaps moving your attention to something outside yourself is a good way to help divert your focus from the pain of RA. Volunteer work might do as much as paid employment to achieve this, and you would be helping others while you help yourself.

*Source:*
*Medical Tribune for the Internist and Cardiologist (36,22:17)*

# Self-help for rheumatoid arthritis

If you have rheumatoid arthritis and the accompanying Sjögren's syndrome, you must deal with dry eyes and dry mouth as well as the other aspects of arthritis. Help for both these problems is right in your own home.

Because of the lack of protective saliva, tooth decay can be a problem that accompanies dry mouth. In a recent study, researchers found that taking small sips of milk throughout the day, as well as drinking milk with meals, helped make people with arthritis more comfortable and helped prevent tooth decay as well.

To combat the dry eyes that sometimes go with arthritis, here are several tips that you should know:

◆ Avoid air conditioning when you can. It dries the air and can irritate your eyes.

◆ Choose glasses instead of contact lenses, which can make your eyes even drier.

◆ When you're outside, wear sunglasses to shield your eyes from dust and wind.

◆ Try artificial tears to moisten your eyes. Just be sure to look for a product without preservatives, which might cause irritation.

*Source:*
*Arthritis Today (10,2:12,50)*

## Promising new discoveries offer hope of arthritis cure

Although there's no cure for arthritis yet, research is being done constantly to learn more about treatments and a possible cure for this condition that affects over 40 million Americans. Two discoveries show particular promise for treating arthritis.

A new synthetic enzyme called *mythionine* promises to relieve arthritis pain without stomach distress. This is a real advantage because many existing arthritis drugs are damaging to the stomach lining and can even cause ulcers. This drug has been very successful in European trials, but it is awaiting more testing in the United States. It should be much less expensive than most other arthritis drugs.

The natural form, *methionine,* is an essential amino acid found in milk, cheese, bread, potatoes, beef, fish, and egg whites. It is one of several enzymes necessary for tissue repair, and it disrupts the process that causes damage and swelling in joints.

Another promising treatment sounds unusual, but it has had good results in clinical studies for a number of years. It's *bovine tracheal cartilage,* taken in pill form or injected. This substance, derived from cows, is composed of the same protein complexes that are found in your joints and connective tissue cells. A shortage of these proteins can cause a number of physical problems, including arthritis.

Bovine tracheal cartilage also stimulates your immune system and increases the ability of white blood cells to help your body fight disease. It is being used more and more as a treatment for cancer.

Bovine tracheal cartilage tablets, especially those that are made without additives, flavorings, and colorings, seem to be safe and without side effects. This treatment is available now from health food stores, and it is worth looking into and discussing with your doctor.

*Sources:*
*AIMplus* (23:24)
*Better Nutrition for Today's Living* (57,5:60)
*Healthy & Natural Journal* (3,1:24)
*The Newnan Times-Herald* (Jan. 13, 1996, 10A)

## Coping with fibromyalgia

If you have the syndrome known as *fibromyalgia,* you know all about fatigue, chronic pain, and tenderness in your joints and muscles. Even though there's no cure, the condition is not life-threatening. Here are some things you can do to manage your symptoms:

◆ Exercise is one of the most effective treatments for fibromyalgia, even though it may cause pain and discomfort at first. Choose the low-impact aerobic type, such as swimming, riding a stationary bike, or using a ski-type machine. Start slowly and build up to at least 20 to 30 minutes of exercise four or more times a week. Then, if you like, you can move to high-impact exercises, such as walking, running, or tennis.

♦ Learn to manage the stress in your life; it is a trigger for fibromyalgia. Decide on your priorities and eliminate those stressful things that are not really important to you.

♦ Get as much sleep as you need. Getting too little sleep can aggravate your symptoms. Alcohol and caffeine can affect your sleep, so you might want to avoid them.

♦ Don't do too much one day, and end up having a bad day the next. Try to plan your activities so that the level is fairly even.

♦ Check out medications. Doctors sometimes prescribe amitriptyline, an antidepressant, to improve sleep and help other symptoms. It does have side effects, however, so discuss the pros and cons with your doctor before deciding if it's right for you.

♦ Contact your local chapter of The Arthritis Foundation to find a support group for people with fibromyalgia.

*Sources:*
American Family Physician (52,3:853)
British Medical Journal (310,6976:386)

# 6 ways to sidestep gout

Called the disease of kings, gout is a form of arthritis with a bad reputation. It is often associated with rich food, overeating, and drinking too much alcohol. But this very painful condition, caused by too much uric acid in the blood, is also influenced by other factors. It is even partly genetic and can be caused by a defective kidney. There isn't a complete cure, but there are several things you can do to keep gout from having too great an influence in your life.

♦ Go to your doctor if you think you have gout, and have it diagnosed. It is one of a few diseases that can be diagnosed with certainty.

♦ Lose weight if you are overweight, and if you drink alcohol regularly, give it up. These two factors increase the uric acid in your blood, and decrease your body's ability to excrete it.

♦ Check with your doctor to see if any of the prescription drugs you are taking could cause excess uric acid to build up in your body. Diuretics, or water pills, are notorious for this. Perhaps there is a substitute drug you can take that won't cause gout.

♦ Decrease your intake of foods containing large amounts of substances called *purines*, which break down to form uric acid. High-purine foods include meat, meat extracts, and gravies; organ meats, such as liver; seafood; yeast and yeast extracts; beer and other alcoholic beverages; oatmeal; spinach, asparagus, mushrooms, and cauliflower; and beans, peas, and lentils.

♦ Increase your intake of fluids. This will help flush the uric acid out of your body.

◆ If preventive measures aren't working and you are having a gout attack, see your doctor immediately. The earlier you catch an attack, the better it can be treated. He can prescribe something to stop the attack in a matter of hours, instead of the two weeks or so that it usually takes to run its course.

◆ Talk to your doctor about the drugs available to prevent gout, as well as those to stop an attack.

Keep in mind, however, that changing your lifestyle to prevent gout is a healthier and less expensive alternative to drug therapy.

*Sources:*
*Arthritis: A Comprehensive Guide to Understanding Your Arthritis,* National Institute of Arthritis and Musculoskeletal and Skin Diseases, 1990
*The New England Journal of Medicine* (334,7:445)

# Beware of the bogus

People are always looking for miracle cures for the diseases that plague us. Arthritis has had more than its share of bogus remedies, including sitting in a uranium mine, wearing copper bracelets, and using vibrating chairs and mattresses. But most of the miracle cures do little more than line the pockets of swindlers and just make people think they're getting some relief.

One of the frustrating things about arthritis is that the pain and inflammation come and go. This makes it easy for people to think that the latest bogus cure really worked, when actually it just happened to coincide with a time when their arthritis improved or disappeared on its own.

Don't let yourself be fooled. Arthritis can be detected, diagnosed, and treated most effectively by your doctor. Early detection and therapy can make a significant difference in the severity of the attacks. Unproven cures don't treat the problem, and they can give false hope and distract you from the treatments that really could help.

If you want to try a remedy you've heard about, ask your doctor what she thinks of it. The bottom line is, if a treatment seems too good to be true, it probably is.

*Source:*
*"Hocus-Pocus as Applied to Arthritis,"* FDA 90-1080, Food and Drug Administration, HFI-40, Rockville, Md. 20857

# Powerful Pain Relief

## Painproof your life

Pain may be simply mind over matter for superheroes, but for most people, it's more a matter of how to get rid of pain quickly. If you're constantly battling chronic pain, try these eight suggestions.

**Turn on the heat.** It relaxes stiff muscles and stimulates blood circulation. Some good sources of heat include warm baths and heating pads. Warming your clothes in the dryer before you put them on also helps. You can warm a damp cloth in the microwave for a few seconds and then apply it to the painful area. Be sure it's not hot enough to burn you. Don't apply any painkilling creams before using heat therapy or you could end up with severe burns.

**Chill out.** Cold relieves pain by numbing pain-sensing nerves and reducing inflammation. Use a commercial ice pack or make your own ice pack by filling a plastic bag with ice. Wrap the cold pack in a towel so you don't freeze your skin. To prevent injuries, never use heat or cold therapy for more than 15 to 20 minutes or apply these treatments to sores or sensitive skin.

**Work out your pain with a massage.** Options include a professional massage therapist, hand-held massagers, foot rollers, massaging shower attachments, or a self-massage. Sore or swollen joints should not be massaged. If you have arthritis, avoid deep muscle massages.

**Give yourself some support.** Braces, splints, and other specially designed devices can help reduce pain and inflammation by stabilizing weak and damaged joints. It is important to be fitted by an occupational therapist or a certified *orthotist* (a specialist who designs and fits these devices) since even slight variations in fit can make a significant difference in how well they work.

**Make your own medicine.** Exercising helps the body produce its own natural painkillers called *endorphins*. Regular exercise also strengthens muscles, improves joint stability, and keeps bone and cartilage tissue strong. You should include aerobics, strength-training, and range-of-motion exercises in your weekly routine. Get a physical therapist to show you range-of-motion exercises appropriate for your condition.

**Try alternative treatments.** Both *transcutaneous electrical nerve stimulation* *(TENS)* and acupuncture can relieve pain by providing stimulation which confuses nerve sensors. These techniques take your mind off your previous pain and focuses it instead on the new, painless sensation. If you'd like to try the TENS technique, talk to a physical therapist. Like exercise, acupuncture may also stimulate the release of the body's natural painkillers — endorphins. If you want to try acupuncture, find a certified acupuncturist.

**Pop a pill for really bad pain.** Acetaminophen relieves pain while drugs such as ibuprofen and aspirin block the production of chemicals that create pain and inflammation. Also, painkilling creams can provide temporary relief when rubbed directly onto the painful area.

*Source:*
*Arthritis Today* (9,6:30)

# Nature's most powerful painkiller

Despite the number of heavy-duty painkillers available today, it may be your brain that produces the most powerful painkiller of all.

Most doctors agree your state of mind affects your ability to handle pain. Since pain affects both body and mind, you'll experience greater relief if you treat both. Learning pain management techniques will give you 20 to 40 percent more pain relief than you can get from medicine alone.

You can learn these techniques at pain clinics or at workshops and classes conducted in your community. Costs range from free to fairly expensive. Sometimes, these classes may be partially covered by health insurance.

In general, an upbeat attitude and an active lifestyle will work wonders for relieving chronic pain. Also, try to avoid fear, anger, and worry thoughts. Work on replacing negative thoughts with positive thoughts and pleasant activities.

If you have a medical condition that often causes you pain, the following mental exercises can increase the effectiveness of painkilling medicine and may eventually eliminate your need for them altogether.

**Reduce pain with relaxation.** Progressive relaxation involves working through all your body's muscles individually, tensing and relaxing each muscle. Start with your toes and then work up to your head.

Meditation is another form of relaxation in which you focus on your breathing or repeat one word over and over to help clear your mind of any pain-related or stressful thoughts. Although you can meditate for as little as one minute, 15 or more minutes will bring deeper relaxation.

**Baby your body with biofeedback.** Biofeedback is a relaxation technique that uses special sensors attached to your body to help you learn to control body functions, such as blood pressure, muscle tension, and heart rate, that you normally control unconsciously. Learning to control these body functions can reduce pain and stress.

**Distract yourself.** As powerful as the brain is, it can only process so much information at once. That's why you'll often stop noticing the pain if you focus all your concentration on another activity, such as playing a board game or card game, enjoying a favorite hobby, recalling a favorite memory down to the very last detail, learning something new, imagining yourself as a hero who succeeds in spite of the pain, listening to music, calling friends to find out what's going on in their lives, or nurturing your mind with nature by watching birds or spending a quiet day in the woods. Any activity at all will work as long as you can lose yourself completely in it for a while.

**Get out and get going.** Getting involved in social activities and a regular exercise program can help take your mind off pain, as well as increasing your self-esteem. Although getting out may seem like the last thing you want to do, it will almost always make you feel better.

**Seek support.** Just talking to others who understand what you're going through because they've experienced it themselves seems to make dealing with pain easier. Sharing solutions for coping with pain is also helpful.

*Source:*
Arthritis Today (9,6:28,50)

# Brain over pain

You can expect plenty of pain after surgery, right?

Not necessarily. The amount of pain you have and how soon you feel better following surgery depend on the thoughts you think.

A recent study of 51 people who underwent abdominal surgery found that those people who visualized themselves coping effectively with the pain and discomforts of surgery actually had less pain and less discomfort than people who didn't imagine themselves coping effectively.

The study participants were divided into two groups. One group listened to an information tape about the hospital. The other group listened to an imagery tape which took them through the stages of surgery and encouraged a positive coping response at each stage of pain they might encounter.

Only the people who listened to the imagery tapes had less pain after surgery. They were able to cope with the pain they did have better than the other group. They also required less medicine.

The imagery tape asked participants to imagine themselves dealing with presurgery and postsurgery discomforts, such as hunger, thirst, dry mouth, pain, nausea, and weakness. While people were imagining themselves in such situations, the tape played positive messages, such as "You can easily manage for the rest of the day." "You feel positive ... knowing that it is necessary and you can easily cope."

The next time you find yourself facing a painful situation, remember that the key to less pain is to acknowledge the pain and then imagine yourself coping effectively with it. Reinforce your efforts by repeating words to yourself that make you feel positive about what you're doing.

*Source:*
Psychosomatic Medicine (57:177)

# Back to work better than bed rest

It's Monday, and your lower back has been aching since you moved those heavy boxes to the attic on Saturday. The pain relievers you've been taking haven't really helped, and now you have to choose between going to work and staying in bed nursing your pain. According to a recent study, you'll recover faster if you go to work.

Researchers studied 186 people in Helsinki, Finland, who were troubled with lower back pain. They wanted to find out which of two treatments, bed rest or exercise, was better at healing back pain. The people were divided into three groups. The first group was treated with two days of bed rest; the second group was treated with back-extension exercises; and people in the third group, called the control group, were not treated at all but were allowed to go about their daily activities as much as their pain allowed. Surprisingly, the people in the control group recovered better than those in the other two groups. People treated with bed rest recovered last.

The researchers concluded that maintaining your ordinary activities, as much as your pain will allow, is the best way to treat your lower back pain. Be sensible, however, and don't exercise strenuously when your back hurts.

*Source:*
*The New England Journal of Medicine* (332,6:351)

## Chiropractic care ranked best

Between 60 and 90 percent of adults suffer from low back pain at some time. If your pain lasts for more than four to six weeks, you should probably consult a doctor, but what kind of doctor? You could choose your family doctor, an orthopedic surgeon, a neurologist, a hospital-based physical therapist, or a chiropractor.

If you go to a neurologist or orthopedic surgeon for acute or chronic back pain, he will usually order tests to determine whether you have a structural problem, such as a herniated disc, that is causing your pain. If the test shows a herniated disc, surgery may be recommended. Some people with herniated discs find relief through surgery, but others recover without it. You can have a herniated disc with no pain at all, so the two conditions are not always connected. The increase in testing and imaging techniques, such as *magnetic resonance imaging (MRI)*, may be responsible for some unnecessary back surgeries to repair herniated discs.

In two separate studies comparing different types of medical care for low back pain, most of the treatments were successful. However, the people who received treatment from chiropractors were the most satisfied with their relief from pain. Chiropractic care requires a greater number of treatments than traditional medical care, and they are usually spread out over a longer time. This may be part of the reason that people were more satisfied with chiropractic care. In the long run, however, the people studied were less satisfied with traditional treatments from doctors and hospitals and more satisfied with the care of a chiropractor.

*Sources:*
*Arthritis Today* (10,1:10)
*British Medical Journal* (311,7001:349)
*The New England Journal of Medicine* (333,14:913)

## Conquer back pain without pills or surgery

Doctors can't explain why some people have back pain. No reason for the pain shows up on an X-ray or MRI scan, and the pain lasts much longer than a damaged muscle would normally take to heal. For some people, even surgery can't stop the pain.

John Sarno, M.D., professor of clinical rehabilitation medicine at the New York University School of Medicine, has an explanation for this kind of pain. He believes the pain is not in your back but in your head. He knows your pain is real, but he blames repressed emotions, such as anger and anxiety, for causing the pain.

These subconscious feelings, especially anger, make your blood vessels constrict. In turn, blood flow is diminished, and your muscles and nerves don't get enough oxygen. The lack of oxygen causes pain, numbness, tingling, weakness, or a combination of these symptoms. Dr. Sarno calls this condition *tension myositis syndrome*, or *TMS*. Since the root of the problem is emotional rather than physical, all the drugs, surgery, and exercises in the world will not cure it without getting at the cause.

The diagnosis of TMS is not widely accepted in the medical community, but people treated by Dr. Sarno often show dramatic improvement when more accepted therapies have failed. How do you know whether your pain is caused by TMS? It could be in the following situations:

- ◆ You can't attribute the pain to a physical incident, like lifting something heavy or participating in athletic activity when your body isn't in proper shape. Even if you can point to an incident that immediately caused pain, it could be TMS if the incident wasn't something out of the ordinary. For instance, if you lean forward at your desk and pain begins, it might be TMS.

- ◆ You have pain in your neck, shoulders, low back, and buttocks. Most pain due to injury is restricted to one area, and it doesn't usually occur on both sides. TMS pain often occurs on both sides, and it affects larger areas.

- ◆ You feel pain in your arms and legs. People often attribute this pain radiating from the back down the arms or legs to disc problems and pinched nerves. But TMS pain can occur at any point on your arms and legs. TMS pain often changes from day to day or even hour to hour. Pain from a condition like arthritis is usually more constant.

If you've tried every back remedy, been to every doctor, or even had surgery and still suffer from chronic back pain, consider these suggestions from Dr. Sarno:

**Try exercise and massage therapy.** Both can increase blood flow to the area, which will help relieve the pain. Of course, since the problem is also emotional, simply treating the symptoms will not offer long-term help.

**Take control of items in your life that cause stress.** That way, you stop stress from getting a foothold in your body. Remember that your body has a strong drive for self-restoration and self-healing, but you have to give your body the opportunity to heal itself.

**Accept the diagnosis.** Take comfort in the fact that there is nothing seriously wrong with your body. The stress of having a major medical ailment alone is enough to make the TMS worse. Dr. Sarno has seen people fully recover after simply understanding that their problems were caused by stress.

*Sources:*
American Health: Fitness of Body and Mind (10,2:23)
*Mind Over Back Pain*, Berkley Books, New York, 1982
*The Newsletter of the American Institute of Stress* (1995,8:3)

## Don't sit still for back pain

Remember all those times your mother told you to sit down and be quiet, or to sit down and do your homework? You got the idea that sitting down and doing your work was the adult thing to do. For many adults, sitting and working at their desks for many hours is accepted behavior. But the habit of sitting for hours can play havoc with your health, especially when it comes to your lower back.

When you sit for a long time, various muscles shorten, pulling your body down into poor postural positions and stretching and weakening other muscles. Take a break every half hour or so to stand up, stretch, or walk around.

Sit up straight in your chair, rather than slumping or leaning forward. Sit with your back firmly against the chair and both feet on the floor. If this posture is not comfortable, you may want to use a *lumbar pillow* for support of your lower back. Putting your feet up on a small footstool can help keep your lower back from arching forward.

Exercises to strengthen your abdominal muscles, such as abdominal crunches, will make your back stronger and better able to support a sitting posture comfortably.

*Sources:*
*Before You Call the Doctor*, Ballantine Books, New York, 1992
*The Secret of Good Posture*, American Physical Therapy Association, 1111 North Fairfax Street, Alexandria, Va. 22314

## How to buy a chair that will baby your back

If you've ever suffered the agony of a backache, you know the value of babying your back. And if you know that sitting places one and a half times more pressure on your back than standing or walking, you know the value of picking the proper chair for your back. Here are some tips to help you choose a chair that will do just that:

- Select a chair with a firm seat that is low enough for your feet to rest comfortably on the floor. Shun soft chairs even though they may seem comfy. They're generally unsupportive and can cause your back muscles to tighten up and go into spasms.
- Look for a chair with a back that fits the curves of your spine and does not cause your back to sway or be overly rounded. Don't pick a chair that has an open space where your lower back will be. Select a chair that is big enough to completely support your thighs.
- Choose a chair that will rock back. This will ease pressure on your spine. Relaxing in a regular rocking chair is very helpful for an aching back. The

rocking motion helps relieve back pain by changing the positions of your muscles and removing some of the strain caused by gravity.

♦ Make sure your chosen chair has armrests and use them. They will reduce the amount of pressure on your spine while you're sitting. Don't forget to use the armrests to shift your weight now and then and to help push yourself out of the chair.

♦ Find yourself a footrest to go with your chair. A footrest will help reduce pressure from your thighs as you sit. If you aren't using a footrest, your feet should rest flat on the floor so the weight of your legs is not supported completely by the front of your thighs.

*Source:*
*The Better Back Book,* William Morrow and Company, New York, 1989

# Best back pain busters

It's much easier to avoid back problems in the first place than to deal with the pain once you have it. Here are some things you can do to steer clear of back pain:

**Get yourself into good physical shape** and maintain your fitness. Be sure to include aerobic exercises, strengthening exercises, and stretches. Swimming, stationary biking, and walking are good choices for your back.

**If you're overweight, lose weight.** A potbelly is especially hard on your back. Your back muscles have to exert 50 pounds of force to balance a 10-pound potbelly.

**Stop smoking.** Doctors are not sure of the exact reason, but smoking seems to aggravate back problems.

**Sleep on a firm mattress.** A weak, sagging mattress will not support your back properly while you sleep. You can always put a board under your mattress if it's too soft. Sleeping on your back with a pillow under your knees or on your side with a pillow between your knees will take some of the pressure off your back.

**Work to improve your posture** while sitting, standing, and walking. Include exercises to strengthen your abdominal muscles, which help support your back.

**Improve your lifting skills.** When you lift a heavy object, keep it close to your body. Squat down, bending your knees and keeping your back straight. Use your arms and legs, rather than your back, to lift the weight.

*Sources:*
*American Family Physician* (52,5:1347)
*Lifetime Encyclopedia of Natural Remedies,* Parker Publishing Company, West Nyack, N.Y., 1993
*Symptoms, Illness & Surgery,* The Berkley Publishing Group, New York, 1995

# New water treatments for back pain

Sometimes an effective treatment for an age-old problem can come from an ordinary source. In searching for a drug-free way to relieve lower back pain in childbirth, doctors in Sweden, Canada, and the United States have found that water does the trick.

In several studies, sterile water, injected just under the skin on the lower backs of pregnant women, relieved severe lower back pain in the first stage of childbirth. The injections were made in four locations on the lower back.

An *epidural block* (anesthetic injected into the spine) is often used to relieve pain in childbirth, but it can have unpleasant side effects, such as a lingering backache or headache. This new water treatment, called *Intracutaneous Sterile Water (ISW)* is easy for doctors and nurses to learn, seems to have no side effects, and lasts for up to three hours. It can be repeated every few hours as necessary to relieve pain.

Doctors are not sure how ISW works, but they think it may have something to do with the body's production of *endorphins*, natural substances in the body that relieve pain. ISW is a simple, effective way to relieve some labor pain without drugs. It has also been tested and shows promise for relieving kidney pain from passing kidney stones and neck and shoulder pain from whiplash.

Water can be used in another way to treat people with low back pain. Dr. Robert P. Wilder of Dallas often treats his patients who are runners by having them run in deep water. After a short period of rest or other treatment, deep-water running can become part of the rehabilitation program. This allows the athlete to maintain his fitness and helps with the transition back to running on dry land.

*Sources:*
*Canadian Family Physician* (40:1785)
*The Physician and Sportsmedicine* (24,4:30)

# Neutralize neck pain

Sitting at a desk or keyboard all day puts lots of stress and strain on your neck. This can reduce your neck strength as much as 40 percent and cause lots of pain as your neck struggles to hold your head properly. Usually the cause of neck pain is tight muscles, so to counteract the pain you need to stretch and strengthen your neck. The best way to avoid neck pain is to take a break every 30 to 45 minutes. Get up from your desk, walk around, and stretch. The next best way is to exercise your neck just as you exercise the rest of your body.

If you work out at a gym or health club, be sure to take advantage of the "neck machine" to exercise your neck. Your instructor can tell you how to use it properly. If you want to do some simple exercises at home, the following ones may help to get your neck pain under control. Be sure to do the exercises only if they are comfortable. If you feel pain, see your doctor or a physical therapist.

Here are three simple stretches to do once a day:

◆ Sit or stand with your neck upright and inhale. Drop your chin down to your chest and exhale. Return your head to its normal position and repeat the exercise 10 times.

◆ Sit or stand with your neck upright and your chin tucked slightly and inhale. Turn your head to the right, keeping your chin level, as far as you comfortably can and exhale. Return your head to its previous position and repeat the stretch to the left. Do each stretch 10 times.

♦ Sit or stand with your neck upright and your chin tucked slightly and inhale. Tilt your head toward your right shoulder as far as you comfortably can and exhale. Return your head to its upright position, then stretch to the left. Repeat each stretch 10 times.

Here are two strengthening exercises to try:

♦ Sit up straight in a chair and clasp your hands behind your head. Push your head back against your hands eight to 12 times.

♦ Sit up straight in a chair with your spine firmly against the seat back. Put your hands together on your forehead and push your head against your hands eight to 12 times.

These exercises can be done one to three times a week.

*Source:*
*American Health* (12,8:94)

## Nighttime remedy for neck pain

If you're bothered by neck pain, here's a simple treatment that may help heal your pain while you sleep. It comes from Dr. Alan S. Kaplan of Potomac, Md. Roll a bath towel into a tube shape and wrap it around your neck. Pin it together in the front with a large safety pin. This makeshift collar will support your chin, hold your head in place while you sleep, and relieve some of the strain on your neck. Try it for a couple of nights to see if it helps your neck pain.

*Source:*
*Emergency Medicine* (27,7;75)

## Spring back from shoulder pain

Hurting your shoulder is easy, especially if you're an active person. Pain usually comes on gradually and is caused by overusing your *rotator cuff* muscles. These muscles attach your upper arm to your shoulder blade, help hold your upper-arm bone in your shoulder socket, and give your shoulder mobility.

You could get a sore shoulder from swimming strenuously, if that's your sport, or from gardening, if that's your hobby. Even carrying heavy packages, backpacks, or books can cause a shoulder strain. Lifting heavy suitcases when you travel can cause or irritate a sore shoulder, too.

So, what can you do if your shoulder is hurting? First of all, see your doctor. If he says your pain is due to problems with your rotator cuff muscles, there are some steps you can take at home to help the healing.

If your shoulder is being aggravated by swimming or other exercises, take aspirin or another anti-inflammatory drug after each workout. Reduce pain and swelling by icing the painful area for 15 minutes after your workout and each night before you go to bed. Ask a coach or trainer to check your technique for mistakes in form that might be causing your pain. Be sure to stretch after you warm up and after you swim, but keep your arms below shoulder height during the stretches.

To help get rid of your shoulder pain and strengthen muscles so you won't be as likely to get hurt in the future, try the following stretching and strengthening exercises. Don't take anti-inflammatory drugs such as aspirin before exercising, since the drug might mask your pain and prevent you from knowing how far to push your body.

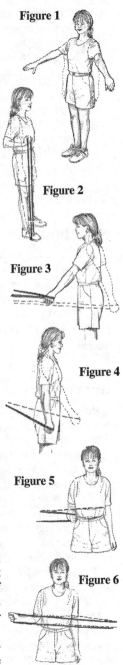

**Figure 1**

**Figure 2**

**Figure 3**

**Figure 4**

**Figure 5**

**Figure 6**

◆ Stand straight with your arms at your sides. With your thumbs pointing downward, raise your arms in front of you, at the 2 o'clock and 10 o'clock positions (Figure 1). Raise your arms as high as your pain allows, keeping them below shoulder level, and don't shrug your shoulders. Begin with two sets of 10 arm raises twice a day, and progress to two sets of 50 twice a day.

The next three exercises require the use of an "exercise band," a thick elastic loop made specifically for resistance exercises and available at sporting goods and department stores. You can work just the injured side, but working both sides of your body will help you develop more consistent muscle strength.

◆ Grasp the exercise band with the hand of your injured arm and hold the band taut by standing on it with your foot. Clench your fist, palm side up, bend your elbow, and pull the band up to the level of your armpit (Figure 2). Begin with a set of five to 15 pulls twice a day and progress to 50 pulls once a day.

◆ Attach an exercise band to a doorknob or other stationary object and stand so it is taut when you grasp it in front and slightly to the side of your body. With your arm straight (Figure 3), pull the band back and down toward your heels, hold for two seconds, and return your arm to the starting position. This works the back part of your *deltoid* muscle, which lies on top of your shoulder. To work the front part of your deltoid muscle, turn around with your back toward the attached band and pull it toward your toes (Figure 4). Begin with a set of five to 15 pulls twice a day and progress to 50 pulls once a day. Once the exercise becomes too easy for you, use a band with more resistance.

◆ Attach an exercise band to a doorknob or other stationary object and stand with your injured side toward the band, your elbow at your side, and your arm bent at a 90 degree angle in front of you. Grasp the band and pull it slowly across your body toward your other arm (Figure 5), then allow it to go back to the starting position. To work more muscles at the back of your shoulder, stand with your opposite side toward the exercise band and your arm across the front of your body grasping the band. Slowly swing your arm outward to stretch the band (Figure 6), then return to the starting position. Begin with a set of five to 15 pulls twice a day and progress to 50 pulls once a day. Once the exercise becomes too easy for you, use a band with more resistance.

*Source:*
*The Physician and Sportsmedicine* (24,2:33)

## Coping with carpal tunnel syndrome

The ability to use your hands for the daily tasks of life is a gift most people take for granted. Sometimes you use your hands too much and don't pay attention when pain and common sense tell you to rest. Spending many hours typing at a computer, doing needlework, assembling products, and many other activities can cause a repetitive strain injury known as *carpal tunnel syndrome* (CTS). In CTS, the *median nerve* in your wrist is compressed by surrounding tissue as it goes through the carpal tunnel. The result can be tingling, numbness, or burning in your hand; shooting pains in your wrist; weakness of your thumb; stiffness or cramping of your hand; frequent dropping of objects; and the inability to make a fist.

If you work at a job that requires strong hand or wrist action, you are at higher risk of developing CTS. You are also at higher risk if you are pregnant; if you have diabetes, hypothyroidism, or Raynaud's disease; if you have gone through menopause; or if you are obese. If your carpal tunnel syndrome doesn't get better, the damage to your median nerve can become permanent along with the symptoms.

There are some things you can do to help prevent CTS, or to treat it if you already have it.

- ◆ Take a break at least once an hour when doing repetitive tasks involving your hands or wrists, such as typing or needlework.
- ◆ If you work at a computer, make sure that your desk, keyboard, and chair are at the correct height for comfortable keyboarding. Your keyboard should be at the height of your hands when your elbows are bent and your forearms and hands are parallel to the floor.
- ◆ Lose weight if you're overweight.
- ◆ Get a handle on your stress as much as possible. Stress seems to make CTS worse.
- ◆ Ask your doctor to prescribe a splint for you that will immobilize your wrist and take some of the strain off the affected area. A splint allows you to continue to work while helping your wrist heal.
- ◆ If you get pain in your hand, especially when you wake up during the night,

hang your hand over the side of your bed and rub or shake your hand to relieve the pain.

◆ Clench your hand into a fist, then straighten your fingers and stretch your hand as wide as possible. Repeat with your other hand.

If nothing else works to relieve your pain, your doctor may recommend surgery.

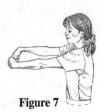

**Figure 7**

*Sources:*
*Complete Guide to Symptoms, Illness & Surgery,* The Berkley Publishing Group, New York, 1995
National Institute of Arthritis and Musculoskeletal and Skin Diseases, Information Clearinghouse, 1 AMS Circle, Bethesda, Md. 20892–3675

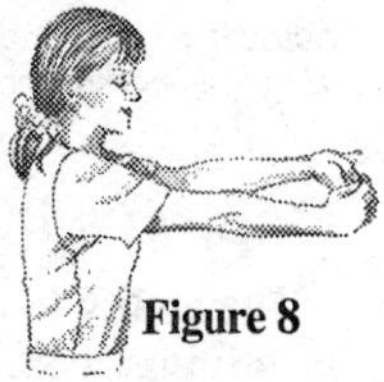

# Erase elbow pain

A pleasant hour of lobbing tennis balls in the sunshine or a day of golf on a lush, green course can have an unexpected cost — several days of intense pain in your elbow. Just resting your elbow won't solve the problem, but some well-planned exercises can help ease your pain and prevent injury in the future. To rehabilitate an injured elbow, you need to stretch your muscles slowly and strengthen them gently. Here are some exercises you can try:

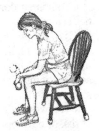

**Figure 8**

**Stretching exercises:**
Do these twice a day to help recover from elbow pain, as well as before and after any sports activity that involves your elbows. Hold each stretch for 20 to 30 seconds, and keep alternating your arms for a period of five minutes.

◆ With your right arm stretched out in front of you and your palm down, use your left hand to pull your right hand gently down and back toward your body (Figure 7). Stretch your left arm and hand the same way. This stretches the muscles on the top of your forearm. If this exercise is very painful, you can do it with your elbow bent.

◆ With your right arm stretched out in front of you and your palm facing up, use your left hand to gently pull the fingers of your right hand down toward the floor (Figure 8). Stretch your left arm and hand the same way. This stretches the muscles on the underside of your forearm.

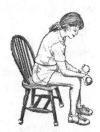

**Figure 9**

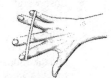

**Figure 10**

**Strengthening exercises:**
Do these next two exercises holding a one-pound weight. Sit in a chair and rest your elbow on your thigh

**Figure 11**

with your wrist extending beyond your knee. Perform three sets of 10 curls once a day.

◆ Holding the weight, bend your elbow with your palm facing the floor and curl your wrist toward the ceiling (Figure 9). Hold the position for 10 to 15 seconds, then relax and drop your wrist. Repeat with other arm. This strengthens your top forearm muscles.

◆ Hold the weight with your elbow bent and your palm facing the ceiling. Curl your wrist to raise the weight and hold the position for 10 to 15 seconds (Figure 10). Relax and let your wrist drop. This strengthens the muscles on the underside of your forearm.

To strengthen your forearm even more, do the following exercise in three sets of 10 once a day, then move to several sessions a day.

◆ Hold your hand with the fingers straight and together. Place a heavy rubber band over your hand at the tips of your fingers. Stretch your fingers outward, pressing against the rubber band (Figure 11). This is a good exercise to do while talking on the telephone.

*Source:*
*The Physician and Sportsmedicine* (24,2:71)

# Turn off TMJ

The terrible pain in your head has been troubling you for months now. It seems to move around, sometimes lodging in your ear, teeth, jaw, or neck, and sometimes turning into a migraine headache. It could take years to track down the cause of this phantom pain. Some people who have it begin to doubt their own sanity when doctors tell them it's all in their heads. One woman with these symptoms had 18 root canals and 13 surgeries before she found the cause. Another woman was so overcome by the pain that she considered suicide. You might not suspect it, but all this pain could be caused by *temporomandibular joint (TMJ)* disorder.

The temporomandibular joints on each side of your head connect your upper and lower jaws to each other and to your skull. They allow your jaws to open and close, rotate, and move back and forth. Some of the other symptoms of TMJ disorder are clicking or popping sounds when you open your mouth or chew, pain when you yawn, and the inability to open your mouth widely.

You can be born with a malformed joint or cause the disorder by unconsciously grinding your teeth or clenching your jaw muscles when you're under stress. If your teeth don't meet correctly to form a good bite, or a blow to your jaw damages the structure of the joint, TMJ can result. Even poor posture in your neck and shoulders or arthritis in your joints can cause TMJ.

To prevent TMJ problems, don't grind your teeth or clench your jaw when you're tense. Learn techniques to relax muscles, such as meditation or biofeedback, and relieve stress by following a regular exercise program. Be sure to see your doctor for his advice.

Learning new ways to channel stress, sometimes using counseling or psychotherapy, is one of the ways a doctor may treat your TMJ syndrome. A dentist or ortho-dontist may be able to help you with braces or a special appliance to wear at night that keeps you from grinding your teeth. Here are some things you can do at home to help soothe the pain of TMJ syndrome:

- Use aspirin or acetaminophen to relieve minor pain.
- Eat a soft diet and avoid chewy foods, such as bagels, when your symptoms are bad.
- Substitute a rolled-up towel under your neck for a pillow while you sleep, and sleep on your back.
- Avoid chewing gum.
- Massage the TMJ area.
- Learn to relax your jaw and limit its movements. You can put your fist under your jaw to block a yawn.
- Try applying ice or heat to the TMJ area to relieve pain. One may work bet-ter for you than the other.

*Sources:*
*Complete Guide to Symptoms, Illness & Surgery,* The Berkley Publishing Group, New York, 1995
*Postgraduate Medicine* (97,5:206)
*The Atlanta Journal/Constitution* (May 3, 1994, E5)

## Peas, no more pain!

If you have sprained your ankle, bruised your arm or leg, or strained a muscle in your knee, neck, back, or shoulder, an ice pack can often relieve the pain and help prevent swelling. If you don't have an ice pack, don't run to the drugstore. There's probably one as close as your freezer.

Dr. Mary Catherine Schniedeknecht of Dallas recommends that you use a package of frozen vegetables as an ice pack. The large plastic bags of peas and corn are especially good at conforming to the area that needs to be iced. Once the bags thaw out, you can refreeze them and reapply them later. Ice that has been crushed in a blender and placed in a heavy plastic bag makes a good ice pack, too.

*Source:*
*Emergency Medicine* (28,10:47)

# Better Hospital and Doctor Care

## How to find the best doctor for your money

How do you choose a doctor? Do you ask your friends for a recommendation? Do you base your selection on the doctor's reputation? Or do you resort to a walk through the yellow pages?

These methods may work, but only if there's a lot of luck involved. By conducting a little research, you can eliminate much of the guesswork and increase the odds of finding the best doctor for your money.

Once you have a name in mind, check a doctor's credentials by taking a trip to the library. Most libraries carry the *American Medical Association's Directory of Physicians*, which contains information regarding each doctor's medical education, board certifications, licensing information, and any disciplinary actions taken against him.

If you are looking for a specialist, you can call the American Board of Medical Specialties Hotline to quickly determine if your doctor is board certified. The number is 1–800–776–2378. Some doctors claim they are specialized in an area of medicine, such as dermatology or pediatrics, but they don't have a board certification. This is legal, but misleading, so you have to check to make sure you are getting a specialist who is qualified in his field.

*Sources:*
Get the Facts on Anyone, Macmillan, New York, 1995
Head Lines, National Headache Foundation (94:7)

## Does your doctor pass the test?

Once you find a doctor, decide on the services you want from him and the traits you want him to have. This will give you a solid basis for deciding who will best meet your medical needs. Here are some good questions to ask:

**Is he friendly and cheerful?** For some people, this is not important as long as the doctor seems capable.

**How emotionally involved does he get?** Many people want their doctors to be understanding and concerned while others prefer their doctors to be detached.

**How formal is your doctor?** Does it bother you to be addressed by your first name? How do you feel about a doctor who touches your shoulder or hand as he talks with you? If you feel your doctor is too familiar, it may get in the way of a productive relationship.

**Does your doctor let you share in the decision making?** Some people want to be involved in the decisions concerning their health care, and some would rather leave all the decision making up to the doctor. If you want to play an active role in your treatment, it's important to find a doctor who is comfortable with your input.

**Do you want or need a specialist?** The nature of your illness may determine how specialized you want your doctor to be. Or, you may think it's important that your doctor be able to treat a variety of illnesses.

**How long do you have to wait to see him?** Does he have convenient office hours? If it's difficult to get away from work, you may need a doctor who has evening and/or weekend office hours. Are you willing to wait an hour or more after your appointment time to see the doctor? It may be worth the wait to see a doctor you trust.

**What age doctor do you prefer?** Do you prefer the recent education of a younger doctor or one who is older and more experienced? Maybe you'd be more comfortable with someone in between.

**Does it make any difference if your doctor is male or female?** According to the 1993 Arthritis Foundation Survey, men tend to choose male doctors, while women seem to be as likely to choose a male doctor as a female doctor.

**Do you want a doctor with admitting privileges at a specific hospital?** If you prefer one hospital over the others, you will probably want a doctor who has admitting privileges there.

**What conveniences does your doctor offer?** If you consider filling out and filing insurance claims a chore, check to see which doctors' offices file them for you. You may also want to check for other services such as on-site labs, pharmacies, and X-ray capabilities.

**Where is his office located?** Are you willing to travel a long distance for a good doctor? If you run on a tight schedule, you may prefer that your health care provider be close to where you live or work.

**Will he answer your questions?** Many people value a doctor who will respond openly to their questions about their health.

Narrow down your choices and get to know prospective doctors so you can select the best one for you. It's important to begin your search for the ideal doctor before you have a medical emergency.

*Sources:*
*Get the Facts on Anyone,* Macmillan, New York, 1995
*Head Lines,* National Headache Foundation (94:7)

# It takes two for top health care

You can be more in control of your health by choosing a doctor that meets your medical needs. From the beginning, establish yourself as an equal partner in your health care, rather than a compliant servant who does whatever the doctor says without question. Medicine is not always an exact science; there are variables in every situation.

Doctors vary greatly in their competence, their philosophies, and their motivations.

You have a right to expect your doctor to explain every diagnosis, every procedure, every test, and every drug that is prescribed for you. If your doctor doesn't volunteer the information, ask for it.

A group of researchers from the New England Medical Center in Boston tested the difference between assertive and compliant patients. Patients who were trained to be assertive, asking questions, expressing their feelings, and taking charge of doctor-patient interactions, stayed healthier than patients who weren't assertive. The assertive people had fewer health problems, lost fewer days from work, and functioned better overall.

Approach your health care as you would any other area of your life. Research any disorder you develop, the drugs prescribed for it, and methods of treatment. You can purchase excellent books on health care written in understandable language, or you can go to your local library and find the information. Choose to be informed in this very important area of your life.

Keep a record of your own medical history. This is useful if you change doctors or have to see another doctor who is on call. The information could also be very important in an emergency. Include any major diagnosis of illness, in medical terms as well as plain English; major test results, along with the date and reason for testing; a list of any medicines you are taking; surgeries you have had; and any allergies to food, drugs, or chemicals. Keep this information with you, if possible, or let a person close to you have quick access to it.

*Source:*
*Public Citizen Health Research Group Health Letter* (11,6:1)

# Wanted: Doctors who talk more and test less

Doctors should talk more and test less, according to a new government study by the U.S. Preventive Services Task Force. For five years, the medical panel studied the effectiveness of testing in preventing disease. Their findings will probably have a strong impact on the behavior of doctors and managed-care systems throughout the United States.

The task force recommended that some tests, such as the PSA blood test for screening against prostate cancer, be used less. They said that this test is costly and does not save lives, but it does encourage many men to have unnecessary biopsies and surgeries that can cause impotence and incontinence. The group also supports mammography screening for women 50 to 69 years old, but not for women between the ages of 40 to 50.

The task force encourages routine cholesterol screening for men age 35 to 65 and women age 45 to 65. They also support screening for colorectal cancer after age 50, and the use of vaccines against chickenpox and hepatitis B. Their strongest recommendation, however, is for counseling of patients.

About 50 percent of deaths in the United States each year are caused by personal behavior problems, such as smoking, alcohol and drug abuse, and diet. If doctors would spend more time talking and advising people in these areas of their lives, these health problems might be avoided.

As long as people look to tests and surgery to solve their health problems, they don't take as much personal responsibility for their behavior. Doctors can change this situation by spending more time talking with their patients and less time ordering tests.

*Source:*
*The Wall Street Journal* (Dec. 13, 1995, B1)

## Smart ways to slash medical bills

The money you shell out when you're sick can make you even sicker. Here's how to develop healthier spending habits:

**Give the doctor as much information about your condition as possible.** That way, he can make a better diagnosis and give you the proper medication the first time, and you'll have fewer doctor visits. Take a list of questions to ask, and question anything you don't understand. You don't want to pay for visits you could have avoided if you'd made sure you understood each other the first time.

**When you go for a second opinion, ask if you can use the same X-rays or relevant tests from the first doctor.** This request is not out of the ordinary, and it can save you a bundle.

**If taking a medication for the first time, ask your doctor for free samples.** You can make sure you are not allergic to the drug and that your system can handle it before you pay for a prescription you won't use.

**Save money at the pharmacy by asking your doctor to increase the quantities on prescriptions he writes for drugs you take regularly.** You'll even save money if you have a prescription drug plan through your insurance. You may be able to get a three-month supply of your medicine at once and pay only one deductible. (Some insurance plans limit you to a 30-day supply while others limit you to a two-week supply. Make sure you maximize your plan.)

**Mail order your drugs.** You mail your prescription to a pharmacy designated by your insurance company and receive your drugs through the mail. Ask your insurance company or the benefits manager at your workplace if mail order is available to you.

**Follow all directions your doctor gives you about your medication.** You don't want to have to buy more just because you didn't take your medicine correctly the first time.

*Sources:*
*How to Pinch a Penny 'Til It Screams,* Avery Publishing Group, Garden City Park, N.Y., 1994
Dell Weaver, pharmacist, Atlanta, Ga.

## Protect your rights: keep medical records private

You may think that information between doctors and their patients is "privileged," as it is between lawyers and their clients. Unfortunately, that's not the case. There is no federal law that protects the privacy of medical records, and state laws vary and are open to interpretation. The transfer of hospital records by computer makes them even less confidential.

When private medical information is made public, reputations, careers, and relationships can be ruined. So, it's important to know when such information is usually released. The most common form of medical disclosure occurs when you apply for life, health, and some other kinds of insurance.

Besides information that you provide, the insurance company may get information from the Medical Insurance Bureau (MIB). Knowledge about any aspect of your life that can affect whether you are a poor risk, such as having a dangerous hobby, can be obtained along with your medical information. If you are denied insurance coverage or charged a much higher premium based on information obtained from the MIB, the insurance company must tell you. Then you are entitled to a free copy of the MIB report to check its accuracy. If you would like to purchase a copy of any information the bureau has on you, you can call (617) 426–3660 or send $8.00 to: MIB, P.O. Box 105, Essex Station, Boston, Mass. 02112.

Although there is no way to keep your medical records completely private, there are a few things you can do to protect yourself. The Privacy Rights Clearinghouse of the Center for Public Interest Law, which is located at the University of San Diego, offers these tips:

♦ When you are filling out an application that has a blanket waiver authorizing all providers (doctors and hospitals) to release everything in your medical records, cross this section out. Write in that you are allowing release of records covering treatment of a specific condition by a particular doctor or hospital.

♦ If you want certain medical information to be withheld from your employer or insurance company, put your request to the doctor in writing. Don't file a claim with the insurance company, and pay for the doctor visit yourself.

♦ If, for some legal reason, your medical records are subpoenaed, ask the court to keep the records closed, or to open only a certain part of them. After the case is settled, you can ask the judge to seal your medical records.

*Source:*
*Medical Update* (19,7:1)

# What doctors don't know can hurt you

According to a recent survey, less than one-third of doctors think they know enough about nutrition to counsel their patients. It's no wonder, since only 20 percent of medical schools require a class in nutrition. Doctors say they would like to know more about nutrition.

With all the books on diet, nutrition, and healthy eating that are available today, perhaps the people who rely on their doctors for nutritional advice should simply educate themselves about nutrition.

*Source:*
*American Family Physician* (52,1:28)

## Hygiene basics your doctor may not do

One important step in health care doesn't get much attention, but it can make a dramatic difference in the control of disease. It's the simple act of hand washing, practiced by doctors and nurses as they move from patient to patient.

Reports in recent medical journals have linked the neglect of this basic practice of hygiene to outbreaks of bacterial and viral diseases in hospitals, nursing homes, and day-care centers. Colds, flu, ear infections, and gastrointestinal illness are easily passed by hand-to-hand contact. Emerging strains of drug-resistant bacteria make the practice of hand washing even more vital for preventing epidemics.

When you are in your doctor's office, expect him and his nurse to wash their hands before they touch you. If they don't, ask them to do so. If you are tactful about your question and your doctor or his nurse is angered by it, you might want to find another doctor.

The same is true in day-care centers. Attendants should not diaper one baby and move on to the next without washing their hands. Using disposable latex gloves is an even better idea. A study in Finland showed that regular hand washing and using some staff members for diapering duty and others for serving snacks was an excellent way to control infection among the children.

It may seem awkward to ask a doctor, nurse, or day-care worker to wash his hands before touching you or your child, but it's much better than getting an illness that could easily have been prevented. Practice good hygiene yourself as a courtesy to others, and expect and demand that people in the health care community do the same.

*Source:*
The Wall Street Journal (Feb. 5, 1996, B1)

## 4 out of 5 doctors spread infection

As your doctor moves from one examining room to another, he usually has that classic symbol of doctoring, the stethoscope, draped around his neck. He uses it dozens of times a day to listen to the hearts of his patients. But how often does he clean that little metal disk that moves from one patient to the next? Probably not often enough.

When stethoscopes in four Houston-area hospitals were studied, 80 percent of the metal stethoscope heads were contaminated with disease-causing bacteria. Dr. Richard Duma, chief of infectious diseases at the Halifax Medical Center in Daytona Beach, Fla., recommends that doctors wash their stethoscopes between patients just as they wash their hands. He estimates that better cleanliness measures, including the washing of stethoscopes, could eliminate as many as 33 percent of hospital infections.

Doctors can wash their stethoscopes with alcohol swabs or antibacterial soap.

This simple action only takes a moment, and it is an effective tool in controlling the spread of disease.

**Sources:**
*American Family Physician* (52,8:2345)
*Medical Tribune for the Internist and Cardiologist* (37,3:1)

# Ease allergy anguish with simple, one-time test

With a simple, new, one-time test, your doctor can determine whether you are allergic to 24 different allergens. The *Thin-layer rapid-use epicutaneous* (TRUE) test checks you for 80 percent of the most common allergens that cause skin rashes. It consists of two self-adhesive pieces of surgical tape that contain 24 allergen patches, and it's applied to your upper back. This convenient, accurate test can help your doctor determine exactly what's causing your allergic reaction.

**Source:**
*Scientific American Medicine Bulletin* (18,10:1)

# Wearing and caring for a cast

That little misstep at the end of your driveway this morning unfortunately ended with a trip to the doctor to set your broken wrist. Now you've been fitted with a cast and told to come back in three days for a checkup. Here are some facts you need to know about wearing and caring for a cast.

Casts are used to help heal broken bones or torn ligaments. The length of time you wear one depends on the type and seriousness of your injury. Your doctor will probably check the cast after three days to make sure everything is beginning to heal.

The cast should relieve some of your pain by restricting movement of the injured area. However, if the pain is worse than it was before the cast went on, you should call your doctor. Increased pain or feeling pain in a new area may mean that the cast is too tight and needs to be redone.

Itching can be an annoying side effect of wearing a cast. Don't stick anything into the cast to scratch, since it could irritate or injure your skin. Try tapping or slapping (not too hard) the outside of the cast instead. Some people say scratching the same spot on the opposite arm or leg helps.

You can bathe or swim in some fiberglass casts without worry, but most casts shouldn't get wet. Getting a regular cast wet can cause irritation and even infection of your skin. To keep a cast from getting wet when you shower, put a plastic bag over it and hold the bag in place with rubber bands. If the cast gets wet, you may be able to use a blow dryer on a low setting to dry it out. First, ask your doctor if this is okay.

**Source:**
*American Family Physician* (52,4:1120)

## Less stressful surgery

Of course, you hope you'll never have to go through the major surgery of having your appendix removed. But it is possible that you might someday face an appendectomy, and then you would need to choose between *open* surgery and *laparoscopic* surgery. Open surgery involves an incision in your lower abdomen, while laparoscopic surgery involves a small hole through which a long tube is inserted.

If you are very overweight, laparoscopic surgery is a better choice for you because open surgery would require a much larger incision to reach your appendix. Also, if your doctor is not completely sure that you have appendicitis, he can get a better view of your abdominal cavity with laparoscopic surgery. For most other people, either kind of surgery works well.

If you choose to have a laparoscopic appendectomy, you may have less pain overall, recover more quickly, and spend less time in the hospital. You'll also have a smaller scar at the incision site. It sounds like a big improvement over the open surgery. The only negative aspect of this surgery is the cost.

With medical insurance as it is today, cost can be a deciding factor in which kind of surgery you choose. An open appendectomy usually costs about $5,700, while a laparoscopic appendectomy costs about $7,500. The difference in cost is due mostly to the expense of disposable laparoscopic equipment, which has to be purchased new for each operation. Even with the shorter hospital stay that accompanies laparoscopic surgery, it is still more expensive.

If cost is not a consideration for you or your insurance company, you may want to choose the less invasive surgery. If cost is a factor in this decision, and you choose the open surgery, you can still feel confident of a complete recovery.

*Source:*
*Emergency Medicine* (27,3:62)

## Easier, safer knee surgery

If you're scheduled for *arthroscopic* surgery to remove damaged tissue in your knee, you may have an easier time than you think. If you're afraid of being put to sleep under general anesthesia, ask your doctor if you can have local anesthesia, which prevents pain only in your knee. This makes the surgery both safer and less expensive and is becoming an increasingly common practice.

*Source:*
*Medical Update* (19,8:6)

## Hidden hazards of hospital beds

When you are in the hospital, you expect the highest degree of care and safety. However, hospital beds with side rails are not always safe for the people who sleep in them. Since 1990, there have been 102 reports to the Food and Drug

Administration (FDA) of people's heads and other body parts becoming trapped in the side rails of hospital beds. The beds were located in hospitals, nursing homes, and private homes. Of these incidents, 22 resulted in injury and 68 resulted in death. Most of the less serious injuries involved breaks, cuts, or scrapes to arms and legs.

Most of the people who had side rail accidents were elderly. People who are restless, lack muscle control, or are mentally unstable, such as people who have Alzheimer's, have the highest risk of injury. If the bed's dimensions are large compared to the user's size and weight, the risk of injury is also higher. All the injuries occurred in the following areas: through the space between split side rails; through the bars of a side rail; between the side rail and mattress; or between the headboard or footboard, side rail, and mattress.

Whether you are using a hospital bed at home, or your loved one is in a bed in the hospital, have the bed checked for safety. Here are some things you can do to make sure the bed is as safe as possible:

- ◆ Inspect the bed frame, side rails, and mattress to check for areas that might cause injury.
- ◆ Check side rails for proper installation and fit.
- ◆ Watch for replacement mattresses that don't fit properly.
- ◆ Don't use side rails as a substitute for protective restraints.
- ◆ Consider additional safety measures for people at high risk of injury.

*Source:*
*FDA Consumer* (29,10:5)

# Home-grown hospital comfort

Being ill and in the hospital can be a difficult, disorienting experience for anyone. For an elderly person who is already slightly confused, it can be even more upsetting. You can help by making the hospital a friendlier, more familiar place for your loved one. Here are some specific steps you can take:

- ◆ Place familiar objects, such as a favorite quilt or photos of family and friends, within sight and within reach, if possible.
- ◆ Provide visual reminders such as a clock, a marked calendar, and a sign stating where the person is.
- ◆ Furnish a night light for after dark.
- ◆ Minimize outside noises and disturbances as much as possible.
- ◆ Encourage the staff to provide reassurance and help the person adjust to his surroundings.
- ◆ Check with the doctor to see if nonessential medication, especially anything that causes confusion, can be stopped.

*Source:*
*Geriatrics* (50,2:42)

## How to handle a hospital problem

If you think you've been mistreated in any way by a doctor or nurse in a hospital, you can get justice without pressing charges. Every hospital has a review process. If you ask for an incident report to be filed against a medical caregiver, it will be.

Besides having a report filed against a nurse, you can complain through the hospital chain of command – first ask to speak to the charge nurse, then to the director of nursing, then to the hospital manager.

*Source:*
Suzanne Wilson, Registered Nurse, Upson County Hospital, Thomaston, Ga.

## 11 smart ways to cut hospital costs

Hospital stays are horribly expensive no matter what you do. Every little bit of saving helps, however. Here are some ways you can save money on your hospital bill.

**Refuse the hospital admission kit.** Take your own supplies instead. If you accept the kit, you'll be charged around $12 for a hospital pillow and $8 for a water pitcher.

**Take it with you when you go.** If the hospital does slip a pillow under you, take it home afterwards. The staff will just throw away anything it uses on you. Those washbasins are great for hand laundry.

**Take your own prescription medicines.** The hospital staff won't like it, but you can insist on using your own prescription eye drops, aspirin, etc. But don't take your own medicine without telling your doctor and nurse. You could have an unpleasant drug interaction. For instance, you wouldn't want to take aspirin if your doctor is giving you Coumadin.

**Ask when the hospital day starts.** The exact time a 24-hour "day" begins varies from hospital to hospital. If you can check in after a day starts or check out before another day starts, you can save money.

**Try to limit your hospital stay to under 24 hours.** Many hospitals consider you an outpatient if you stay for less than 24 hours. Insurance companies often pay the entire bill for outpatient care instead of charging you a copayment.

**Inquire about a semiprivate room.** Does your insurance company only pay for a semiprivate hospital room? You may be able to get privacy without paying for it yourself. All you have to do is ask if any of the semiprivate rooms are unoccupied. The hospital staff will put you in an empty room if there's one available, but only if you ask for it. If all the semiprivate rooms have an occupant, ask the hospital what it charges for private rooms. Being alone may be worth the extra $15 or so a day.

**Don't let the hospital issue you another pair of crutches** if you or a friend have a set at home.

**Never get any care in an emergency room that can be provided in a doctor's office.** Emergency-room care is expensive.

**Ask to have your medicine by mouth instead of by injection.** Unless you can't keep your medicine down or there's some other reason you need shots or an I.V., try to start taking your medicine orally as soon as possible. It's a lot less expensive.

**Provide your own blood.** If you're having elective surgery, you may be able to store your own blood ahead of time.

**Examine your final bill very carefully.** Make sure you aren't charged for treatment and equipment you didn't receive.

*Source:*
Suzanne Wilson, Registered Nurse, Upson County Hospital, Thomaston, Ga.

## Painkilling secrets nurses won't tell you

Picture yourself in the hospital after surgery, in severe pain, begging your nurse for medicine to kill the throbbing ache – because that's exactly where you'll be if you don't make other post-surgery arrangements.

It's not the nurse's fault. Most pain medicines are listed on your chart as *PRN*. That means "repeat as requested." You have to ask for it before you get it. However, the nurse will usually give you your medicine on a regular schedule, every four hours or so, if you make it clear that that's what you'd prefer. Or, you can ask for your medicine 20 minutes before you think you'll really need it.

Even better, ask for a *PCA* (Patient Controlled Analgesia). With this handy system, you can give the pain medicine to yourself. If you aren't getting adequate relief, ask your nurse to see if your doctor can prescribe another painkiller. Medicines have different effects on different people.

One of the most common mistakes people make during hospital stays is waiting until they are in severe pain before asking for medicine. It's very rare to become addicted to a painkiller during a short hospital stay. Besides, nurses say, it takes more medicine to relieve pain than to prevent it. So, don't try to be a hero. Take the medicine you need, when you need it.

*Source:*
Suzanne Wilson, Registered Nurse, Upson County Hospital, Thomaston, Ga.

## Avoiding hospital medication errors

A stay in the hospital for an illness or operation usually brings with it the need to take new and different types of medicine. To be sure you get the medicine you're supposed to, and nothing else, the Institute for Safe Medication Practices, in Warminster, Pa., offers these tips:

◆ When the nurse comes in to give you medicine, have her check your identification bracelet to be sure she has the correct patient.

◆ If you're routinely taking medicine, make sure it's the same color, size, and shape as before. If not, ask why. It might be a generic form of the same thing.

◆ Before you take a new medicine, ask for the name, what it does, and any possible side effects.

◆ If you're scheduled for tests, ask whether they require any drugs or dyes, and which ones. If you've been allergic to these substances before, tell the staff.

*Source:*
*FDA Consumer* (29,9:8)

# Making the Most of Your Medicine

## Preventing prescription disasters

No matter how healthy you are, the time may come when you have to take a prescribed medicine for some ailment. Prescription drugs can be helpful, healing, and even lifesaving. But less than 60 percent of people get the benefits they're supposed to from the drugs they take.

Many people get sick as a result of taking drugs they don't need or from misunderstanding how to take their drugs properly. Better communication between you, your doctor, and your pharmacist can help keep you from becoming one of those statistics.

Here are some questions you need to ask your doctor when he prescribes any medicine for you:

◆ What is the name of this medicine, and what exactly is it supposed to do?
◆ How should I take this medicine, how much should I take, what time of day should I take it, and for how long?
◆ What are the possible side effects of this drug, and what should I do if they occur?
◆ Is this drug compatible with other medicine I am taking?
◆ Are there any specific foods, drugs, or activities I should avoid while taking this drug?
◆ Do you have any written information, such as a pamphlet, that you can give me about this drug?

When you get your prescription filled, read the label and be sure it's the same as your prescription. Or you may want to repeat back to the pharmacist the name of the drug, dosage, and the reason you are taking it, just to be sure it is correct.

Be sure to take your medicine exactly as it is prescribed. Don't assume that it's okay to skip a dose, or double a dose if you missed the previous one. Never take more than the recommended dose of any drug. It may take a while to see results, so be patient. Consult your doctor if you have any questions or problems with any medicine.

*Sources:*
*Archives of Internal Medicine* (155,18:1949)
*Geriatrics* (50,2:15)

## Cracking the prescription code

The first prescriptions for medicine were written in the 1400s. They were written in Latin, which made sense at the time, since it had been one of the main languages of Western Europe for centuries. It also was a language that didn't change, and it was very exact in its meaning.

Today, however, Latin is used only on the portion of a prescription that gives directions for taking the drug. Since Latin is not currently a second language for most people, it would be difficult to interpret these instructions even if they weren't in abbreviated form. Many of the abbreviations are similar and can be easily confused, so doctors are using them less often.

Meanwhile, you may get a prescription that has instructions in Latin. Here's a list of these terms, with abbreviations, and their meanings:

| LATIN TERM | ABBREVIATION | MEANING |
|---|---|---|
| ante cibum | ac | before meals |
| bis in die | bid | twice a day |
| gutta | gt | drop |
| hora somni | hs | at bedtime |
| oculus dexter | od | right eye |
| oculus sinister | os | left eye |
| per os | po | by mouth |
| post cibum | pc | after meals |
| pro re nata | prn | as needed |
| quaque 3 hora | q 3 h | every 3 hours |
| quaque die | qd | every day |
| quater in die | qid | 4 times a day |
| ter in die | tid | 3 times a day |

*Source:*
*FDA Consumer* (29,6:27)

# Getting the best buy on your prescriptions

Most people will spend valuable time looking for bargains in clothing, appliances, cars, and anything else they purchase. Did you know you can also save money on your prescription drugs? There are several ways you can cut the cost of your medicine, but you may have to do a little research in your area to find the best deals. Here are some tips on how to begin the bargain hunt:

◆ Compare costs around town. Neighborhood drugstores usually base their prices on what sells most in their area, and prices can be as much as 25 percent higher than at a large discount chain. It may be worth the drive to get a better deal.

◆ Ask for a "senior-citizen discount." Many drugstores give good discounts to people over 65.

◆ Buy the generic. This is the form of the drug that is not specified by brand name, and it can be considerably cheaper. Check with your doctor to see if he thinks that you can take the generic form of the drug just as well.
Some generic drugs may not be the same quality as brand-name drugs, and sometimes the formulation is slightly different. You can ask your pharmacist to check on the generic drug in the "Orange Book," a Food and Drug Administration publication which tells you how much a particular generic drug varies from the brand name.

◆ Buy in bulk. You can often save money by buying larger quantities of drugs that you use all the time. If you are using an insurance card that underwrites the cost of the drug, you may be able to get a larger quantity for the same price as a smaller amount.

◆ Ask for free samples. Your doctor may have free samples of the medicine that you can try without investing any more money. If there are no samples, ask for a smaller prescription. This will allow you to be sure that you tolerate the drug well before you pay for a larger prescription.

If you can't afford your prescription, you may qualify for free medicine under a special prescription drug program. Check with your doctor.

◆ Fill your prescriptions by mail order. This service is usually available through health-care programs from your employer. It takes longer to get your medicine this way, sometimes more than a week. You also need to be aware that no one will be monitoring your prescriptions the way a local pharmacist might. But if you are a careful consumer, you may be able to get a good discount this way.

*Source:*
*The Atlanta Journal/Constitution* (Aug. 15, 1994, E1)

## Best ways to keep prescription drugs safe and effective

While you are taking medicine, the flip side of taking it properly is storing it correctly and making sure it's safe for you to take. Here are some ways you can help assure that your medicine will do what it's supposed to do:

◆ Keep a written record of any medicine you are taking, including the reason you are taking it, times and instructions for doses, and any problems or side effects you are having. (Unexpected side effects should be reported to your doctor.) If you become ill, or have any severe side effects, take this list with you to the doctor's office or hospital.

◆ Keep your medicine in its original container, which has the name, dose, and directions for use. If you choose to put it in a daily pill dispenser for convenience, ask your pharmacist if its stability would be affected. Don't put different kinds of pills in the same bottle or same compartments of a pill dispenser. They can react chemically to form harmful substances, or they can become inactive.

◆ If your medicine comes in a brown glass container, don't transfer it to a clear one. The dark container protects the drug from light.

◆ Never store medicine near any dangerous substance that could be taken by mistake.

◆ Don't store medicine in the bathroom. Heat and humidity can cause many substances to break down, and they won't dissolve properly when you take them. If you're carrying medicine, don't put it in a pocket next to your body; it can get too warm. Medicine should be stored in a cool, dark, dry place.

◆ Look for expiration dates on over-the-counter drugs. Don't take a medicine if it's expired, or if it seems deteriorated in any way. For example, aspirin gives off a vinegar odor when it breaks down.

◆ Read label instructions about tamper-proof features. Inspect the package carefully for any signs of broken seals, holes, or damaged wrappings. If your medicine is in pill form, check to be sure all the pills look exactly alike. Look carefully at your medicine, and if it looks discolored or seems suspicious in any way, return it to your pharmacist.

◆ Be sure to keep all medicine out of the reach of children at all times.

*Sources:*
*Arthritis Today* (10,2:13)
*FDA Consumer* (29,9:8)

# 14 tips for taking your medicine

Once you have your medicine in hand, whether it's prescription or over-the-counter, you have to take it properly. Some drugs don't work if you don't take them a certain way, and some can even be harmful. Here are some hints to ensure that you get the most from your medicine:

◆ Be sure to keep your medicine in the bottle it came in. Moving it to another container could cause a mix-up. Read the label before you take a drug to be sure it is the correct one, and you are taking the correct dose. If you are taking medicine at night, turn on a light and read the label before you take it

◆ Take your medicine at the right time. If the label says something like, "take three times a day," ask your doctor exactly when to take it. Find out if it should be taken on an empty stomach or after meals.

◆ Never take medicine prescribed for someone else.

◆ If the medicine is something that you apply, be sure you know how, where, and how often to apply it.

◆ Make a chart to keep track of your medicine. This is especially important if you are taking more than one type of drug. Note on the chart when you take each dose.

◆ Take your pills standing up, if possible, so that gravity can help the medicine go down. Never take a pill while you are lying down; it could get stuck in your windpipe.

◆ Ask your doctor's or pharmacist's advice before you break, crush, or split any pill. Some can be absorbed too quickly if they are split or broken and must be swallowed whole. Also, be sure to swallow pills instead of chewing them. Chewing can affect the rate of absorption, too.

◆ Unless your doctor tells you otherwise, take pills with water. It will help them go down more smoothly, and it won't upset your stomach or interact with the drug.

◆ To take a pill, first take a drink of water to wet your throat. Place the pill on the back of your tongue and take several swallows of water. After a few minutes, take another drink of water. If you think the pill may be stuck in your throat, try a few bites of banana to coax it down.

◆ If you cannot swallow a prescribed pill, no matter what you do, talk to your doctor. The medicine may come in another form that could be easier for you to take.

◆ If you are taking a liquid medicine that separates, shake it up before pouring out the dose.

◆ Don't measure a dose of liquid medicine with a household spoon. If the medicine comes with a measuring cup, use it. If it doesn't, ask your pharmacist about purchasing a special spoon, dropper, or oral syringe to measure the drug accurately.

◆ Double-check the dose of liquid medicine before you take it. It is easy to confuse lines marking teaspoons and tablespoons.

◆ Don't stop taking medicine your doctor has told you to finish just because your symptoms disappear. Certain drugs, such as antibiotics, must be finished completely to ensure that the illness doesn't return in an even stronger form.

◆ Never take medicine prescribed for someone else.

*Sources:*
*FDA Consumer* (29,9:8)
*The Diabetes Advisor* (4,1:22)

## Important precautions for people taking pain relievers

When you run into the drugstore for a little something to relieve those aches and pains you got from working too much in your garden, you may be in for even more aggravation when you reach the pain-relief section. With such a vast array of pain relievers to choose from, it's easy to get confused about which one to choose, whether you need relief from muscle pain or a simple headache. Knowing a little about each type of pain reliever may help you decide what to buy. There is a description of each kind of OTC (over-the-counter) pain reliever in articles that follow.

No matter which over-the-counter pain reliever you choose, remember that it is intended for short-term use only. Usually, a label warns that children should take the medicine no longer than five days, and adults should take it no longer than 10 days. If you are taking medicine for fever, the time limit should be three days. The reason is that long-term use might mask a serious condition. If fever or other symptoms get worse, pain continues, or there is redness or swelling, you need to see your doctor.

*Source:*
*FDA Consumer* (29,1:11)

## NSAIDs defined

Any information you hear or read about over-the-counter pain relievers will probably contain the term *NSAID*. So, what exactly is an NSAID? The abbreviation stands for "nonsteroidal anti-inflammatory drug." It describes drugs that work by blocking the production of hormone-like *prostaglandins*, which cause pain and inflammation in the body. Aspirin, ibuprofen, and naproxen sodium in all their different forms are NSAIDs. Acetaminophen is an *analgesic* (pain-relieving) drug, but it is not an NSAID.

*Source:*
*Arthritis Today* (9,4:30)

## All-star relief for aches and pains

Aspirin (acetylsalicylic acid) has been a favorite pain reliever for almost 100 years. It works partly by slowing your body's production of *prostaglandins*, hormone-like substances that play a number of roles in the body.

Prostaglandins cause pain and inflammation in damaged tissue. They also affect body temperature, blood vessel constriction, blood clotting, metabolism, and uterine contractions. Prostaglandins protect the lining of the stomach and small intestine against ulcers. That's why overuse of aspirin can cause irritation of the stomach — the protective prostaglandins in the stomach are not being produced.

Aspirin comes in different strengths. "Regular" strength aspirin contains 325 milligrams (mg) per tablet, and "extra" or "maximum" strength contains 500 mg. The usual adult dose (for people age 12 years and older) is one or two 325-mg tablets every four hours.

Some aspirin also contains caffeine. There isn't any evidence that caffeine relieves pain, but it may enhance the effects of aspirin by lifting your spirits when you take it. You can get the same effect by taking plain aspirin and drinking a cup of coffee.

Some brands of aspirin are "buffered" with antacids to prevent stomach irritation, or coated so that the pills don't dissolve until they reach your intestines. These may be helpful to people with sensitive stomachs, or those who have to take a lot of aspirin. The problem with coated aspirin is that it takes longer to dissolve, and it may take up to twice as long to provide pain relief.

Certain people should not take aspirin. Don't take it if you have any of these conditions:

◆ ulcers, since aspirin can make symptoms worse
◆ asthma, since aspirin can trigger an attack in some people
◆ liver or kidney disease, because aspirin can make these conditions worse
◆ bleeding disorders, or any condition for which you are taking anticoagulant medication, since aspirin may cause bleeding
◆ uncontrolled high blood pressure, because of an increased risk of stroke

If you are a person who takes high doses of aspirin regularly, you may develop hearing loss or *tinnitus* (ringing in the ears). If you are a heavy drinker, aspirin may cause gastrointestinal bleeding.

Other people who should not take aspirin are pregnant women in the last trimester of pregnancy, and children or teen-agers who have chickenpox or flu-like symptoms. In pregnant women, aspirin can increase the risk of stillbirth and maternal or fetal bleeding during delivery. In children and teen-agers, the use of aspirin during illness increases the risk of Reye's syndrome, a rare disorder that can cause serious illness and even death.

*Sources:*
*FDA Consumer* (29,1:11)
*The American Medical Association Encyclopedia of Medicine,* Random House, New York, 1989

## Alternatives to aspirin

Here are three other kinds of over-the-counter pain relievers to try if you want an alternative to aspirin.

**Acetaminophen** relieves pain, but doctors are not sure exactly how it works. One theory is that it acts on nerve endings to suppress pain. For reducing fever and relieving mild-to-moderate pain, acetaminophen works well. But it's not as effective for relieving the pain of soft-tissue injuries, such as muscle aches or sprains. It can be helpful in preparations for relieving menstrual cramps, but most of these preparations also contain other ingredients, such as diuretics or antihistamines. These added ingredients aren't harmful, but they may not be effective at relieving cramps.

The usual adult dosage for acetaminophen is two 325-mg tablets every four hours. It may not be any faster or better than aspirin at relieving pain, but acetaminophen is gentler on your stomach, and doesn't carry the risk of Reye's syndrome for younger people.

There is one serious risk associated with acetaminophen: Even in moderate doses, it can cause liver damage in heavy drinkers. In 1994, a Virginia man, Antonio Benedi, won an $8.8 million verdict against the makers of Tylenol acetaminophen after he had to have an emergency liver transplant. A jury was convinced that Tylenol destroyed the liver of Mr. Benedi, who habitually drank two or three alcoholic beverages a day.

**Ibuprofen** and **naproxen sodium** used to be available only by prescription. Now both come in 200-mg tablets, a much lower dosage than the prescribed versions. One 200-mg tablet of ibuprofen can be taken every four to six hours, or one 200-mg tablet of naproxen sodium can be taken every eight to 12 hours.

Both ibuprofen and naproxen sodium work, like aspirin, by suppressing the production of prostaglandins. They are especially effective at relieving menstrual cramps, minor arthritis, toothaches, and injuries with inflammation, such as tendinitis. They are also somewhat gentler on the stomach than aspirin.

However, people who have ulcers or get gastrointestinal upset from aspirin should also avoid ibuprofen and naproxen sodium. The same is true for people with asthma and people who are allergic to aspirin. Heavy drinkers run the risk of gastric bleeding and impaired liver function if they take these products.

No matter which over-the-counter pain reliever you choose, remember that it is intended for short-term use only. Usually, a label warns that children should take the medicine no longer than five days, and adults should take it no longer than 10 days. If you are taking medicine for fever, the time limit should be three days. The reason is that long-term use might mask a serious condition. If fever or other symptoms get worse, pain continues, or there is redness or swelling, you need to see your doctor.

Refer to the following *"Over-the-counter pain relief primer"* prepared by the

Food and Drug Administration for information on specific pain relievers and what each one does.

**Sources:**
*FDA Consumer* (29,1:11)
*The American Medical Association Encyclopedia of Medicine*, Random House, New York, 1989
*The Atlanta Journal/Constitution* (March 23, 1996, E12)

## Over-the-counter pain relief primer

| TYPE/ DOSAGE | COMMON BRANDS | WHAT IT DOES | POSSIBLE SIDE EFFECTS |
|---|---|---|---|
| aspirin 325 mg 500 mg | Anacin Ascriptin Bayer Bayer Plus Bufferin Ecotrin | Relieves mild to moderate pain from headaches, sore muscles, menstrual cramps, and arthritis; reduces fever. | Prolonged use may cause gastrointestinal bleeding, especially in heavy drinkers; may increase the risk of maternal and fetal bleeding and cause complications during delivery if taken in the last trimester; can cause Reye's syndrome if given to children and teenagers who have the flu or chickenpox. |
| acetamin- ophen 325 mg 500 mg | Anacin-3 Excedrin Pamprin Midol Tylenol | Relieves mild to moderate pain from headaches and sore muscles; reduces fever. | May cause liver damage in drinkers and those taking excessive amounts (more than 4,000 mg daily) for several weeks. |
| ibuprofen 200 mg | Advil Motrin-IB Nuprin Pamrin-IB | Relieves mild to moderate pain from headaches, backaches, and sore muscles; re- lieves minor pain of arthritis; provides good relief of menstrual cramps and toothaches; reduces fever. | Gastrointestinal bleeding, especially in heavy drink- ers; stomach ulcers; kidney damage in the elderly, those who have cirrhosis of the liver, and people taking diuretics. |
| naproxen sodium 200 mg | Aleve | Relieves mild to moderate pain from headaches, backaches, and sore muscles; re- lieves minor pain of arthritis; provides good relief of menstrual cramps and toothaches; reduces fever. | Gastrointestinal bleeding; stomach ulcers; kidney damage in the elderly, those who have cirrhosis of the liver, and people taking diuretics. |

**Source:**
*FDA Consumer* (29,1:13)

## Antibiotics losing battle against bacteria

The discovery of antibiotic drugs was a true breakthrough in medical history. For the first time, doctors had an effective weapon against the raging infections that sickened and killed so many people. But as antibiotics became commonplace, they began to be prescribed for many less serious illnesses.

It's not unusual today for a person with a bad cold or flu to go to his doctor and ask for a prescription for an antibiotic. Over the years, many doctors have prescribed these drugs in just such situations, but they really don't help. What many people don't realize is that colds and flu are caused by viruses, and antibiotics are only effective against infections caused by bacteria.

More antibiotics are prescribed today for childhood ear infections than for any other illness. In spite of this, the number of doctor visits for this ailment has doubled since 1975. Antibiotics are also widely prescribed for bronchitis, sore throat, sinusitis, and acne, even though their effectiveness against these problems is questionable.

People often take a medicine for an illness until they feel better, and then stop taking it. Normally, that's a sensible course of action, but not for antibiotics. When an antibiotic is prescribed for a bacterial infection, it is vitally important to finish the entire prescribed amount. When you don't succeed in killing all the organisms (germs) causing the infection, you may suffer a relapse, or you may allow the bacteria to change into another strain of organism that resists the antibiotic.

Because so many antibiotics have been overprescribed, and because people have left their medicine unfinished so many times, new, antibiotic-resistant strains of bacteria are growing. In 1994, there were medical reports of antibiotic-resistant strains of the bacteria that cause pneumonia, tuberculosis, gonorrhea, pertussis (whooping cough), and salmonella (food poisoning). These reports are occurring more frequently throughout the country.

New medicines called "broad spectrum antibiotics" kill more than one type of organism at a time, and they are being used against antibiotic-resistant bacteria. More antibiotics are being invented to combat the new types of bacteria. The question is whether new medicines can be invented fast enough to keep up with the changing, growing bacteria. These new strains of bacteria pose a threat to us all.

*Sources:*
*Journal Watch* (15,1:6)
*The Atlanta Journal/Constitution* (Jan. 18, 1995, A1 and Nov. 8, 1995, E3)

## An antibiotic plan of action

Here's what you can do to join the fight against new strains of antibiotic resistant bacteria:

- ◆ Don't ask your doctor for an antibiotic when you have a cold or the flu.
- ◆ Ask questions if your doctor does prescribe an antibiotic for an illness. Be sure it is necessary for you to take it.
- ◆ Listen to or read your pharmacist's instructions about taking any antibiotic. Take your medicine on schedule, and take all of it.

315

Antibiotics are some of the most important weapons in the medical arsenal for fighting disease. You can do your part to keep our defenses strong.

**Sources:**
*Journal Watch* (15,1:6)
*The Atlanta Journal/Constitution* (Jan. 18, 1995, A1 and Nov. 8, 1995, E3)

# New antihistamines don't cause drowsiness

In the tissues of your body, *histamine* has several roles. It's one of the substances responsible for redness and swelling in reaction to an injury, and it's released during an allergic reaction. It also stimulates the production of stomach acid and narrows the airways of the lungs. *Antihistamines* are drugs that counteract the effects of histamine on your body.

The first antihistamine was discovered in 1944. Antihistamines that have been in use for a number of years are called "classic agents." These include Dimetane, Chlor-Trimeton, Polaramine, Clistin, Tavist, Dramamine, Benadryl, Unisom, PBZ, Periactin, Optimine, Nolahist, Atarax, Vistaril, and Antivert. The main drawback of these drugs is that they may cause drowsiness and dizziness. Some other possible side effects are dry mouth, retention of urine, very low blood pressure, weight gain, and *tinnitus* (ringing in the ears). Most of these side effects should decrease within three or four days of use.

New antihistamines that don't cause drowsiness have recently been developed. These include Hismanal, Claritin, and Seldane. They are more expensive than the classic ones, and they also take longer to work. Classic antihistamines take effect in 15 to 30 minutes, while the new ones may take from one hour up to 48 hours to achieve the desired effect. Increased appetite and weight gain can be side effects of some new antihistamines. The worst side effect, however, is the possibility of potentially fatal cardiac *arrhythmias* (irregular heartbeat). People who are elderly, who have problems with liver function, or who take medicine for their hearts should not take the new antihistamines.

Whether you use a new antihistamine or one of the classic ones depends on which type is most appropriate for your situation. Check with your doctor to be sure the drug's side effects are ones you can live with.

**Sources:**
*American Family Physician* (52,2:593)
*The American Medical Association Encyclopedia of Medicine*, Random House, New York, 1989

# Antihistamines from A to Z

It may surprise you, but antihistamines play a variety of roles in helping care for your health. Here are some of the things antihistamines can do for you:

◆ Relieve swelling, itching, and redness of *urticaria* (hives) and other allergic skin rashes, and soothe insect bites.

◆ Dry up secretions in your nasal passages to make you more comfortable when you have a cold. Diphenhydramine is the antihistamine that actually suppresses coughs by controlling the cough center in your brain.

- Control itchy, watery eyes; sneezing; and runny nose of hay fever and other respiratory allergies.
- Rescue victims of *anaphylactic shock*, a severe, life-threatening allergic reaction. An antihistamine is administered by injection for immediate results.
- Reduce the symptoms of tremor, rigid muscles, and drooling in some people with Parkinson's disease. Diphenhydramine has been most widely used to treat these symptoms.
- Prevent and treat motion sickness, dizziness, nausea, and vomiting. Dramamine (dimenhydrinate) is a popular remedy with queasy travelers.
- Work to stimulate your appetite and promote weight gain. They can help people with anorexia or growth problems. This can also be an unwanted side effect if you are taking the antihistamine to treat some other problem. The drug Hismanal (astemizole) has been reported to cause increased appetite and weight gain in some people who take it.
- Help prevent asthma brought on by cold air or exercise by helping open your air passages. The newer antihistamines seem particularly effective.

Specific antihistamines can be prescribed for each of these conditions. Your doctor knows best which antihistamine may help with your specific problem.

***Source:***
*American Family Physician* (52,2:593)

# Food and drug interactions

Most of us realize that the medicines we take can affect each other. But did you know drugs also frequently interact with vitamins and minerals in your body?

In fact, some drugs commonly cause nutritional deficiencies. In some cases, taking nutritional supplements cancels out a medicine's intended effect. Even eating food that normally is good for you, such as yogurt and broccoli, can be harmful if you're taking certain drugs.

Here are some things to look out for if you take any of these medicines:

- Prednisone and similar drugs such as cortisone (Cortone), betamethasone (Celestone), dexamethasone (Decadron), prednisolone (Delta-Cortef), and methylprednisolone (Medrol) can rob you of potassium, as well as vitamins B6, B12, folic acid (a B vitamin), and D3. Because you need vitamin D to absorb and use calcium, these drugs may cause bone loss and eventually osteoporosis.
- Phenytoin (Dilantin), used to treat epilepsy, is another vitamin D thief.
- Cholestyramine (Questran), a cholesterol-lowering drug, latches onto cholesterol and bile acids from your gallbladder and escorts them out. Unfortunately, it also leaves with a whole party of critical nutrients including essential fatty acids, iron, vitamin B12, folic acid (a B vitamin), and the fat-soluble vitamins A, D, E, and K. If you take extra vitamins and minerals, be sure to take supplements and the drug at different times.
- Mineral oil laxatives (Agoral, Milkinol, Neo-Cultol) used too frequently prevent your body from absorbing fat-soluble vitamins A, D, E, and K. A better strategy is to combat constipation by eating lots of fruits and vegetables. For additional fiber, try a psyllium product such as Metamucil, Fiberall, or Modane Bulk

◆ Antibiotics kill off unwanted bacteria, but they also sterilize your digestive tract, destroying the good intestinal bacteria that produce vitamin K and biotin, a B vitamin. Eat yogurt or take acidophilus supplements found at health food stores and many drugstores to replenish your supply.

◆ Thiazide (Aldoril, Diuril) and HCTZ (HydroDIURIL, Ser-Ap-Es, Esidrix, Oretic) are diuretics, or water pills, that often are prescribed to treat high blood pressure. Unfortunately, they also wash out minerals including potassium, sodium, and magnesium. Solution? Eat potassium-rich foods including potatoes, peppers, spinach, bananas, and oranges and magnesium-rich foods like nuts, whole grains, dark green vegetables, and seafood.

Even short-term, using these drugs can increase your cholesterol, so have it checked regularly. Monitoring your blood sugar is important, too, because high blood fats play havoc with the way your body responds to insulin, the hormone that helps your cells take in sugar.

◆ INH, used to treat tuberculosis, nearly always steals vitamins B6 and niacin. The result is irritability, sleep disturbance, and even convulsions. But don't take a supplement without checking with your doctor. Too much B6 interferes with the drug. Do eat plenty of vitamin B-rich foods, such as milk, eggs, beans, and whole grains.

Be sure to ask your doctor or pharmacist about taking your medication with food or between meals, as well as what foods or beverages you should avoid with certain drugs. Here are some examples:

◆ Glipizide (Glucotrol) helps control the boost in diabetics' blood sugar following a meal. It works best if you take it about 30 minutes before eating.

◆ Griseofulvin (Fulvicin, Grifulvin, Grisactin), a fungus fighter, is actually absorbed better when taken with a high-fat meal.

◆ Tetracycline antibiotics (Achromycin, Aureomycin, Minocin, Panmycin, Terramycin) lose half their punch if you take them with dairy products or with iron or calcium supplements. Wait at least two hours between the time you take the medication and the time you eat dairy products or take mineral supplements.

◆ Warfarin (Coumadin, Panwarfin), a blood-thinner commonly used to prevent blood clots, can be overwhelmed by too much vitamin K in your diet. Rather than avoid healthy foods high in this vitamin, such as asparagus; broccoli; cabbage; brussels sprouts; liver; and green, leafy vegetables like spinach, eat them in moderation, keeping daily intake fairly constant.

◆ Ibuprofen (Motrin, Advil, Nuprin, Medipren, Rufen) is frequently used to relieve arthritis pain. Always take it with food or milk to avoid stomach irritation and ulceration.

◆ Metronidazole (Flagyl, Femizole, Metizol, Metryl, Protostat) is used to treat a multitude of infections, including the vaginal infection *Trichomonas*, amebic dysentery, and bacteria-caused ulcers. Combining this drug with alcohol spells disaster.

Always ask your doctor and pharmacist about possible interactions between nutrients and your prescription and over-the-counter medications. Alert them to all drugs and nutritional supplements you routinely use.

*Sources:*
*American Family Physician* (51,5:1175)
Joe Graedon, author of *The People's Pharmacy*
*Journal of the American College of Nutrition* (14,2:137)
*The Nutrition Desk Reference,* Second Edition, Keats Publishing, New Canaan, Conn., 1990
*The Nutrition Desk Reference,* Third Edition, Keats Publishing, New Canaan, Conn., 1996
*The People's Guide to Deadly Drug Interactions,* St. Martin's Press, New York, 1995
*The People's Pharmacy: Completely New and Revised,* St. Martin's Press, New York, 1996

## Special trick makes taking common heart drug easier

If you are taking the drug cholestyramine to lower your high cholesterol level, here's a tip to make taking it much easier. This comes from Dr. Mikhail Y. Imseis of Ness City, Kan.

Doctors usually recommend dissolving cholestyramine in orange juice, but try using prune juice instead. The mixture tastes a little better than it does with orange juice, and it has the added benefit of helping you avoid constipation, which is one of the side effects of this drug.

If you warm the mixture in a microwave oven for just a few seconds, it will dissolve even better. Also, try using a small whisk instead of a spoon to stir the cholestyramine and make it dissolve faster.

*Source:*
*Emergency Medicine* (27,2:115)

## Deadly drug risk

If you are at risk of getting blood clots, you are probably taking an anticoagulant drug to prevent them. There are a number of drugs that might react with your anticoagulant medicine, so you must be very careful which other drugs you take. However, there is one everyday hazard that you might not know about.

It's quinine, the flavoring in tonic water. Quinine reacts with anticoagulant drugs to make them more powerful, which can cause dangerous bleeding. If you are taking an anticoagulant drug, do not drink tonic water or anything containing quinine.

*Source:*
*The People's Guide to Deadly Drug Interactions,* St. Martin's Press, New York, 1995

## Severe stomach bleeding triggered by drug duo

You may think that washing down your blood pressure medicine with a little glass of wine won't hurt a thing. After all, you've heard that red wine is supposed to be beneficial for your heart. But mixing alcohol with any drug, either prescription or over-the-counter, could be a dangerous mistake.

Many older people take medicine, and some take several different kinds for different ailments. The side effects of consuming alcohol with sedatives, antidepressants, anticoagulants, or prescription drugs for high blood pressure include dangerous bleeding, changes in blood pressure, and serious stomach irritation. It only takes a small amount of alcohol to cause these reactions, especially in elderly people.

Taking over-the-counter NSAIDs (nonsteroidal anti-inflammatory drugs), such as aspirin and ibuprofen, can cause bleeding in your stomach. If you take them with alcohol, you're four times as likely to have severe stomach bleeding.

*Sources:*
*Medical Abstracts Newsletter* (15,11:7)
*Medical Tribune for the Internist and Cardiologist* (36,22:19)

## Over-the-counter overdose danger

Many over-the-counter antacids, laxatives, and pain relievers contain salts of magnesium. If you are elderly, these remedies pose a danger to you that you may not be aware of.

Magnesium toxicity is caused by a buildup of magnesium in your body. Magnesium is excreted from your body by your kidneys, and the function of your kidneys decreases with age, making elderly people more susceptible.

Lightheadedness, low blood pressure, muscle weakness, confusion, heart rhythm disturbances, nausea, and vomiting are symptoms of magnesium toxicity. It can even cause coma and respiratory failure. The danger is that these symptoms are common to many illnesses, so you may not know when they're caused by too much magnesium.

If you're taking over-the-counter medicines, you may not think to mention them to your doctor when he asks you to list all your medications. They should definitely be mentioned, especially if you are having any of the symptoms listed.

When you are buying over-the-counter products, be sure to check the label for magnesium. Avoid taking products containing magnesium every day, and don't combine products that contain it. If you have kidney problems, ask your doctor what products are safe for you.

A natural alternative to antacid tablets, papaya tablets contain the natural enzyme papain, which gives a boost to your digestion. Chamomile tea is a traditional cure for chronic indigestion. It is most effective when you take it three or four times a day for an extended period of time. Its medicinal effects are cumulative. Kelp (dried seaweed) is another herbal remedy for indigestion, and it's available in tablet or capsule form. Perhaps these herbal remedies for indigestion will do away with your need for over-the-counter antacids altogether.

*Sources:*
*Archives of Family Medicine* (4,8:718)
*Miracle Medicine Herbs,* Parker Publishing Company, West Nyack, N.Y., 1991
*Pharmacy Times* (62,5:106)
*The Good Herb,* William Morrow and Company, New York, 1995

## Common additive causes drug reaction

Several people in England taking the drug enalapril were troubled by skin rashes. Enalapril (Vasotec) is an ACE inhibitor prescribed for high blood pressure. The problem occurred when people taking this drug switched from a lower-dose form of the drug that does not contain artificial coloring to a higher dose.

The higher-dose pills contain iron oxides, artificial colorings that sometimes cause allergic reactions. The skin rashes of the people taking enalapril were caused by the artificial colorings, and the rashes went away when they switched back to taking the lower-dose pills. They were able to get the higher dose by taking more of the lower-dose pills.

If you are having an unusual reaction to a prescription drug, check with your doctor. If it's being caused by artificial coloring, maybe he can switch you to a form of the drug that is color-free.

**Source:**
*British Medical Journal* (310,7014:1204)

# Eye problems linked to popular heart drug

If you are taking digitalis to regulate the rhythm of your heart, you probably know the symptoms of overdose to look for. The best-known visual symptoms are disturbances in the way you see color. Seeing too much yellow or green is an especially telling sign.

The artist Vincent Van Gogh, who painted halos of color around many subjects and used an abundance of yellow and green in his paintings, is thought to have suffered from digitalis overdose.

In a recent New York study, a small group of people ages 66 to 85 years went to eye doctors with complaints of blurred, snowy vision; flashing spots of light in their outer fields of vision; or decreased visual sharpness.

All of these people were taking normal or below-normal doses of digitalis, but it turned out that digitalis was the cause of their visual problems. When their doctors took them off digitalis, these eye problems went away.

If you are having problems with your eyes and you are taking digitalis, check with your doctor to see if the problem is in your eyes or in your medicine.

**Source:**
*Annals of Internal Medicine* (123,9:676)

# The latest word on calcium channel blockers

Calcium channel blockers are popular drugs used to treat high blood pressure. However, three recent medical studies questioned the safety of these drugs.

Calcium channel blockers come in both short-acting and slow-acting formulations. The short-acting kind is taken three or four times a day and releases the medication immediately. The slow-acting kind is taken only once a day. In the studies, people taking short-acting calcium channel blockers were found to have a 60 percent higher risk of heart attack than people taking other types of drugs to lower blood pressure.

One particular drug, short-acting *nifedipine*, was shown to be especially dangerous to people being treated for heart disease. People taking more than 80 milligrams a day tripled their risk of death. A statement issued by The National Heart, Lung, and Blood Institute recommended that this drug should only be used with "great caution (if at all)."

If you are currently taking calcium channel blockers to lower high blood pressure, don't stop taking your medicine. If you are concerned about the drug's safety, be sure to discuss this with your doctor. He may be able to recommend another drug that's safer.

Don't forget, there are also natural things you can do, such as losing weight, exercising regularly, and keeping your diet healthy, to help control your high blood pressure.

**Sources:**
*Journal Watch* (15,18:141)
*The Journal of the American Medical Association* (274,8:620)
*The Wall Street Journal* (Jan. 25, 1996, B1)

# AIDS breakthrough offers new hope

It's finally ending. We're waking up from the nightmare that made us shrink away from a hurt stranger, hesitate before helping a bleeding friend, and fear more than ever the consequences of surgery and blood transfusions.

After 15 years of a worldwide AIDS epidemic, researchers have found a "drug cocktail" that turns AIDS into a treatable disease like high blood pressure or diabetes. The drug cocktail is a combination of three drugs that work together to keep the human immunodeficiency virus (HIV) from reproducing and attacking your immune system.

There are three parts to this drug breakthrough:

First, one of the drugs in the three-part combo was finally created after 10 years of research.

Second, two brilliant doctors finally figured out that HIV couldn't fight all three drugs at once. Before, doctors had always assumed that HIV would quickly mutate into new virus particles that were resistant to any drug you used to fight it. But it can't produce enough mutations to survive against the three-drug mix.

Third, one of the doctors — Dr. David Ho of the Aaron Diamond center in New York — discovered that we weren't treating the infection fast enough. Doctors thought that HIV was dormant for years after you were infected. They would actually wait as long as possible to give you a drug because they thought the virus would have more time to mutate and beat the drug if they gave it to you early. Dr. Ho realized that HIV begins spreading right away, and the only reason you don't notice AIDS immediately is because your immune system does an incredible job of fighting the virus.

Nobody is ready to say so, but fighting HIV immediately with the drug AZT, the drug 3TC, and one of the new protease blockers may actually *cure* AIDS. A little more time in the scientific laboratories will tell.

Already, people with AIDS are calling the new treatment a miracle. In one study, eight out of nine people with advanced AIDS who've taken the drugs for a year have absolutely no signs of HIV infection in their blood. People with AIDS now have hope for a normal life, and the rest of us have a lot less to fear.

**Source:**
*The Wall Street Journal* (June 14, 1996, A1)

# Alternative Healing

## Homeopathic healing

"A hair of the dog that bit us" is a hangover remedy that's been around for over 400 years. Taking a tiny nip of an irritant applies to the 200-year-old practice of homeopathic medicine, too. A homeopathic cure for allergies may contain minuscule amounts of the allergen that's causing you problems.

After studying your symptoms, the classical homeopathic doctor would just give you a single dose of a single remedy. A nonclassical homeopath may give you many doses of a multi-remedy formula.

Homeopathic medicine can't hurt you because the doses are so small. In fact, homeopaths believe that the smaller and more diluted the dose, the more powerful the healing.

The tiny size of the dose is the reason scientific researchers have always doubted the powers of homeopathy. Recently, scientists set out to prove that a fake solution (a placebo) would work just as well as the homeopathic solution for a group of people with allergic asthma.

Much to their surprise, the placebo didn't work as well. The people who took the homeopathic brew began to cough less and breathe easier than the people who took the placebo.

After four weeks, the people using the ancient treatment had reduced their asthma and allergy symptoms by one-third. When the scientists measured their lungs' responses to allergy triggers, they found an improvement of over 50 percent.

Another controversial scientific study showed that a homeopathic treatment helped treat children with diarrhea.

If you want to experiment with the healing powers of homeopathy, don't let your regular doctor discourage you. Inform him that homeopathy is gaining respect and reports can be found in medical journals such as *The Lancet*.

For the best results, find a homeopathic M.D. with a proven track record. Or, you can try to treat yourself with the solution-soaked sugar pills found in health-food stores.

*Sources:*
Medical Tribune (36,1:11)
Pediatrics (93,5:719)
The Lancet (344,8937:1601)

## Mind control speeds recovery

If you can relax and focus, then you have the ability to use your mind to lift pain, tiredness, and depression out of your body.

Recently, hypnotherapists taught a group of people having bypass surgery the next day to relax and visualize a speedy return to a painfree, comfortable, normal life. The people who used the exercises later were six times more energetic and three times less depressed than the people who didn't.

Hypnotherapists are most successful at helping you overcome bad habits and control pain or stress, but some people believe hypnotherapy can cure diseases like multiple sclerosis or ulcerative colitis.

We know that stress can cause all sorts of diseases, but the extent of the connection between the mind and the nervous system is a mystery. A hypnotherapist may be able to help you harness your far-reaching mental powers.

To find a certified hypnotherapist near you, you can call the International Medical and Dental Hypnotherapy Association at 1-810-549-5594.

**Source:**
*Journal of Alternative and Complementary Medicine* (1:3)

# Prayer: a prescription for healing

A loved one is ill. You're struck by crushing chest pain. Or your dog is hit by a speeding car.

What do you do?

Seek medical care, of course. And, if you are like millions of Americans, you'll also quickly turn to prayer.

Gallup polls have consistently shown that about 95 percent of us believe in God, and most believe in miracles. Now the medical profession is taking a serious look at how prayer and religious beliefs can produce a powerful prescription for healing.

For example, there have been three national conferences held recently — including one sponsored by the National Institutes of Health's Institute on Aging — where doctors and scientists discussed the latest findings that prayer and religious beliefs promote health.

There's mounting evidence that the effects of prayer can actually be scientifically measured. Santa Fe, New Mexico, internist Dr. Larry Dossey has collected the results of dozens of controlled studies that demonstrate the power of prayer.

One dramatic example involved 393 heart patients. Half, picked randomly by a computer, were prayed for by a home prayer group, but the patients themselves weren't aware of this. The results? The prayed-for group was five times less likely to need antibiotics, three times less likely to have complications, and fewer died.

Other experiments have suggested that prayer positively affects high blood pressure, wound healing, anxiety levels, headaches, and heart attacks. Prayer, in fact, has been shown under laboratory conditions to exert a positive influence on all kinds of living things — from shrinking tumors in mice to speeding the growth of seeds.

At the National Institute for Healthcare Research conference "Spiritual Dimensions in Clinical Research," held in Leesburg, Virginia, Dr. Jeffrey Levin of Eastern Virginia Medical School noted that in 26 out of 27 studies, evidence of religious involvement (like church attendance) was linked to a positive effect on health problems ranging from cancer to heart disease.

Other research presented at the conference concluded that when faced with serious health problems, you are much less likely to be seriously depressed about your plight if you use prayer and your religious faith to help you cope.

The bottom line, according to psychiatrist Harold Koenig of Duke University, is something a lot of us have long believed ... there is no longer any question that spirituality and religion have important health benefits.

*Sources:*
*Healing Words: The Power of Prayer and the Practice of Medicine,* HarperCollins, New York, 1993
*The Journal of the American Medical Association* (273,20:1561)

## Hands-on headache remedy

Next time your head begins to throb, press the webbing between your thumb and your index finger with the thumb of your other hand. That point is known as *ho-ku*, and Chinese practitioners of acupressure have been connecting it to headache relief for 5,000 years.

Acupressurists believe you can manipulate the flow of energy in your body by pressing certain points. That may sound far-fetched, but however it works, the technique has been proven effective.

Start by using your right thumb to press the webbing on your left hand. Press slightly toward the bone that connects with the index finger (Figure A). Hold for one minute. Then switch hands.

Pregnant women should not try this technique. This pressure point can supposedly cause premature contractions.

Other headache pressure points are at the base of your skull and in your eye sockets (Figures B and C).

First, use your thumbs to press the hollow areas behind your head, at the base of your skull, two to three inches apart. Close your eyes and tilt your head slowly back. Take deep, long breaths and hold for one to two minutes.

Next, press the center hollow at the base of your skull with your right thumb. With your left thumb and index finger, press the upper hollows of your eye sockets, near the bridge of your nose. While you press these points, again tilt your head back and breathe deeply, for one to two minutes.

**Acupressure Points**

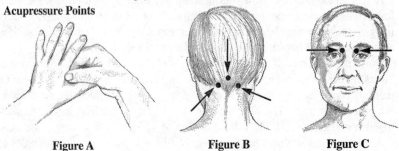

Figure A          Figure B          Figure C

*Source:*
*Alternative Medicine The Definitive Guide,* Future Medicine Publishing, Puyallup, Wash., 1993

## Pressure-point nausea relief

Those wrist bands with a plastic button really seem to work to control nausea, if you use them correctly, a new study shows. The wrist bands are based on an ancient medical therapy known as acupressure.

A few people have used the bands for years to control motion sickness and morning sickness. Doctors recently tested them on people undergoing surgery, since you usually feel nauseated when you wake up from anesthesia. And they worked!

Far fewer people who wore the acupressure band felt nauseated (six out of 19), and none of them vomited. The other 22 people in the study wore a wrist band that fitted too loosely or had the plastic button on the wrong side. Ten of them felt nauseated and six vomited.

A specialist can puncture the same spot on your wrist with a needle to prevent nausea, say acupuncture practitioners. But you don't need a specialist to treat yourself with the pressure of a plastic button.

*Source:*
*Medical Tribune* (34,21:20)

## Body work: Treat yourself to a tuneup

"Body work" sounds like something your car needs after smashing into your grandson's bike parked just behind the rear bumper, but it's also a term for the therapeutic use of touch. Body work is more than massage: It's a total-body tuneup.

Dr. Andrew Weil, an authority in natural and preventive medicine, recommends four of his favorite types of body work.

*Feldenkrais work* is a gentle and effective system of floor exercises and massage. It is meant to retrain the central nervous system to find new pathways around blocked or damaged areas. To put it simply, Feldenkrais teaches you to move easier.

Here's an easy lesson: Turn your head slowly to the right until it stops. Face forward again, close your eyes, and imagine doing the same movement. Vividly imagine the movement becoming smoother and easier over 10 or 15 times. Now actually turn your head to the right. Has the movement improved?

Don't be concerned if a friend tells you she's "Getting Rolfed." Someone *is* "working her over," but in a good way. *Rolfing* is a firm massage. It can even be painful. You usually go through a series of massages, each focusing on a different part of the body. The idea is to break up tissues that have begun to stick together and grow rigid. The release of tension you feel can be very emotional.

A *shiatsu* masseuse uses her fingers only. She will use them at right angles to your body to improve your energy and blood circulation. That's called *tonification. Calming* is a gentle, rocking motion of the masseuse's fingers. *Dispersal* is a very active motion to distribute energy and break up blood blockages. This healing art is from Japan.

If you want to relax and feel good about yourself, try *Trager work*. The practitioner will gently rock, cradle, and rotate your body parts, releasing tense muscles and increasing your flexibility. Trager work has helped people with traumatic injuries, disabilities, polio, and other problems involving the nerves and muscles.

Some Trager practitioners will also teach you dancelike exercises to help you move more easily. One exercise is simply letting your arms drop freely to one side, and another is adding a shaking motion to your foot while you walk.

*Sources:*
*Alternative Medicine: The Definitive Guide*, Future Medicine Publishing, Puyallup, Wash., 1993
*Nursing Times* (89,46:38)
*Spontaneous Healing: How to Discover and Enhance Your Body's Natural Ability to Maintain and Heal Itself*, Alfred A. Knopf, New York, 1995

# Chiropractic care helps 1 in 3

If you've been suffering with low back pain and can't find relief in any drug, exercise, or mind control technique, you may be considering what a chiropractor could do for you. It's understandable — 1 in 20 Americans had chiropractic treatment last year. Some of them may be your own friends and relatives. And according to one major study, most of them are happier with the outcome than people who were treated in traditional hospitals.

Your doctor may not think it's a great idea though. Many traditional doctors don't think much of chiropractors, labeling them quacks and discrediting their approach. It doesn't help their credibility when some chiropractors claim to be able to cure everything from bed-wetting to cancer. It can be very confusing. So, if you're considering chiropractic care, it pays to ask questions.

**How are chiropractors different from medical doctors?** Chiropractors are the third largest group of health professionals, right behind doctors and dentists, with over 45,000 practicing in the United States. Most chiropractic colleges offer four- and five-year degrees and require two years of previous college experience. While these standards are not as tough as those required for a medical degree, chiropractic colleges are accredited, and chiropractors must be licensed by the state. Unlike regular medical doctors, chiropractors are not allowed to prescribe medicine or perform surgery.

**How does chiropractic work?** Here's the theory in a nutshell: You have 33 individual bony vertebrae in your spinal column. Hundreds of nerves branch off the spine through openings in the vertebrae. Chiropractors believe that tiny misalignments in the vertebrae, called subluxations, can pinch these nerves. The body parts that are served by the nerves can't function correctly. By adjusting your vertebrae and eliminating the subluxations, chiropractors relieve the pressure on your nerves and allow your body to heal.

**Does chiropractic help back pain?** Research has shown that chiropractic care can be effective in treating low back pain. Studies have shown that chiropractic care relieves low back pain better than outpatient hospital care.

The people treated by chiropractors were also less likely to suffer a relapse. In a study that followed people over a three-year period, the people treated by chiropractors showed a 29 percent greater improvement in their symptoms than those treated by hospital therapists.

In another survey, people being treated for low back pain were asked to rate their satisfaction with the care they received from their doctors. People being cared for by a chiropractor were three times more likely to report that they were very satisfied than those who were being treated by a family doctor.

**Can chiropractic also help my headaches?** There are many different types of headaches. Chiropractic can't help with all types, but it may help with tension headaches. Sometimes muscle spasms in the neck and shoulders cause tension headaches. Chiropractic therapy can help loosen and relax the muscles and allow your spine to move normally again.

**Does chiropractic cure diseases and infections?** Some chiropractors say that spinal adjustments are necessary for the health of every part of your body. They claim to be able to cure ear infections, allergies, bed-wetting, infantile colic, and asthma. A few even suggest that chiropractic care may be the key to curing cancer. But there's no real scientific evidence to support these claims, and not all chiropractors agree with them. A group of chiropractors in Canada has formed an organization whose professionals only use chiropractic adjustments to help with back and neck pain. Some chiropractors in the United States want to establish professional guidelines that outline which ailments chiropractors should be allowed to treat.

**How do I choose a chiropractor?** If you decide to see a chiropractor, call your state's Chiropractic Board of Examiners before you make an appointment. (Look in your telephone book under state government.) They can tell you if the chiropractor is licensed, and whether or not people have complained about him or his practices. It might also be a good idea to call the chiropractor himself and ask questions. Does he only treat bone and muscle problems like back and neck pain? Is he willing to refer you to a doctor if necessary? Does he recommend long-term treatment? Will he take extensive X-rays? (Because there are risks associated with getting too many X-rays, they should be used sparingly.)

**How many treatments are necessary?** Seven to 12 treatments per injury should be enough to relieve back pain. If you don't see an improvement in three weeks, chiropractic therapy may not work for you.

Chiropractic can be a safe, natural alternative to drugs or surgery for back pain. It may lead to a quicker, longer-lasting recovery for many people. Just remember to use caution when considering chiropractic care for any ailment, and don't hesitate to ask questions.

*Sources:*
*American Health* (11,3:41)
*British Medical Journal* (300,6737:1431 and 311,7001:349)
*Canadian Medical Association Journal* (152,3:329)
*Health* (7,4:45)
*National Headache Foundation* (Fall 1994, Number 90)
*The Atlanta Journal/Constitution* (Dec. 18, 1995, B5)
*The Western Journal of Medicine* (150,3:351)

## Top 10 healing herbs

Based on centuries of experience plus scientific evidence, these herbs are likely to be true healers, experts say.

**Chamomile** — for indigestion
**Echinacea** — for boosting immunity
**Feverfew** — for migraine headaches
**Garlic** — for lowering cholesterol
**Ginger** — for nausea
**Gingko** — for circulation, especially to brain
**Hawthorn** — for heart disease (consult your doctor before using)
**Milk thistle** — for liver damage (consult your doctor before using)
**Saw palmetto** — for enlarged prostate
**Valerian** — for sleep problems

*Source:*
Varro Tyler of Purdue University and Norman Farnsworth of the University of Illinois, cited in *Consumer Reports* (60,11:700)

## The best time to use herbs

When you pay attention to your body, you learn that you have a certain rundown feeling before the cold symptoms furiously strike, you feel the itch before the cold sore erupts, and you have a vague sense of unrest before the infection takes hold.

That's the ideal time to use herbs, says Master Herbalist Debra St. Claire. In our Western society, we tend to use drugs and herbs to treat symptoms. With Ayurvedic medicine (the oldest recorded healing system, originally from India), you use herbs to give your body strength and restore your imbalances before you get sick.

Once you're sick, you may need prescription drugs, which can interact dangerously with herbal treatments.

Using mild herbs in your food and drink is just one of the many ways you can keep your body free from tension, daily pain, and disease. And that may be the key to avoiding such killers as cancer and heart disease.

*Source:*
*Healthy & Natural Journal* (2,1:116)

## Boost brain power with gingko

One of the oldest surviving tree species can turn your brain cells into survivors, too. Recently, people aged 50 to 70 took part in a study which showed that the fan-shaped leaves of the gingko tree increased blood flow to their brains by 70 percent. Better blood flow boosts brain power, improves short-term memory, and may fend off Alzheimer's disease.

In a 1993 study, a group of elderly men with age-related memory loss took gingko supplements. The supplements significantly sped up how fast their brains processed information taken in by their eyes.

The older you are, the more gingko does for you. Gingko does get blood flowing better to your brain when you're under 50, but only by 20 percent, the recent study showed.

In the United States, you can buy the concentrated extract of the gingko leaves in herb shops, but German pharmacies sell the gingko extract as a drug, both over-the-counter and prescription. Doctors there write millions of gingko prescriptions for older people who need improved blood circulation to the brain.

Improving circulation to the brain can help more than your memory. It can help prevent dizziness, headaches, tinnitus (ringing in the ears), mood swings, depression, and anxiety.

Many Germans also take gingko for intermittent claudication. That's the cramping pain you feel in your calves when you walk if you have poor circulation in your legs.

Better blood flow is good news for people with Raynaud's disease, too. Raynaud's is the numb, tingling, freezing feeling in the fingers that some people have as a sudden reaction to cold or stress, and it happens when blood vessels in the fingers contract too much.

Gingko improves blood flow in several ways. It makes the blood less sticky, it expands the blood vessels, and it strengthens tiny vessels so that they don't leak. It also helps keep the bad LDL cholesterol from clumping up on blood vessel walls.

All these benefits really kick in after you've been taking gingko for a while. The recommended dosage is one tablet three times a day with meals, and it's well-suited for long-term use. Some people experience mild side effects, such as an upset stomach or a headache. Very large doses may cause restlessness, nausea, diarrhea, and other unpleasant effects.

You can't harvest the herb yourself — any tea you could make from the leaves would not be strong enough to help you. Besides, touching and eating the fruit causes severe allergic reactions in some people. Simply enjoy the beauty of the tree and let the marketers do the harvesting work. You can reap the benefits at the herb shop.

A gingko tree can live for 1,000 years and survive on the side of a traffic-jammed city street. Perhaps whatever keeps that tree sap running can get your blood flowing for a long, healthy, and memory-filled life.

**Sources:**
*Herbs of Choice: The Therapeutic Use of Phytomedicinals*, The Haworth Press, Binghamton, N.Y., 1994
*Pharmacy Times* (62,1:77)
*The Honest Herbal*, The Haworth Press, Binghamton, N.Y., 1993
*The Lawrence Review of Natural Products*, Facts and Comparisons, St. Louis, Mo., 1995

## Easing nausea is a snap with ginger

Which would be worse — being strapped into a tilted chair rotating at high speed or being locked into the back seat of a car driven by your most reckless family member?

Whichever situation you find yourself in next, consider taking along some ginger capsules. In a recent study, ginger prevented motion sickness better than Dramamine.

Researchers subjected 36 college students with a strong tendency to motion sickness to a torture test in a tilted rotating chair. A dose of 940 mg of powdered ginger taken 25 minutes before the test helped prevent nausea more than a 100 mg dose of dimenhydrinate (Dramamine).

German health authorities have approved ginger as a treatment for motion sickness at a daily dose of 2 to 4 grams.

Ginger may also lower cholesterol, make your blood less sticky and likely to clot, and improve arthritis symptoms. Seven people with rheumatoid arthritis had less pain, swelling, and stiffness when they took ginger for a clinical study. One person ate 50 grams of lightly cooked ginger every day. The other six took 5 grams of fresh ginger or 0.1 to 1 gram of powdered ginger every day.

Gingersnaps and gingerbread may be the yummiest ways to get ginger, but the best way to get a large dose is the 500 mg capsules. You can also make ginger tea or eat candied ginger (easily found in an Oriental food market).

Of course, you shouldn't overdose on ginger. Very large amounts could cause central nervous system depression and heart rhythm disturbances.

**Source:**
*Pharmacy Times* (61,11:50)

## Proven power in a purple flower

Before modern antibiotics came along in the 1930s, some of the most popular products made by drug companies were Echinacea products. These creams and pills were sold as anti-infectives.

These days, your typical doctor would never prescribe the native American plant known as the Purple Coneflower, but the healing member of the daisy family seems as powerful as ever.

You can use it internally to boost your immune system and ward off colds and flu, prostatitis, and possibly rheumatoid arthritis. The creams and oils seem to help heal wounds, eczema, burns, psoriasis, and herpes.

An important warning: It's possible that using Echinacea for a long period of time can actually depress your immune system. It seems safe to take it for a few weeks, then stop for a few weeks. Even better, you may just want to take the liquid or tablet form of Echinacea when you feel the first hint of a cold or other infection.

Growing Echinacea yourself isn't practical because it takes such a concentrated extract to do any good, but you may find the flower growing wild in your backyard, especially if you live in Kansas, Nebraska, or Missouri. It has narrow leaves, a single purple flower, and a sturdy stem that can be 3 feet tall. Chewing the strong, bitter plant makes your lips and tongue tingle.

No one has reported any bad effects from taking Echinacea, but when you take any herb, you should watch yourself for allergic reactions.

Many scientific studies on this herb are under way — researchers are hoping to prove its good immune system effects — so keep looking for news about purple flower power.

*Sources:*
*Pharmacy Times* (61,10:73)
*The Lawrence Review of Natural Products,* Facts and Comparisons, St. Louis, Mo., 1995

# No comfort from comfrey

Comfrey tea sounds harmless and, well, comforting, but don't be fooled. It contains enough toxins to permanently damage your liver, and even cause death. It could put you at risk for liver cancer, too.

Using comfrey as a wound-healing poultice is probably safe, but why risk it. The Henry Doubleday Research Association says that unless future research shows comfrey is safe and effective, "no human being or animal should eat, drink, or take comfrey in any form." For now, consider the herb poisonous.

*Source:*
*The Lawrence Review of Natural Products,* Facts and Comparisons, St. Louis, Mo., 1995

# Ginseng: miracle cure or major myth?

Ginseng. No doubt you've heard of it. Advertisers rave that this miracle root can cure everything that ails you, including colitis, cancer, concentration problems, impotence, and lost energy.

What you may not know is that despite the mass of material written about ginseng, this well-known root remains shrouded in superstition. Very little scientific support backs up advertisers' claims.

Ginseng's most famous claim to fame is its reputed ability to help men overcome impotence. According to Dr. Tony Lee, professor of pharmacology at

Southern Illinois School of Medicine, this claim could be true.

He's found ginseng contains compounds that stimulate nerve cells in the penis, which may help men maintain an erection. While Lee's research gives some credibility to this age-old claim, it's still not proven.

His research also indicates that ginseng is an antioxidant, which means it may help slow the aging process. It may also help keep your heart healthy by dilating your blood vessels and helping to lower your blood pressure.

Other scientists believe that ginseng helps the body cope more effectively with stress, preventing illnesses that stress can cause. Many animal studies appear to confirm this theory. Unfortunately, scientists have yet to prove that ginseng has the same effect on humans.

The bottom line about ginseng is that there aren't enough studies to back up these claims. Even the proper dose and duration of treatment are debatable.

One analysis of 54 ginseng products (such as powders, capsules, tablets, teas, candies, cigarettes, extracts, etc.) found that 60 percent of the products analyzed were worthless. Twenty-five percent contained no ginseng at all.

If you want to purchase quality ginseng, your best bet is to buy an entire ginseng root. With a little practice, these roots are easy to recognize. However, this can be expensive. The very best roots with a humanlike shape (a common characteristic of ginseng) can cost thousands of dollars. If you can't afford or choose not to buy the root, you'll simply have to try to find a reputable manufacturer.

Another problem with purchasing ginseng, even by the root, is that any benefits it has to offer are likely to be affected by the age of the root, where it was grown, and the harvesting and curing methods used. Right now researchers don't know which conditions produce the best ginseng.

If you do decide to buy, be careful not to confuse true ginseng — called Panax ginseng (also known as Asian or Oriental ginseng) — with the popularly marketed Siberian ginseng. Siberian ginseng was introduced by Russian scientists about 30 years ago as a cheap substitute for the real stuff.

There are two other types of authentic ginseng you may run into. One is called Panax quinquefolius (also known as American ginseng). The other is Panax pseudo-ginseng. In general, the effects of all three types of ginseng are similar. However, most scientific studies have been done on Asian ginseng.

Ginseng probably won't hurt you, but it could pose a very serious risk to your pocketbook, without giving you much in return, except maybe a little diarrhea or insomnia. Even though ginseng may offer some healing properties, you're more likely to be ripped off than experience any real benefits.

***Sources:***
*Herbs of Choice: The Therapeutic Use of Phytomedicinals*, The Haworth Press, Binghamton, N.Y., 1994
*The Atlanta Journal/Constitution* (Jan. 19, 1995, H3)
*The Lawrence Review of Natural Products,* Facts and Comparisons, St. Louis, Mo. 1995

# Indian herb lowers cholesterol better than drugs

An herb the Indians have used for centuries in the practice of Ayurvedic medicine has just appeared in American herb shops, and it may lower cholesterol as effectively as the prescription drug clofibrate, researchers say.

You may feel like you're returning to babyhood when you say the name of the plant, but guggul actually has an impressive background. It is a relative of the myrrh of the Bible, and the Asiatic Indians have treasured it as a treatment for arthritis, obesity, and other disorders.

Eighty percent of the people in a recent study lowered their cholesterol by an average of 24 percent with an extract of the guggul plant. They took 500 mg of "gugulipid" for 12 weeks.

A later, larger study compared gugulipid with the cholesterol-lowering drug clofibrate. The average decrease in cholesterol with gugulipid was 11 percent. With clofibrate, the average decrease was 10 percent. The gugulipid therapy also raised many people's good HDL cholesterol, and the clofibrate didn't.

So far, no real negatives have been reported about the guggul plant, except for a few stomach upsets, but the safety profile for humans hasn't been well-described.

By the way, in animal studies, a mixture of guggul and garlic was more effective in reducing blood fat levels than guggul alone, and garlic's safety has been proven.

*Source:*
*The Lawrence Review of Natural Products,* Facts and Comparisons, St. Louis, Mo., 1995

# A dangerous fungus among us

There's a hot new craze hitting America and it's called *kombucha*. Pronounced kom-boo-cha, it sounds like the latest moves on a Latin dance floor, but it's not. It is a fungus tea that is definitely sweeping people off their feet, but it could land them in the hospital.

Kombucha, also called Manchurian or Kargasok tea, looks like a giant mushroom. You may even hear some people call it a mushroom. It's actually a mixture of bacteria and yeasts that forms a patty. The patty grows in a bowl containing a black or green tea and sugar mixture. The liquid mixture is the part you drink — not the mushroom.

As the tea begins to ferment, a new layer of the fungus grows on top of the original or "mother" layer. It takes seven to 10 days for the new "baby" to mature. Then just like friendship bread, the new baby is passed on to a friend or put in its own bowl to grow and reproduce. Those who dare to drink it say kombucha tea tastes like hard cider gone sour.

Kombucha has been touted as a miracle cure for anything that ails you, ranging from memory loss, premenstrual syndrome, cancer, and flatulence to arthritis, psoriasis, aging, multiple sclerosis, baldness, and even AIDS.

Although praises for this cure-all tea are rampant, no scientific tests have validated any of these claims. One leading health authority not only won't recommend the tea to others but has gone on record to say he won't drink it either.

More important than its wondrous claims are the dangers of kombucha tea. In Iowa, two women who regularly drank kombucha tea were hospitalized with excessive acid in their blood. One woman eventually died from the condition. Doctors are not sure if it was the tea or a contamination of the tea that caused the poisoning.

The most dangerous health threat to kombucha tea drinkers is its potential contamination by bacteria and mold. Aspergillus, an airborne mold, can grow in the tea, leading to serious adverse effects in people with immune system problems as well as those allergic to antibiotics. Another danger is that drinkers may rely on kombucha's so-called healing powers instead of seeking necessary medical treatments.

Although kombucha tea may be a trendy new craze you're tempted to try, this is not your best partner in staying healthy. For your health's sake, pass this one by.

*Source:*
The Lawrence Review of Natural Products, Facts and Comparisons, St. Louis, Mo. 1995

# Herbs vs. prescription drugs
## What's the difference between an herb and a drug?

The answer isn't as clear-cut as you might think. An herb is simply a plant that is used to flavor foods or a plant that has medicinal value. And, the main ingredient in about a quarter of the prescription drugs sold in the United States comes from plants. For instance, the drugs digoxin and digitoxin come from the herb digitalis.

Drug companies know that plants can heal, and they would love to profit from selling herbs like ginger or garlic, but our government's Food and Drug Administration makes that almost impossible. The FDA began to lay down the law in the early 1900s when a series of deadly food and drug scandals rocked the United States. The final straw was the 1950s tragedy when the "safe" sleep aid Thalidomide caused serious birth defects in thousands of children. At that time, the FDA passed a law that said drugs must be proven safe and effective before they are sold.

That sounds simple and fair, but to get through the FDA drug approval process, drug companies must spend years of research and millions of dollars to prove the safety and effectiveness of a drug. No drug company is going to spend that kind of money unless they can get a patent on a drug. A patent means nobody else can sell the drug, at least until the patent runs out.

Healing herbs can't be patented. Anyone can go out into his backyard and grow an herb. So, drug companies pinpoint the ingredient in the herb that has medicinal value, they play with it in their laboratories to make it chemically unique and possibly more effective than before, then they patent drugs made out of these "new" chemicals.

Selling a drug made out of an herb is profitable, but selling the herb itself as a medicine usually isn't.

Why is it so hard to get information on what herbs do for you?

Since most herbs haven't gone through the FDA approval process, they can't be sold as medicine. They are sold as food supplements instead. The FDA standards for food supplements are much less strict. But the food supplement status means that people who sell herbs can't make any healing claims for them. In the recent past, they couldn't even warn you about possible side effects.

That's why a bottle of herbal supplements sold in the United States has almost no information on it.

In 1994, the government passed the Dietary Supplement Act, which allows companies to use reputable and unbiased books and journal articles that discuss their products, as long as the articles don't mention a brand name. Herb shops can display the scientific information, but not right next to the supplements. Also, package labels can now state how the herb will affect your body.

Perhaps the FDA will continue to ease the unnecessarily rigid standards for selling herbs, especially when the plants have been used as remedies for centuries. Concerned citizens should encourage the government in this direction.

**Why would you use an herb instead of a drug, especially since so many drugs are made out of plants?**

One obvious advantage to using drugs instead of herbs is that the drugs have gone through that strict FDA approval process. They have the government stamp of approval that says they are safe and effective.

But many herbs are long-time remedies, and while they haven't been through hundreds of clinical trials, you can be reasonably sure that they work and they are safe

Herbs can be much cheaper than prescription drugs, and some have fewer side effects. Garlic seems to lower cholesterol as well as many prescription drugs, with fewer side effects. Garlic costs about 15 cents per day, compared with approximately $4 for a prescription drug.

Some herbs for migraines cost cents a day instead of the dollars you'd spend on prescription drugs.

Using herbs can save you money and give you more control over your health care. But since you are in control, you need to use extra caution to stay safe.

◆ Learn as much as you can about the herbs you plan to take. (The American Botanical Council has published English translations of excellent German descriptions of herbs. These reports combine historical traditional use with modern scientific information.)

◆ Buy herbs with labels that say they've been "standardized." That means the manufacturer has tried to get a consistent amount of the healing herb in each pill.

◆ Don't use more of an herb than the experts recommend. You may even want to use lower-than-normal doses, especially if you are older.

◆ Pay attention to your body's reaction to the herbs you take. Know the symptoms of toxicity.

◆ Tell your doctor that you are using herbs, especially if you also take prescription drugs.

*Sources:*
*Medical Tribune for the Internist and Cardiologist* (36,2:11)
*The Honest Herbal*, The Haworth Press, Binghamton, N.Y., 1993
*The Journal of the American Medical Association* (273,8:607)

## How to grow your own herbs

Herbs are most flavorful when fresh, and, fortunately, some of the best herbal seasonings are the easiest to grow. Basil, sage, parsley, chives, and rosemary will thrive indoors and out. They just need at least six hours of sunlight a day.

It's easiest to buy the small herb plants and transfer them to your own large container. If you think that's cheating, you can buy the packets of seeds. Fill tiny containers with a light potting soil mix, moisten it, then sprinkle on some seeds. Cover the seeds with a bit more soil and water. When leaves begin to grow, transfer your plants to a bigger container.

To grow herbs in your outdoor garden plot, pulverize the soil at least 8 inches deep, fertilize, and lime the soil. Cover seeds with a thin (1/8 to 1/16 inch) layer of soil, then cover with 2 inches of pine or wheat straw. Water gently every day if possible, wetting the soil 1 to 2 inches deep.

After the plants grow, you can begin to snip off leaves and just-opened flowers. Make your herbs happy by doing your snipping in the morning sunshine. Your herb plants will be more full if you pinch them back after harvesting the first usable leaves.

Parsley tastes best fresh. Store it or other herbs in a zip-locked bag in the refrigerator and use within a week. Chopping or mincing the herbs before cooking will release their full flavor.

You can also put bags of herbs in the freezer. The color may change but the taste will still be fresh. To preserve chives, freeze them instead of drying them.

To dry your herbs, put them on a covered plate in a dark place for a few days. When they crumble easily, put them in airtight jars in a dark place. Some herbs, like oregano, actually taste best when dried.

*Sources:*
*Abercrombie's Family Nursery News* (4,2:2)
*American Institute for Cancer Research Newsletter* (47:1)

## Tip-offs to rip-offs

Unfortunately, experimenting with alternative medicine can be like leaping into murky waters filled with hungry piranhas. Don't be a victim of health fraud. Watch out for these red flags of fraud:

◆ A claim that the product works by a "secret formula."

◆ Ads in the back pages of magazines, phone solicitations, editorial-style newspaper ads, and 30-minute television commercials.

◆ A claim that the product is an amazing or miraculous breakthrough. Real medical breakthroughs are rare. Most alternative medical practices that work have been around for a while.

◆ Easy-weight-loss promises.

◆ Guarantees of a quick, painless cure.

Steer clear of any alternative medicine doctor who wants you to quit seeing your regular doctor. He should want to work along with your regular doctor. Also, ask any practitioner of alternative therapy if he is certified.

Before you begin a treatment, try to find people who've gone through it already. Most people will be honest about their experience.

Be open-minded, but be wary, too.

*Source:*
*FDA Consumer* (29,5:10)

# Complementary Cancer Care

## Cancer survival secret

Every year, over 100,000 Americans die of cancer who shouldn't. These people would live if they could only spot their cancers at an early enough stage to be treated and cured.

Your odds of surviving cancer are excellent if you know the early warning signs and you ask for regular cancer screenings. The American Cancer Society says that about two-thirds of the people who get cancer survive to the important five-year mark. By spotting cancer early on, about 92 percent would survive. The warning signs for the most common cancers are listed below:

**Lung cancer.** Look for a cough that won't go away, blood in your sputum, chest pain, an unpleasant sweet taste to your food, and repeated bouts of pneumonia or bronchitis. Your chances of survival are almost 50 percent if you detect the cancer early enough, much better than the standard five-year survival rate of 13 percent.

**Colon and rectal cancer.** Watch for blood in your stools and for changes in your bowel habits. Even if you don't have symptoms, the American Cancer Society recommends that you get tested for this common cancer.

Get a digital rectal exam every year after age 40, a stool blood test every year after age 50, and a sigmoidoscopy every three to five years after age 50. Five-year survival rates for colon cancer are over 90 percent if you catch it early.

**Breast cancer.** Danger signs are a change in your breast, such as a lump; a thick, swollen, or dimpled area; irritated or scaly skin; a painful, tender, or distorted nipple; or discharge from the nipple.

Women age 20 and older should have a doctor examine their breasts every three years. Women over age 40 should have a mammogram every one to two years. Women 50 and over should have a mammogram every year. The five-year survival rate is 94 percent if you detect it early, compared with 18 percent if the cancer has already spread when diagnosed.

**Prostate cancer.** Signs include weak urine flow; inability to urinate; difficulty starting or stopping urination; a frequent need to urinate (especially at night); blood in your urine; pain or burning when you urinate; and constant pain in your lower back, pelvis, or upper thighs.

Men 40 and over should have a digital rectal exam every year, and men over 50 should have a prostate-specific antigen (PSA) blood test every year. Survival rates are 94 percent if you detect prostate cancer early.

**Uterine cancer.** There are two types of uterine cancer — cervical cancer and endometrial cancer. For both, look for abnormal bleeding or spotting and abnormal vaginal discharge. Women over 18 should have a Pap test every year, and women over 40 should have a pelvic exam every year.

The Pap test is very effective in detecting cervical cancer, but it can miss endometrial cancer. Women at high risk of endometrial cancer should have an endometrial tissue sample tested at menopause. Survival rates for both types of uterine cancer are over 90 percent if discovered at an early stage.

**Leukemia.** Some danger signs are fatigue, pale skin, unexplained weight loss, repeated infections, easy bruising, and nosebleeds. Early on, doctors often mistake leukemia symptoms for other less serious conditions.

**Skin cancer.** Examine yourself once a month for changes in the size or color of a mole; scaly, oozing patches of skin; bleeding; unusual bumps or lumps; and itchy or tender spots.

The most dangerous kind of skin cancer, malignant melanoma, can spread quickly, but your survival chances are 93 percent if you detect it early.

**Ovarian cancer.** Especially if you are over 40, watch for unexplained stomachaches, gas, and bloated feelings. The most common sign is an enlarged belly, caused by fluids. You may have abnormal vaginal bleeding. You need a thorough pelvic exam every year if you are over 40. The survival rate is 90 percent if you detect it early, compared with the average 42 percent survival rate.

**Bladder cancer.** Signs are blood in the urine and the need to urinate frequently. The five-year survival rate is 92 percent if detected early.

**Oral cancer.** Watch your lips, tongue, mouth, and throat for bleeding sores that won't heal, lumps or thick areas, and red or white patches that don't go away quickly. Later signs are difficulty chewing, swallowing, or moving your tongue or jaw.

If you think you're at risk for a particular type of cancer, let your doctor know and ask him to examine you on a regular basis. Over a million Americans are diagnosed with cancer every year. If you're one of them, you want to make sure you're a survivor.

*Source:*
*Cancer Facts & Figures – 1995,* American Cancer Society, 1599 Clifton Road N.E., Atlanta, Ga. 30329–4251

## Foods that fight cancer

About one-third of all the deaths caused by cancer may be related to the food you put in your mouth. That's good news because you can (usually) control that.

It boils down to a few basic pieces of nutrition advice:

1) Eat more high-fiber foods.
2) Cut down on fatty foods.
3) Eat fewer salt-cured, pickled, and smoked foods.
4) Eat more fruits and vegetables.

Other food choices may affect your chances of getting cancer — such as garlic, soy, fish oil, coffee, calcium — but compared with the big four listed above, these are like tiny raindrops in a tropical storm.

One of the most fun choices you can make is to eat more fruits and vegetables.

The cancer protection they offer is proven and incredible. Here's what a few of the studies show:

- Healthy genes need *methionine* and *folate* — two substances found in fruits, vegetables, poultry, fish, and dairy products. Your body needs methionine and folate to make methyl groups, which genes need to work properly. A diet low in these substances may cause cancerous genes to form or may cripple natural tumor suppressors. By the way, alcohol can also interfere with the formation of methyl groups, putting you at risk for cancer if you drink regularly.

- Healthy lungs need *lutein* — a protective carotenoid found in leafy, dark-green vegetables. People on the South Pacific island Fiji get very little lung cancer even though they smoke, and researchers think it's because they eat so many of these cancer-fighting vegetables.

- Tomatoes fight against prostate cancer. You don't even have to like vegetables to get this benefit. Pizza and pasta are usually loaded with a tomato-rich sauce.

- Green and yellow vegetables seem to stop tumor growth. The best ones may be cauliflower, cabbage, brussels sprouts, and broccoli. All these contain the cancer-fighting substance *brassinin*.

- Broccoli may be one of the top cancer protectors you can eat. The American Institute for Cancer Research recommends that you fight the effects of carcinogens with foods rich in fiber, vitamin C, and vitamin A. Broccoli is a great source of all three.

- Vitamins C and E offer strong protection against cancer, if you get them in fruits and vegetables instead of in supplements. If you look at all the scientific studies that have been done, you'll see that nobody really knows yet if taking vitamin supplements will help prevent cancer. On the other hand, all the studies averaged together show that eating at least five fruits and vegetables a day reduces your risk of gastrointestinal and respiratory cancers by 40 percent. In other words, people who eat fewer than two servings of fruits and vegetables a day are almost twice as likely to get these cancers.

Scientists think that all the nutrients in various fruits and vegetables work together to prevent damage to your body structures. For instance, vitamin C (a water-soluble vitamin) does its antioxidant work more in the watery parts of blood and tissues, and vitamin E (a fat-soluble vitamin) works in the fatty substances. The two vitamins need each other, along with other nutrients, to work properly.

Eating a variety of fruits and vegetables will offer you the best cancer protection. Add broccoli to your macaroni and cheese, snack on carrot sticks, and finish off lunch with an apple. You'll find that eating at least five fruits and vegetables a day is much more fun, and filling, than taking a vitamin supplement.

*Sources:*
*American Journal of Clinical Nutrition* (62,6:1385S)
*Diet & Cancer ... What's the Link?,* American Institute for Cancer Research, 1759 R Street, N.W., Washington, D.C. 20069
*Food Safety Notebook* (6,3:19)
*Journal of the National Cancer Institute* (87,4:265)
*Medical Abstracts Newsletter* (16,2:3)
*Nutrition Research Newsletter* (15,1:6)

## How to get unconventional cancer treatments for free

Every day, scientific researchers study new cancer treatments, searching for breakthroughs that really work to fight the growth and spread of tumors.

Every day, people with cancer search for treatments that haven't been proven in scientific laboratories, hoping against hope to find the miracle that will cure their disease.

These two groups can help each other. If you are interested in trying an unconventional, unproven treatment for cancer, don't go to a quack who claims to have a secret cure. Instead, ask your doctor if you are eligible to participate in a *clinical trial*.

Researchers use clinical trials to find out if promising new treatment methods really work. If you participate in one of these treatment studies, you (along with many others with cancer) will be given the new treatment and carefully watched. All your reactions will be written down and compared with others.

When the study is over, the researchers will gather all their findings, publish them in medical journals, and discuss them at scientific conferences. If the study results are positive, the unconventional experiment you were a part of may become a common treatment for millions of people who have cancer.

Being a guinea pig in a trial is a safe way to try out unproven cancer treatments. Don't be bamboozled by people offering unconventional treatments who may either waste your money or, worse, waste the valuable time you need to take advantage of therapies that can really work.

When you're deciding whether to try an unproven remedy, take these steps:

♦ Ask a librarian to help you find out if the treatment has been reported in reputable scientific journals.

♦ Be wary of any treatment that is mainly dietary or nutrition therapy. Scientists don't believe right now that you can get rid of cancerous cells in your body simply by changing your diet.

♦ Watch out for treatments that supposedly have no side effects. Cancer treatments have to be powerful, so it's not likely that you'll find an effective therapy with no side effects.

If you're interested in participating in a clinical trial, ask your doctor to use PDQ (Physician Data Query) to get information for you. PDQ is a computer database of information from the National Cancer Institute (NCI).

You can also call the NCI's Cancer Information Service to request information about clinical trials. The staff will tell you about cancer-related services in your area. The toll-free number of the Cancer Information Service is 1-800-4-CANCER (1-800-422-6237).

By the way, you don't have to have cancer to take part in a clinical trial. People without cancer can contribute to medical science by helping researchers find new ways to stop the disease before it starts.

*Source:*
National Cancer Institute, Office of Cancer Communications, 31 Center Drive, MSC 2580, Bethesda, Md. 20892-2580

## Microwave cooking and cancer

Have you ever stuck a tub of margarine into the microwave to soften it? That's a bad idea. You should never microwave food in the package you bought it in unless the directions tell you to do so. The high temperatures can cause cancer-causing substances in plastic or paper containers to leach into your food.

Don't reuse the plastic microwavable dishes manufacturers provide, either. The container may be safe the first time around, then begin to break down the more often you use it.

The safest containers to use in the microwave are glass and ceramic, even though not all of these are microwave-safe either. Here's a quick test for glass: Microwave the empty container for one minute. If it's warm, it's not safe for the microwave. If it's lukewarm, you can use it safely to reheat foods. If it's cool, you can use it for actual microwave cooking.

*Source:*
*FDA Consumer* (24,2:17 and 29,8:14)

## Ancient cure receives cancer researchers' support

People in the Orient have been singing the praises of the man-shaped ginseng root for thousands of years. Lately, Americans have jumped on the ginseng bandwagon and sent sales of the expensive root rocketing into the millions.

Ginseng's reputation as a cure-all has very little scientific evidence to back it up (see *Alternative Healing* chapter for more information), but Korean researchers believe that using ginseng regularly protects you from cancer.

The researchers asked almost 4,000 people, half of whom had cancer, whether they had used ginseng in the past. The people who had used ginseng had half the cancer risk as people who didn't use it at all.

The longer people had used ginseng, the lower their cancer risk seemed to be. Using ginseng for one year offered some protection, but using ginseng for 20 years really lowered cancer risk.

For some unknown reason, fresh ginseng slice, fresh ginseng juice, and white ginseng tea didn't seem to offer any cancer protection. Most other ginseng products were linked with reduced cancer risk, including fresh ginseng extract, white ginseng extract, white ginseng powder, and red ginseng.

Using ginseng meant fewer cancers of the mouth, pharynx, esophagus, stomach, colon, rectum, liver, pancreas, larynx, lung, and ovary. Ginseng had little effect on cancers of the breast, uterus, bladder, and thyroid.

*Source:*
*Cancer Epidemiology, Biomarkers & Prevention* (4,4:401)

## Tasty tofu fights cancer, too

Have you ever tried to be helpful but just felt as though you were getting in the way?

That's the life of a *phytoestrogen*. These natural substances are very weak estrogens, maybe 100 to 1,000 times weaker than the estrogen hormone you produce in your body.

Phytoestrogens all by themselves seem to do what estrogen does, although not very well. However, when you put the weak phytoestrogen beside your body's estrogen, the little phyto just gets in the estrogen's way.

That sounds like a bad thing, but it's not. The estrogen in your body encourages certain kinds of cancer, such as breast and prostate cancers. Eating foods that contain phytoestrogens may help protect you against cancer.

The best source of phytoestrogens is food made with soybeans. Some soy foods contain more of the cancer-fighting phytoestrogen called *genistein* than others.

A graduate student experimenting with genistein found that it works best to block cancer before it starts. In his lab experiments, genistein was 10 times more effective in discouraging cancer growth in normal, noncancerous cells than in cells where cancer growth had already started.

Genistein-rich foods include:

◆ Tofu — sold in blocks, looks and feels like a soft cheese. You can buy soft or extra firm tofu. For safety and for better-tasting tofu, only buy refrigerated brands. Rinse and pat dry before using. Cover leftover tofu with water and store in the refrigerator. Change the water daily and use within one week.

◆ Tempeh — a chewy cake made from soybeans. It can be grilled or added to soups and casseroles.

◆ Soy milk — used like cow's milk. A plus for people who don't digest milk well: It's lactose-free.

◆ Soy flour — ground from roasted soybeans. In recipes, replace about one quarter of the regular flour with the nutty-flavored soy flour. Don't try it in recipes that contain yeast, though. Your bread won't rise.

◆ Soy protein (to replace ground meat), soy beans, soy burgers and hot dogs, soy-based frozen desserts, soy margarine, and soy cream cheese. Make sure these foods aren't high in fat.

Here are some tips for cooking with tofu:

◆ Marinate extra-firm tofu in barbecue sauce (or any marinade) and grill with vegetables such as onions, green peppers, and tomatoes.

◆ Cube firm tofu and use it to replace meat in soups, chili, stews, and casseroles. Add the tofu during the last 15 minutes of cooking.

◆ Use tofu to replace some of the cheese on pizza and in lasagna. Silken tofu will work best in lasagna.

◆ Add tofu cubes to stir-fries and fajita recipes. Add during the last two minutes of cooking.

Not only is tofu rich in phytoestrogens, it's also full of calcium and protein. Experiment with this healthy vegetable protein. It's so versatile, you're sure to find some soy recipes you truly enjoy.

**Source:**
*American Institute for Cancer Research Newsletter* (49:6)

## Get omega-3 protection from the sea

The sunny shores of Greece and the cold tundras of Alaska have one thing in common: The people who live there have a low risk of certain types of cancer. That could be because they eat lots of fish.

Fish contain omega-3 fatty acids, and cancer researchers everywhere believe that this powerful substance stops the growth and spread of cancers of the breast, prostate, and colon.

In a recent German study you can be glad you weren't involved in, researchers studied the stools of 24 healthy volunteers. They found that people who took fish oil capsules excreted less of a substance suspected to cause colon cancer.

Buying fish oil capsules is one option, but your best protection will come from eating more fish. The richest sources of omega-3 include mackerel, striped bass, lake trout, herring, salmon, lake whitefish, anchovy, bluefish, and halibut.

Cooking fish is easy, so don't be afraid to experiment. Mackerel, salmon, and trout are fattier fish. They'll taste good grilled, baked, or broiled. Ten minutes on a piece of foil in a 400 degree oven will do for most fish fillets. Add spices and a splash of lemon or lime juice.

Poach or microwave leaner fish such as bass and halibut. For another moist cooking method, place fish fillets on individual pieces of foil with juice or wine, spices, and some thinly sliced vegetables — onions, snap peas, and carrots, for instance. To seal in the juices and flavor, tightly fold up the edges of the foil packages. Cook for 10 to 15 minutes in a 450 degree oven.

Be careful when choosing frozen fish meals. The saturated fat in the breaded and deep-fried varieties can cancel out the good effects of the omega-3 fatty acids. At restaurants, you can ask for "dry-grilled" fish to get a healthy, low-calorie dish.

*Sources:*
*American Institute for Cancer Research Newsletter* (48:11)
*Controlling Your Fat Tooth,* Workman Publishing, New York, 1991
*Nutrition and Cancer* (25,1:71)

## Trim the fat to cut cancer risk

What's for dinner? If you are trying to choose between a baked chicken breast, a steak and vegetable stir-fry, or rice and beans, you may be at a lower risk for cancer than someone who plans to eat a hamburger, prime rib, fried chicken, or pork spareribs.

There's nothing wrong with enjoying a piece of meat, but study after study is showing that diets high in fatty red meat raise your risk of all kinds of cancer — breast and prostate cancers, colon cancer, even skin cancer. A new study says that women who eat lots of red meat almost double their risk of non-Hodgkin's lymphoma.

You don't have to become a vegetarian, although a life of pasta primavera, bean burritos, vegetable soup, and "loaded" baked potatoes sounds appealing to some of us. Meat can be good for you. A three-ounce serving of beef provides:

◆ Iron — approximately 15 percent of the RDA for women, 25 percent for men.

◆ B vitamins — 40 percent of the RDA for vitamin B12, a nutrient vegetarians have trouble getting enough of.

◆ Protein — 50 percent of the RDA for women, 40 percent for men.

Unfortunately, meat, especially fatty meat, is a problem food for most Americans because we eat too much of it. Compounds in the red meat and fat in the meat may combine to increase our risks of cancer. Meat contains heterocyclic amines that seem to cause DNA damage, which increases cancer risk. Heterocyclic amines are brought out even more by certain cooking methods, such as frying, broiling, and grilling.

Also, your body has to work extra hard to metabolize fat, and the process can produce damaging free radicals that promote cancer. Too much fat in your diet may also keep your immune system from recognizing precancerous changes in your body.

One new study from Texas shows that people with a history of skin cancer are able to reduce their chances of developing tumors five times by eating less fat. The people in the study ate the same amount of calories because they increased their intake of complex carbohydrates, but they decreased their fat intake from 40 percent to 21 percent of calories.

Over a two-year period, the 38 people eating a low-fat diet developed an average of three skin tumors each. The 38 people eating high-fat foods developed 10 tumors each.

To eat a healthy, low-fat diet that includes meat, think portion control. Three ounces of meat is plenty. That's about the size of a deck of cards.

The leanest beef cuts are labeled "loin" or "round." Compare 3 ounces of roasted eye of round at 155 calories and 5.5 grams of fat with 3 ounces of braised short ribs at 400 calories and 35.7 grams of fat. And forget about finding a lean hamburger patty.

Look for pork, lamb, and veal labeled "loin" or "leg." A 3-ounce serving of broiled pork tenderloin has 4.1 grams of fat and 141 calories. The same amount of pan-fried pork top loin has 28.3 grams of fat and 333 calories. When you cook, trim away all the fat you can see.

Watch out for cold cuts and sausages. If you eat them at all, look for low-fat versions.

Chicken and turkey are healthy choices if you eat the light meat and remove the skin. Most of the fat in poultry is found just under the skin. Three ounces of skinless chicken breast has 3 grams of fat and 140 calories. A thigh, which is dark meat, with skin has 13.2 grams of fat and 210 calories.

Picture yourself as a healthy and cancer-free 90-year-old enjoying a delicious, low-fat turkey dinner with your family. Maybe that will help you resist your next Big Mac attack.

**Sources:**
*American Journal of Epidemiology Supplement* (141,11:S62)
*Controlling Your Fat Tooth,* Workman Publishing, New York, 1991
*Diet, Nutrition & Cancer Prevention: The Good News,* NIH Publication 87–2878, National Cancer Institute, Bethesda, Md. 20892
*Medical Tribune for the Internist and Cardiologist* (36,21:17)

## Walk away from cancer

Heaven help you if you don't know by now that taking a daily stroll builds a stronger heart and reduces your chances of dying from heart disease. What you may not have heard is how much influence a little exercise has over the second biggest killer of American men and women — cancer.

In fact, a man who walks a couple of hours a week or plays a weekly game of tennis is 30 percent less likely to develop colon cancer. In other words, he's reduced his chances of developing the cancer he's most likely to get after prostate and lung cancer by almost one-third.

And the good news marches on. Harvard researchers say you could cut your colon cancer risk in half by putting more oomph into your exercise program. For that kind of risk reduction, you'd need to run for four or more hours a week or walk 12 or more hours a week.

Of course, you're not limited to walking or running. You can do any type of exercise you enjoy — whatever keeps you slim and active. (The Harvard study of almost 50,000 men also showed that gaining more than 40 pounds after age 21 makes you twice as likely to develop colon cancer.)

Nobody is sure exactly why exercise reduces cancer risk, but it could have something to do with the insulin in your body. Animal studies have shown that insulin is a factor in tumor growth. Both weighing too much and being inactive tend to raise your insulin levels.

*Sources:*
*Annals of Internal Medicine* (122,5:327)
*Medical Tribune for the Internist and Cardiologist* (36,7:19)

## Garlic: a cancer-suppressing clove

It's a proven fact that garlic fights heart disease. Researchers are less certain about the spice's protective effects against cancer, but numerous studies keep showing positive results.

Garlic seems to stop or slow the development of tumors in the breast, liver, lungs, and colon. Studies show that garlic keeps your body from producing carcinogens and keeps carcinogens from binding to your genetic material.

You'll get the most protective benefits from garlic if you don't overdose on protein and saturated fat. Too much fat or too much protein in your diet may suppress garlic's ability to act against carcinogens.

The extra flavor added by a dash of garlic can help you forgo fattier flavorings such as butter, margarine, and oil.

*Source:*
*American Institute for Cancer Research Newsletter* (48:10)

## Natural, no-fuss way to protect against colon cancer

Want to outfox the fat you eat? You can repair the damage fat does to your colon by supplementing your diet with a half-ounce of wheat bran or a calcium tablet a day.

When you eat a high-fat diet, your body secretes extra bile acids to help digest it. Too many bile acids in the intestines are thought to cause or contribute to colon cancer.

A new study done in Arizona over a 9-month period showed that people who supplemented their diets with 13.5 grams (about a half-ounce) of wheat bran daily reduced the bile acids in their colons by half.

In the same medical study, researchers gave another group of people calcium supplements of 1,500 mg per day. These people showed a one-third reduction in their bile acids. So keeping up with your calcium intake will now have two benefits: You'll be reducing your risk of osteoporosis and colon cancer.

If you're concerned about colon cancer, it's easy to supplement your diet in a healthy way. You'll find wheat bran at your nearest grocery or health food store. It comes ready to eat, and can be added to almost any food, not just baked goods, for a pleasant, nutty flavor.

You'll need to take a calcium supplement to get the 1,500 mg amount used in the study. Good food sources of calcium are low-fat dairy products and leafy green vegetables.

Since colon cancer is the second most common type of fatal cancer in America today, it's worth your best effort to do whatever you can to prevent it. Adding wheat bran or calcium to your diet is an easy, inexpensive way of providing "health insurance."

*Sources:*
*Journal of the National Cancer Institute* (88,2:67 and 88,2:81)
*The Atlanta Journal/Constitution* (Jan. 17, 1996, D4)

# Colon cancer self-defense

Looking like the Bobsey twins can be fun, but one trait you don't want to share with your siblings is a tendency for cancer. If you have just one first-degree relative with colon cancer, your risk for the cancer is doubled.

Once you hit age 50, the American Cancer Society strongly urges you to undergo a flexible sigmoidoscopy every three to five years. You need a total colonoscopy only if a polyp is found.

If you have colon cancer in your family, though, you may want to have a total colonoscopy when you reach age 50 and every three to five years after that. Your colon cancer risk is high, and a regular, thorough test will help you detect the cancer early and get rid of it.

*Source:*
*Geriatrics* (51,2:63)

# Dump coffee and chocolate to lower cancer risk

A cup or two of coffee a day is a perfectly fine pick-me-up. Four cups of coffee a day may cause cancer. French researchers say that people who drink more than four cups of coffee a day are four times more likely to develop colon and rectal cancer than people who don't drink coffee.

Plus, their study of about 500 people said that eating a chocolate candy bar every day doubles the risk of colon and rectal cancers.

"Moderation in all things," the ancient Romans said.

*Source:*
*Medical Tribune* (36,12:8)

## Cancer prevention as close as your medicine cabinet

In the early 1800s, German and Italian chemists in old-fashioned laboratories tinkered with white willow bark and meadowsweet flower buds to pull out their powerful healing ingredient, salicin. In 1860, chemists created a stronger version of salicin — acetylsalicylic acid. They named the new drug aspirin.

Then everyone forgot about the experiments for 50 years until a German chemist, searching for anything to relieve his arthritic father's pain, stumbled upon the old reports. That chemist worked at the Friedrich Bayer pharmaceutical company.

Now, researchers firmly believe that the aspirin in your medicine cabinet not only relieves pain, reduces fever and inflammation, and helps protect your heart, but it may also prevent cancer in your digestive tract, especially cancers of the esophagus and colon.

Colon cancer is the third most common and most deadly cancer for both men and women. Esophageal cancer is much less common, but, like many of the other cancers, it's on the rise. Twice as many people die from it today as 30 years ago.

A recent study compared thousands of people who took aspirin occasionally with people who never took the pain reliever. The people who took aspirin every once in a while were 90 percent less likely to develop esophageal cancer over a 16-year period.

Another group of researchers looked at the questionnaires from the huge Nurses' Health Study to determine if taking aspirin was connected with a lower cancer risk. They found that women who took at least two aspirin tablets a week for 10 years or more lowered their risk of colon cancer. Taking four to six tablets a week seemed to lower the risk even further.

Taking lots of aspirin is very likely to damage your stomach lining, so you wouldn't want to take it to reduce your chances of cancer. Unless, that is, your doctor agrees that you have a very high risk of cancer. It runs in your family, for instance.

The researchers who analyzed the Nurses' Health Study for aspirin's effect on cancer recommend that people at risk for colon cancer take a 325 mg aspirin tablet every other day.

People who have already had a tumor removed from their colons should consider taking a small dose of aspirin every day or two. Taking aspirin frequently seemed to cut the risk of developing a new tumor in half for a group of 750 people who already had colon tumors removed.

You could try to get cancer protection from the herbs that gave us aspirin, but the attempt may make you appreciate the powers of the chemistry lab. You'd have to drink around 5 1/2 gallons of bitter willow bark tea a day to equal a 4.5 gram dose of aspirin. Fortunately, Mother Earth and modern medicine combined their strengths to give us the miracle of an aspirin tablet.

*Sources:*
*Cancer Facts & Figures – 1995*, American Cancer Society, 1599 Clifton Road N.E., Atlanta, Ga. 30329-4251
*Herbal Medicine*, Beaconsfield Publishers, Beaconsfield, England, 1988
*Herbs of Choice: The Therapeutic Use of Phytomedicinals*, The Haworth Press, Binghamton, N.Y., 1994
*Medical Tribune for the Internist and Cardiologist* (36,11:7 and 36,21:17)
*The New England Journal of Medicine* (333,10:609)

## An early sign of lung cancer

The most frightening thing about lung cancer is that almost nine out of 10 people who get it die from it within five years of being diagnosed. That's mainly because lung cancer is so hard to detect at an early stage. By the time you start having symptoms like coughing, pneumonia, chest pain, or blood in your sputum, it's usually too late. Even regular lung X-rays don't always pick up the signs of cancer in time.

But now, four doctors have discovered a previously unreported, very early warning sign of lung cancer. It's an unpleasant sweet taste to the food you eat, and you may experience it long before you have any other symptom of cancer.

The doctors noticed a pattern when three of their patients came to them complaining about an annoying sweet taste. The three (all heavy smokers) later turned out to have small cell carcinoma of the lung.

Everything tasted so sweet to one 63-year-old woman that she felt nauseated and began to eat only salty foods. Another man just noticed that his daily banana tasted unpleasantly sweet.

Apparently, the cancer tumor causes your body to secrete a hormone that increases the amount of water you retain and lowers the level of sodium in your blood. The sweet receptors in your tongue need sodium to work correctly, so that's why you end up with an unpleasant taste.

If your food starts tasting supersweet, see your doctor immediately. One of the men who waited three weeks before seeing his doctor about the taste died one year later.

Watching closely for this early sign of lung cancer and acting quickly could save your life.

*Sources:*
*Archives of Internal Medicine* (155,12:1325)
*The American Medical Association Encyclopedia of Medicine*, Random House, New York, 1989

## Bare it all to beat cancer

Shut the blinds, turn up the lights, and get naked. It's skin cancer survival time — time to check your skin for the tiny spots and funky moles that could mean a deadly, unstoppable bout with cancer is on the way. This simple exam is guaranteed to reduce your chances of dying from skin cancer, maybe by 50 percent.

The first step is to look at both sides of your hands and at your lower and upper arms.

Then stand in front of a full-length mirror and look at your whole body, front and back. Raise your arms so you can check under them. You're looking for anything new, especially a change in a mole or a new mole. Use a hand mirror for any back parts you can't see.

Next, use the hand mirror to examine your scalp and the back of your neck. Part your hair or use a blow dryer for a closer look.

Now check out the backs of your legs and the bottoms of your feet with the mirror. Look between your toes, too.

Melanoma, the kind of cancer that comes from the cells that give color to your skin, can show up in a mole or in normal skin. It can be hard to tell the difference between a melanoma and a mole. The danger signs are:

A= Asymmetry. That means one half of a mole doesn't match the other half. The mole isn't round or oval.

B= Border. The border, or edges, of a mole are uneven instead of smooth.

C= Color. A mole has different colors in it. It may be shades of tan, brown, and black, or it may even be red, white, and blue.

D= Diameter. A mole larger than a pencil eraser may be a sign of cancer.

See your doctor immediately if a mole grows, bleeds, changes color, or becomes scaly, itchy, or painful. You should also know that most people think flat moles or patches are harmless, but that's not necessarily true.

Melanoma is the most dangerous type of skin cancer, but you should scan your skin for basal and squamous cell skin cancers, too. These cancers can look like a pale, waxlike, pearly bump or a red, scaly, sharply outlined patch.

Catching melanoma in its earliest stages can save your life. Dr. Perry Robins, president of the National Skin Cancer Foundation, says, "The difference between life and death is a quarter of an inch. If you catch it early, nobody need die." That's worth a few bare minutes with your mirror.

*Sources:*
*American Family Physician* (49,1:91)
*Cancer Facts & Figures – 1995*, American Cancer Society, 1599 Clifton Road N.E., Atlanta, Ga. 30329–4251
*Cutis* (56,6:313)
*Medical Tribune for the Internist and Cardiologist* (35,1:2 and 37,2:11)

# Tanning bed tragedies

When a red-haired, freckled 43-year-old woman found a reddish-brown, scaly patch on her arm, she immediately went to her doctor. Diagnosis: skin cancer. Over the next eight years, the woman developed skin cancers on her leg, her temple, her chest, her buttocks, and her breast. Cancer did not run in her family, she was not overly sensitive to ultraviolet A radiation, and the last two body parts had never been exposed to the sun.

This native of overcast northern England was the victim of a tanning bed. For the three years before she was diagnosed with skin cancer, she had used a tanning bed once or twice a week, 30 minutes a session.

She'd never been able to tan in the sun, but in the tanning bed, she was able to turn a light brown. She was always careful not to burn herself, so she thought she was safe.

No one who uses tanning beds is safe from skin cancer, and people who tan poorly or have many moles, freckles, a previous severe sunburn, or lowered immunity for any reason are particularly at risk.

Don't be tempted by the tanning salons, even if tanning is included in a fitness and beauty package you purchase. The tanned look may appeal to you, but the look of skin cancer lesions certainly won't.

**Source:**
*The New England Journal of Medicine* (332,21:1450)

## Cure your ulcer to prevent possible cancer

If you have an ulcer or even the beginnings of one, you may have had a bellyful of the *Helicobacter pylori* bacteria, both literally and figuratively. The bacteria was discovered in the early 1980s, but it took until the '90s for many doctors to accept that most ulcers are caused by *H. pylori* instead of stress or poor eating habits. Some doctors still haven't accepted it, but these days, it seems like everyone is talking about it.

You may have somehow missed the bacteria bandwagon, but now is the time to jump on. Not only is *H. pylori* at the root of most ulcers, it may put you at risk for stomach cancer, a new study shows.

If you've been thinking about being tested for the presence of *H. pylori* in your stomach, don't put it off any longer. The newest blood tests for *H. pylori* are very accurate and very inexpensive.

If the tests show that you have the bacteria, your doctor can prescribe certain antibiotics along with bismuth subsalicylate, the main ingredient in Pepto-Bismol. In two weeks or less, you can cure your ulcer and lower your risk of stomach cancer.

**Sources:**
*Geriatrics* (50,10:57)
*The Lancet* (345,8964:1525)

## How to prevent the deadliest cancer of all

You won't meet many people with pancreatic cancer — not because the cancer is rare, but because most people die quickly after being diagnosed. Only 3 percent of people with pancreatic cancer are still alive five years after diagnosis.

Because it's so rapidly fatal, nobody knows much about what causes the cancer. You don't even have any symptoms until it's too late. Fortunately, researchers in Montreal and in Shanghai have recently managed to pinpoint some food habits that may lead to the disease. To lower your risk, take this nutrition advice:

◆ Eat as many "natural" foods — foods without additives or preservatives — as possible.

◆ Eat foods raw or cooked in a pressure cooker, microwave oven, or by electricity.

◆ Eat fruits and vegetables.

Eating habits that may increase your risk of pancreatic cancer are:

◆ Eating lots of salt, smoked meat, dehydrated food, preserved food, fried food, and refined sugar.

◆ Preparing food by deep-frying, grilling, curing, or smoking, or cooking with firewood.

*Source:*
*Nutrition Research Newsletter* (15,1:7)


## Special warning to canker sore sufferers

Some people don't think twice about drinking scalding coffee, sucking on lemons, or biting their lips. For others, a tiny mouth injury can turn into a nasty, painful canker sore that lasts for 10 to 15 days. Even a stressful week or a vigorous toothbrushing can lead to a sore.

Why some people are plagued by the sores and others aren't is a mystery, but canker sore sufferers may be naturally more susceptible to nitrates in foods. Nitrates may be more likely to turn into cancer-causing compounds called nitrosamines in their bodies.

So, if you've always been a canker-sore sufferer, a meal of beans and franks or chipped beef on toast, especially if you wash it down with beer, could put you on the road to esophageal cancer.

Beer and processed meats and fish are all foods you need to watch out for. Processed meat includes ham, bacon, pastrami, bologna, corned beef, dried beef, pickled loaf, sausages, hot dogs, and other luncheon meats. Try to eat fresh meat instead.

To help keep nitrates from breaking down into dangerous nitrosamines, add tea and vitamin C to your diet. In fact, it's a great idea to keep a salt shaker filled with vitamin C sprinkles on your dinner table. You can find the sprinkles at most health food stores.

Sprinkle on the vitamin C at the table or, as your final cooking step, add a half teaspoon of vitamin C per six servings of any cured or smoked meat dish.

By the way, meat packers know that nitrosamines cause cancer in animals and may cause cancer in humans. When they add nitrates to keep the meat from spoiling, they also add vitamin C to delay the formation of nitrosamines. The vitamin C just isn't as stable as the nitrosamines. That's why you need to add more before you eat the meat.

*Sources:*
*Medical Update* (14,3:5)
*Nutrition Research Newsletter* (14,2:23)

## The hazards of heartburn

If you have antacid tablets in a drawer by your bed, in bathroom and kitchen cabinets, and in the glove compartment of your car ... if your significant other, tired of pink and white globs on all your clothes, searches through your pants pockets for tablets before doing the wash ... you may have heartburn.

The burning pain you suffer daily may be harming you more than you think. It may be putting you at risk for esophageal cancer — a cancer that has rapidly become more common over the past 15 years.

Instead of just popping antacid tablets, you may need to lose weight. Not everyone with heartburn is overweight, but losing a few pounds would help most sufferers. The extra weight squeezes your belly and forces the acidic digestive juices back up into your windpipe.

That *reflux* of stomach acid is a known risk factor for the development of cancerous tumors in the esophagus.

Smoking is another cause of heartburn. Researchers at the Fred Hutchinson Research Center in Seattle say that smoking, alcohol, and obesity account for more than half of the cases of esophageal cancer.

This news isn't meant to add stress to any heartburn sufferer's life (especially since stress is another common cause of heartburn). It's just meant to encourage you to take your heartburn seriously.

Don't eat right before bedtime. Don't bend over immediately after you eat. Wear clothes that fit loosely at your waistline. Avoid fatty and spicy dishes, peppermint, and chocolate. Drink liquids an hour before or after meals to prevent bloating. Cut down on coffee and tea. And most importantly, lose extra pounds and quit smoking.

*Sources:*
*Before You Call the Doctor,* Fawcett Columbine, New York, 1992
*Cancer Epidemiology, Biomarkers & Prevention* (4,2:85)
*Environmental Nutrition* (18,2:1)
*Food Safety Notebook* (6,3:28)
*Medical Update* (15,8:5 and 17,6:1)

# For Men Only

## Prostate primer

If you've noticed that you spend more time running back and forth to the men's room as you get older, you're not alone. The reason for this could be that mysterious part of a man's anatomy called the prostate. The prostate is a walnut-sized gland located around the urethra at the point where it leaves the bladder. Urine and semen travel through the urethra, and the prostate's main job is to contribute fluid to the semen. When the prostate becomes enlarged, it can squeeze off the urethra, making it difficult to urinate. Symptoms of an enlarged prostate include:

- Difficulty beginning the urine stream
- Frequent urination
- Incomplete bladder emptying
- Incontinence
- Weak urine stream

*Benign prostatic hyperplasia* (BPH) or enlarged prostate is a natural part of the aging process. This enlargement could be due to hormonal changes as a man ages. It affects most older men to some degree, whether or not they ever experience symptoms.

Usually an enlarged prostate is not a serious problem. However, if it causes urine retention, it can lead to a bladder or kidney infection. Occasionally, the bladder will fail completely from the constant exertion of trying to expel urine through a blocked passageway.

If symptoms of BPH become too bothersome, treatments are available. You have to weigh the potential side effects of the treatments with the degree of discomfort you're experiencing. The most common treatment for BPH is surgical removal of the prostate. However, side effects include incontinence, impotence, and *retrograde emission* (ejaculation backs up into the bladder rather than exiting the penis).

The drug most often prescribed for BPH is *finasteride* (Proscar). It helps about 40 percent of the men who take it, but it could be six months before you see an improvement. It also may produce side effects of impotence, incontinence, and decreased sexual desire.

A newer treatment for BPH is *balloon dilation*, which involves inserting a small balloon catheter into the urethra and inflating it for about 10 minutes to expand the constricted passageway. It isn't always as effective as surgery, but it has fewer side effects.

Many men with less severe symptoms opt for "watchful waiting," which is merely monitoring symptoms carefully while postponing treatment as long as possible.

*Sources:*
*Emergency Medicine* (27,7:20)
*The American Medical Association Family Medical Guide*, Random House, New York, 1982

## Put your prostate to the test

People fear anything that threatens their sexuality. Of all diseases, women probably fear breast cancer most, because it attacks their femininity. Men, though perhaps less willing to admit it, fear prostate cancer.

Prostate cancer is the second leading cause of cancer deaths among men, right behind lung cancer. Because it is so common among older men — those over age 60 — many of those diagnosed die from other causes before the prostate cancer has time to grow. It has been said that you're more likely to die with

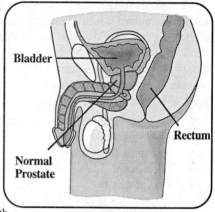

prostate cancer than from it. However, people do die from it, approximately 35,000 a year in the United States alone.

In 1986, a new testing method for *prostate specific antigen* (PSA) changed the way prostate disease is diagnosed. A PSA test measures a substance emitted by a normal prostate as well as cancerous tissue in the prostate. Because a healthy prostate releases very little of this substance, an elevated PSA could mean cancer is present. A PSA below 4 is considered normal. Although this test can detect prostate problems much earlier than rectal exams, it isn't always accurate.

Prostate cancer tends to grow more slowly than many other types of cancer, and since it occurs mostly in older men, some doctors think that PSA testing causes needless alarm for many men. They say that a man is more likely to die from other causes, and there is no proof that early detection increases survival rates from prostate cancer. Therefore, according to critics, PSA testing does nothing but feed a man's fear and make him anxious to seek treatment that may cause him more problems than the disease.

Despite the controversy, the American Cancer Society recommends that men over age 50 have a rectal exam and a PSA test done every year, as well as men over age 40 who have risk factors. Risk factors include race (African-Americans have a two to three times higher risk of prostate cancer) or a relative who has had prostate cancer.

*Sources:*
*Emergency Medicine* (27,7:20)
*Fortune* (133,9:73)

## Making sense of prostate options

Being diagnosed with prostate cancer can lead a man into a confusing whirlpool of options and decisions. Do you simply put your trust in your doctor and follow whatever he recommends? Or do you investigate treatment options on your own?

**Prostatectomy.** Urologists, the specialists who usually deal with prostate problems, have long considered prostatectomy (surgical removal of the prostate) the "gold standard" of treatment. However, prostatectomy is major surgery, with serious potential side effects. Though the numbers vary, some surveys say that as many as half the men who have prostatectomies experience incontinence and as many as 88 percent experience impotence.

**Cryosurgery.** This technique involves inserting probes filled with liquid nitrogen into the tumor, freezing and destroying it.

**Radiation.** External radiation bombards the general vicinity of the prostate in order to destroy the cancer cells. It causes fewer side effects than surgery, but it may be less effective. However, new techniques for radiating the cancer with "seeds" implanted in the prostate have increased radiation's effectiveness.

**Watchful waiting.** This is a strategy being used by more and more men as PSA tests make early detection possible. Monitoring your condition regularly is also easier and more accurate with PSA testing. The down side of this is that tumors can sometimes grow rapidly, and by the time you make the decision to act, it could be too late.

Whatever strategy you decide to use to cope with prostate cancer, know your options and weigh them carefully.

*Source:*
*Fortune* (133,9:55,73)

## Lose jelly belly to protect prostate

According to the poem, "A Visit From St. Nicholas," Santa had a "round little belly that shook when he laughed like a bowlful of jelly." If so, Santa probably also had urinary problems.

A study of 25,000 men in Boston found that increased abdominal fat raised the risk of developing urinary problems. An increase in waist circumference of 7 inches was associated with a 75 percent increase in urinary problems after age 50.

Another study found that almost half the men with a waist circumference of more than 43 inches had severe urinary problems or had undergone prostate surgery. Only about a third of the men with waists smaller than 43 inches had similar problems. Researchers say that waist size is an indication of internal abdominal fat which could be pressing against your prostate, eventually resulting in urinary obstruction.

Researchers have also found that prostate death rates are higher in countries where people eat diets high in fat. A recent study on rats found that a low-fat diet slowed the growth of prostate tumors.

Fat on your waistline and fat in your diet seem to add to your chances of experiencing prostate problems. Santa may have been jolly, but if he'd lost that jelly belly, he would have been a lot healthier.

*Source:*
*Medical Tribune for the Internist and Cardiologist* (36,1:16 and 36,20:16)

## Pizza protection

If you think pizza can't be a health food, think again. Pizza was among three tomato-based foods (along with tomatoes and tomato sauce) in a Harvard study that was associated with a reduced risk of prostate cancer. Tomato sauce was associated with the greatest protective benefit. Of the other foods studied, only strawberries showed a protective effect.

Researchers found that the risk of prostate cancer was reduced by 45 percent among men who ate at least 10 servings of tomato-based products a week. This reduction was attributed to *lycopene,* the substance in tomatoes that gives them their red color.

Tomato juice was not associated with a reduced risk. Researchers speculated that heating the tomato products in oil makes the lycopene more easily absorbed by your body. This might explain why tomato sauce has such a high protective benefit, and tomato juice has none.

An apple a day may keep the doctor away, but two tomatoes a day can provide you with powerful prostate protection.

*Source:*
*Geriatrics* (51,2:21)

## Swollen testicles — no sweat

The swelling of one of your testicles can certainly be upsetting, but it doesn't necessarily mean that you have a serious health problem. It could be a common condition called a *hydrocele.*

A hydrocele is a swelling in the scrotum that is usually soft and painless. It's caused by too much production of lubricating fluid in the membranes that cover the testicles. Hydroceles are common, especially in older men, and are considered harmless. They may be caused by an inflammation or an injury to your testicle, but usually the cause is unknown.

If a hydrocele causes you pain or grows very large, you may need to have your doctor drain the fluid. This is a simple procedure done with a needle and syringe under local anesthetic. If you have a hydrocele that recurs frequently and causes you discomfort, your doctor may recommend surgery to tighten or remove the membrane and prevent the accumulation of the lubricating fluid.

*Source:*
*The American Medical Association Family Medical Guide,* Random House, New York, 1994

## A hidden hurt: epididymitis

One part of the male reproductive system that you may never have heard of is the *epididymis*. The epididymis is a long, oval-shaped tube attached to the back of each testicle.

If an epididymis becomes inflamed, you may feel pain and swelling at the back of one of your testicles, and the area may feel hot and tender. Your scrotum will develop painful swelling and stiffness, and you may get fever, chills, and pain in your groin area.

This condition is called *epididymitis*. It can result from a urinary tract infection, mumps, tuberculosis, prostatitis, a sexually transmitted disease, prostate surgery, or long-term use of a urinary catheter. In younger men, the most common cause is a urinary tract infection.

See your doctor immediately if you think you have epididymitis. The infection can usually be identified by lab tests, and the treatment can begin. Antibiotics will usually cure the problem.

To get some relief from the pain of epididymitis, rest in bed and use some sort of support for your scrotum, such as snugly fitting briefs. Ice packs may help relieve the pain and swelling.

*Sources:*
*Taber's Cyclopedic Medical Dictionary,* F.A. Davis Company, Philadelphia, 1989
*The American Medical Association Family Medical Guide,* Random House, New York, 1994

# Dealing with male menopause

At a certain age, women go through "the change." At around the same age, many men also go through a change. It isn't as recognizable, with clear-cut physical symptoms, but it happens nonetheless, and it can have serious consequences on a man's life and emotional health.

**Erection difficulties.** This problem goes to the heart of male menopause. One study found that half the males between ages 40 and 70 had problems with their erections. Though this is a normal part of the aging process, and is usually only an occasional problem that can be treated, it can still cause great distress and worry for men and their partners.

**Coincidence with female menopause.** When women hit menopause, among their symptoms is an *increase* in sex drive as well as vaginal dryness that can make intercourse painful. When this happens at the same time a man is beginning to have erection difficulties, it can really strain a relationship. It helps to keep the lines of communication open, and work together to solve your problems.

**Feelings of depression.** A man experiencing male menopause may have general feelings of depression and anxiety for no obvious reason. While not as severe as clinical depression, because you are able to work and function, these feelings still interfere with your enjoyment of life.

**Awareness of aging.** You may become overly aware of your age, feeling those little aches and pains more acutely. You may spend a lot of time dwelling on the past and thinking how much better you felt when you were younger.

**Personality changes.** Male menopause can have a profound effect on your personality. You may become more withdrawn, hostile, or unable to make decisions

Male menopause may not be the easiest time of your life, but it's not fatal. If you are experiencing male menopause, here are some things you can do.

**Take a break.** You may require time to shift your life and your thinking in a new direction to sort out your personal life, career, and financial priorities. A vacation could be just what you need to break your routine and make a fresh start.

**Increase your fitness.** This could be the perfect time to take control of your health and fitness. Eat right and exercise to look and feel younger.

**Face facts.** Accepting the fact that you're not the young stud you once were may be painful. However, it is the first step in learning to make the most of your life.

**Perfect your foreplay.** If your partner is also going through menopause, she may need more time for natural lubrication of the vagina to occur, and you may need more stimulation to achieve an erection. Take your time and experiment. You may not have sex as frequently as you did 20 years ago, but it can be much more satisfying.

Male menopause may be a time of change, but it can be a change for the better. The second half of your life can be just as rewarding as the first.

*Source:*
*Look 10 Years Younger, Live 10 Years Longer — A Man's Guide,* Prentice Hall, Englewood Cliffs, N.J., 1995

# Sexual security

Very few situations cause men to feel as frustrated and helpless as impotence. In fact, the word impotent has come to mean a lack of power or control. Most men will have an occasional encounter with impotence sometime in their lives, especially as they get older. Impotence is not a personal failing, and over 80 percent of the cases can be traced to physical causes, such as:

◆ Alcohol or drug abuse
◆ Diabetes
◆ Kidney disease
◆ Neurological disorders such as multiple sclerosis, epilepsy, and Parkinson's disease.
◆ Physical injury
◆ Problems with blood flow, such as hardening or blockage of the arteries, thickened blood, and abnormal leakage of blood in the penis.
◆ Side effect of prescription drugs or surgery

The remaining 20 percent may be due to unidentified physical causes or to psychological factors like stress.

Though impotence may be viewed as an inevitable result of the aging process, you can exert a little control to prevent or delay its appearance.

**Eat right and watch your weight.** A healthy, balanced diet contributes to your sexual well-being in three important ways. First, a diet high in fat and salt can contribute to high blood pressure. Many drugs used to control high blood pressure may cause impotence. Second, excess fat and cholesterol can cause blood flow problems, like hardening of the arteries, that may lead to impotence. Third, a diet that contributes to obesity can increase your risk of developing diabetes, a major cause of impotence.

**Get your vitamins.** Unstable molecules in your body called *free radicals* may damage cells, leading to heart disease or other physical problems that cause impotence. *Antioxidants* can fight the effects of free radicals. The most common antioxidant vitamins are vitamin A (especially in the form of beta carotene), vitamin C, and vitamin E. Foods rich in vitamin A include carrots, sweet potatoes, cantaloupe, apricots, and spinach. Vitamin C can be found in citrus fruits, broccoli, strawberries, and brussels sprouts, and vitamin E is found in vegetable oils, fruits, and vegetables.

**Exercise.** Regular exercise can help prevent impotence by improving your heart health, lowering your cholesterol, and helping you control your weight.

**Limit alcohol.** Though an occasional drink may not be harmful, excessive drinking can cause nervous system damage and alter hormone levels. Male alcoholics often have low testosterone levels and high estrogen levels.

**Avoid harmful drugs.** Unfortunately, impotence can sometimes be a side effect of prescription drugs, such as those used to treat high blood pressure. However, avoiding illegal drugs and some over-the-counter drugs, such as many cold and sleep remedies, may help you steer clear of impotence.

**Practice sensible sex.** Attempting to have sex when the possibility of failure is high can contribute to anxiety, adding to the problem. Make sure you are relaxed and free from distractions. Testosterone levels are highest first thing in the morning, which could increase your chances of success.

*Source:*
*Overcoming Impotence,* Prentice Hall, Englewood Cliffs, N.J., 1994

## Sexercise

You may have heard your female friends mention Kegel exercises, but it seemed like one of those personal feminine things that men aren't supposed to hear. However, Kegel exercises aren't just for women anymore.

Dr. Arnold Kegel invented these exercises to help women maintain better bladder control. These exercises can also help men achieve firmer erections, improve orgasms, and increase sexual stamina.

The muscles involved control urine flow. Imagine that you're trying to stop the flow of urine after it has begun. Tense those muscles and hold for a count of three. Relax and repeat about 10 times. Next, tense and relax the muscles as quickly as you can. Then, imagine that you are trying to force out the last few drops after urinating.

Practice these exercises in sets of 10, five times a day, and soon you'll be more in control of your erections and enjoy longer-lasting orgasms.

*Source:*
*Look 10 Years Younger, Live 10 Years Longer,* Prentice Hall, Englewood Cliffs, N.J., 1995

## Hair today, gone tomorrow

It has been the boast as well as the bane of men since the beginning of time. Some call it "folliclely" challenged, others call it beautiful, but most of us know it as baldness. It is an age-old condition that affects two out of three men, yet experts are still perplexed on how to effectively treat hair loss.

Although the majority of baldness is a result of aging, several other factors can cause hair to bail out early. It is important to get the proper diagnosis for hair loss since it could indicate a more serious medical problem.

Rapid weight loss, stress, chemotherapy, and tight-fitting hats can cause hair loss that may not become obvious until several months later. This kind of hair loss is a temporary condition and usually doesn't need to be treated. Your hair will eventually grow back.

Hair loss can also be caused by drugs such as blood thinners and thyroid medications as well as large doses of vitamin A. It can also indicate other medical problems such as infections, anemia, or exposure to pesticides or toxins. A hair sample or scalp biopsy may help reveal the cause.

Unfortunately, baldness due to aging is inevitable. Most men are partially or completely bald by the age of 60. Fortunately, there are many clever ways to combat hair loss.

Trying to pick through the slew of products claiming to restore hair is enough to make you pull your hair out. Your options range from natural to surgical and permanent to temporary. No one treatment is right for everyone. With millions of men looking for hair loss cures, there are bound to be people who want to take advantage of you. To protect your health, wallet, and self esteem, carefully check out the pros and cons and consult experts before you buy.

Although most oral and topical hair loss treatments have not proved effective, you may find an herbal mixture that works for you. Royal jelly, nettle, and jojoba oil all claim to stimulate hair growth. A mixture of lavender oil, calamus oil, gentian tincture, and rosemary spirit rubbed on your scalp is said to put hair on your head.

Topical minoxidil is a popular prescription for baldness but has not received rave reviews. Only a third of the men who have tried the ointment had any regrowth. This ointment is expensive, and little is known about its long-term effects.

A permanent solution is hair transplants. Patches of skin with your own hair are transferred to thinning or bald areas. This can be a good option for men who don't want a daily treatment routine. But, as with any surgery, make sure the person who performs the transplant is well-qualified. Hair transplantation is not well policed, and unqualified practitioners abound. Reported problems of infection, scarring, and the need for a second transplant have increased dramatically.

Of course, there are always hairpieces and creative hair styling. Although temporary solutions, these have no side effects and are relatively inexpensive.

If you are dreading the thought of losing your hair, remember that beauty is in the eye of the beholder. Many men have embraced the inevitable and proclaim the beauty of baldness. They have started clubs and organized special events promoting the shiny look. And if you prefer the look of a thick mane on top, you have many choices. Baldness can be bad or beautiful. It's really how you look at it.

*Sources –*
*American Family Physician* (51,6:1513)
*Health News* (12,6:4)
*Herbal Medicine*, Beaconsfield Publishers, Beaconsfield, England, 1988
*The Columbia University College of Physicians and Surgeons Home Medical Guide*, Second Edition, Crown Publishers, 1989
*The Honest Herbal*, The Haworth Press, Binghamton, N.Y., 1993
*The Journal of the American Medical Association* (273,11:897)

## Scratch out jock itch

You don't have to be a football or baseball star to suffer from jock itch. This irritating fungal infection got its name from its association with jock straps. And even though a jock strap can contribute to jock itch, you don't have to wear one to get it.

Fungi, like the kind that causes jock itch, thrive in warm, moist environments. The groin area is particularly susceptible because the scrotum rubs against the thighs. Sweating during physical activity, especially in warm weather, can lead to a red, scaly, itchy area on your skin next to your scrotum. In severe cases, blisters appear, usually around the edges of the affected area. Fortunately, the infection rarely spreads to the penis or the scrotum itself.

Fungal creams and ointments can treat jock itch, but here's how you can avoid this annoying, painful, and embarrassing itch.

◆ Wear loose, absorbent clothing — preferably natural fabrics like cotton rather than synthetic fabrics.

◆ Bathe as soon as possible after any activity that causes you to sweat.

◆ Make sure you rinse soap completely from your groin area and dry thoroughly after bathing.

◆ Wet bathing suits can contribute to jock itch, so towel off well after swimming and change into dry clothes as soon as possible.

*Source:*
*The Physician and Sportsmedicine* (18,8:63)

## Get it off your chest

Are you afraid to take your shirt off at the beach because your breasts are so large they embarrass you? Enlarged male breasts may be a simple matter of too much fat. Occasionally, however, they may be a symptom of a greater problem.

*Gynecomastia* is the swelling of a man's breasts due to an imbalance of male hormones (androgens) and female hormones (estrogens). It can be a sign of testicular cancer, or even lung, liver, or kidney cancers. In rare cases, it can be a symptom of male breast cancer.

Gynecomastia often occurs as a side effect of drugs like antibiotics, ulcer medication, antidepressants, or hormone therapy. This can usually be corrected by changing your medication. Alcohol, steroids, and drugs like marijuana can sometimes cause gynecomastia.

Most men who have gynecomastia aren't aware they have it and probably think they have just put on a few pounds. If you have abnormal breast swelling, especially if it is tender to the touch, see your doctor. If it is an indication of a more serious problem, the sooner you find out, the better.

*Source:*
*Forbes* (155,10:172)

# Exclusively for Women

## Why women need chocolate

If you created an organization of "Chocoholics Anonymous," meetings would probably be filled with women only. Researchers recently discovered what women have known all along. Women need chocolate.

Certain foods affect chemical levels in our brains, which in turn can affect our moods. Sugar and starch, for example, increase the level of a brain chemical called *serotonin*. A high level of serotonin produces a feeling of calmness and contentment. Fats increase levels of *endorphins*, another brain chemical, which create feelings of energy and well-being.

Women crave sugar and fat because of the way estrogen affects brain chemicals and blood sugar levels. Food cravings usually occur whenever estrogen levels fluctuate, like in puberty, during pregnancy, and just before your menstrual period. Women experience many different types of food cravings, as any expectant father who's ever trudged out in the middle of the night for sardines and cheesecake can tell you. However, chocolate accounts for the most common and powerful food craving of all. Chocolate contains about half sugar and half fat, which makes it the perfect choice for quenching two of women's cravings at once.

In addition, a Polish researcher recently confirmed what men have probably known all along. Chocolate produces an aphrodisiac effect in women. Chocolate contains a substance which works on the brain's "mood center" to create a sensation similar to falling in love. This explains all those huge heart-shaped boxes of chocolates on Valentine's Day.

Do women now have a legitimate reason for eating tons of bon-bons and drinking gallons of hot chocolate with whipped cream? Sorry, but too much fat and sugar still causes too much fat on the body and too much stress on the heart. That little craving tells you that you need a little chocolate, but don't overdo it. If you eat a balanced diet, you can indulge your "chocolate tooth" in small amounts and feel no guilt. You really do need that chocolate bar.

*Sources:*
*The Journal of the American Medical Association* (275,6:491)
*Why Women Need Chocolate,* Hyperion, New York, 1995

## Self-defense against second leading cause of death

One out of nine women will battle breast cancer sometime during her life. Breast cancer is the second leading cause of cancer deaths among women. Though your family history plays a part in determining your risk of developing breast cancer, you are not completely helpless. There are things you can do to prevent this disease from adding you to the statistics.

**Perform monthly breast self-examinations.** If you discover breast cancer early, the five-year survival rate is about 85 to 90 percent. However, if the cancer has time to grow and spread, the survival rate drops sharply. Monthly self-examinations provide the best method of early detection.

**Have regular exams by your doctor.** Between the ages of 20 and 40, you should have a breast exam by your doctor every three years. After the age of 40, you should have your doctor examine your breasts every year.

**Get mammograms.** The American Cancer Society recommends that you have your first mammogram between the ages of 35 and 39. Between the ages of 40 and 49 have one every two to three years and have one every year after age 50.

**Exercise.** Regular, moderate physical activity may reduce your risk of breast cancer by 60 percent. On the other hand, excess weight raises your risk of breast cancer. This seems to be especially true if you gain weight steadily over several years. A 30-year-old woman who is 20 pounds overweight increases her breast cancer risk over 50 percent. Regular exercise helps control your weight and reduces breast cancer risk.

**Try olive oil instead of butter or margarine.** Greek women, who eat a lot of olive oil, have a much lower risk of breast cancer than other women. This led Harvard researchers to do a study which found that women who consume olive oil more than once a day lower their risk of breast cancer by one-fourth.

**Limit stress as much as possible.** One study found that women who had severe life stress were more than twice as likely to develop breast cancer. Those who dealt with stress they had no control over, such as a serious illness in the family or the death of a relative, by directly confronting it were more likely to develop breast cancer than those who didn't.

*Sources:*
British Medical Journal (311,7019:1527)
Medical Tribune for the Internist and Cardiologist (36,4:14 and 36,15:21)
Reducing Your Risk of Breast Cancer, American Institute for Cancer Research, Washington, D.C. 1993
The Saturday Evening Post (267,6:22)

# Lower cancer risk: learn to love your mirror

Women spend countless hours in front of a mirror, fixing their hair and make-up, but most won't spend a fraction of that time examining their breasts. No woman wants to face the chilling discovery of a potentially cancerous lump in her breast. Perhaps that's why very few women practice breast self-examination. By the year 2,000, if the current trend continues, breast cancer will account for over half a million deaths a year worldwide.

Early detection greatly increases your chance of surviving breast cancer, and over 90 percent of breast lumps are discovered through self-examination. So, what's your excuse for not examining your breasts once a month? Maybe you just don't know what to look for, or when you try to examine your breasts, they always feel lumpy. If you examine your breasts monthly, you'll know what they feel like normally. Here are some things to watch out for:

◆ New lumps
◆ Puckering or dimpling of the skin
◆ Thickening or hardening of the skin
◆ Bleeding or discharge from your nipple
◆ Retraction of the nipple

Okay, now you know what you're looking for, so get in front of the mirror and look. Raise your arms above your head and look again. Do you see any changes in size or shape since your last exam? Is there any puckering, dimpling, or changes in skin texture, such as scaliness? Squeeze your nipples gently and look for a discharge. Now you can lie down on the job. Place a folded towel under your left shoulder and your left hand under your head. Using your right hand, gently examine your left breast thoroughly, and then change sides and examine your right breast. Most women use a circular motion, gradually spiraling inward toward the nipple. However, straight lines or another method may work better for you. Just be sure to examine your entire breast, including the armpit area, which also contains breast tissue.

Before you turn on your curling iron or your makeup mirror, take the time to examine your breasts. The few minutes it takes could save your life.

*Sources:*
*The Lancet* (346,8979:883)
*Breast Cancer: Early Detection is a Woman's Best Protection,* National Breast Cancer Awareness Month, Zeneca HealthCare Foundation

## Everyday painkillers slash risk of breast cancer

Nonsteroidal anti-inflammatory drugs (NSAIDS), like aspirin and ibuprofen, can do more than ease your aching muscles or relieve that pounding headache New research shows that NSAIDs can slash your risk of breast cancer. Researchers at Ohio State University found that women who took aspirin or ibuprofen at least three times a week for five years reduced their risk of breast cancer by one-third. More research needs to be done to confirm these findings. However, the chance that an inexpensive tablet could help prevent a disease that kills thousands of women each year is exciting news

*Source:*
*Science News* (149,8:116)

## Less is more when it comes to this surgery

Finding a lump in your breast can quickly bring a lump to your throat. If you were smart enough to catch it early, your chances of survival are good· However, the prospect of losing your breast to a mastectomy may still terrify you. New research shows that a lumpectomy (removing only the lump, rather than the whole breast) is as effective as a mastectomy in treating breast cancer. The study, which followed over 2,000 women for 12 years after their breast cancer treatments, found that the survival rate was the same for women who had lumpectomies (with or without radiation treatments) as for the women who had total mastectomies.

*Source:*
*Medical Tribune for the Internist and Cardiologist* (36,24:15)

## Bone up on osteoporosis protection

When you were a kid, did your mother make you drain every drop of milk from your glass before you left the dinner table? If so, she did you a big favor. Getting enough calcium helps prevent osteoporosis, a bone loss disease that affects more than 20 million people over age 45.

Women, especially, need lots of calcium because they are much more likely than men to suffer from osteoporosis. However, a recent study found that about one-third of the women surveyed thought that they were getting enough calcium when they were actually getting less than 60 percent of the amount they needed. The recommended daily allowance for calcium is 800 mg, but many experts suggest that you get as much as 1,000 mg. Your body absorbs calcium from food better than from supplements, so try to get your calcium from your diet. Choose foods from the following list to boost your daily calcium intake.

| SOURCE | QUANTITY | CALCIUM (MG) | CALORIES |
|--------|----------|--------------|----------|
| Whole milk | 1 cup | 291 | 150 |
| Skim milk | 1 cup | 302 | 85 |
| Cheddar cheese | 1 oz. | 204 | 115 |
| Cottage cheese | 1 cup | 155 | 200 |
| Yogurt | 1 cup | 350-400 | 140-230 |
| Salmon | 3 oz. | 167 | 120 |
| Broccoli | 1 cup (cooked) | 354 | 45 |

*Sources:*
*Journal of the American College of Nutrition* (14,4:336)
*Medical Tribune for the Internist and Cardiologist* (36,18:8)

## Calcium robber

You eat lots of calcium-rich foods to protect your bones. However, if you're also eating foods high in sodium, all that calcium may be going down the drain. Research shows that sodium levels over 2,600 mg a day can steal as much as 891 mg of calcium from your body. Considering most experts recommend 1,000 mg of calcium a day, that's almost a whole day's worth of calcium.

Salt and calcium compete for absorption into your body. If you take in too much salt, you stack the odds against calcium. If you want a sturdy skeleton, you should skip the salt or beef up the calcium. Better yet, do both ... for your bones' sake.

*Source:*
*The American Journal of Clinical Nutrition* (62,4:740)

## Quick and painless osteoporosis tests

The National Osteoporosis Foundation telephone hotline at 1-800-464-6700 can help you find the nearest place to get bone mass tests that are accurate at any age.

◆ **DEXA** – Dual Energy X-ray Absorptiometry. This is a very accurate and advanced test that delivers only a small radiation dose. It checks specific sites like the hip or spine and takes 5 to 15 minutes.

◆ **DPA** – Dual Photon Absorptiometry. This is the earlier generation of DEXA and is now in limited use.

◆ **SXA** – Single-Energy X-ray Absorptiometry. This is a low-dose X-ray that measures wrist or heel bone density.

◆ **QCT** – Quantitative Computer Tomography. This is a type of CT (CAT) scanner with special computer software. It measures spine bone density. It delivers a higher radiation dose than DEXA, and it is usually more expensive.

◆ **RA** – Radiographic Absorptiometry. This is a specialized X-ray of the hand.

*Source:*
*Act Against Osteoporosis,* National Osteoporosis Foundation, P.O. Box 96616, Washington, D.C., 20077

## Northerners need more of this essential vitamin

Living in the North may mean you should consider taking extra vitamin D in the winter and spring when you get less sunlight. The RDA of vitamin D, 200 IU (international units), wasn't enough to cut hip bone loss in a study of 247 older women in Boston, even though they took 500 mg of calcium each day. Those taking more vitamin D lost less hip bone. Researchers recommend 800 IU of vitamin D a day to minimize bone loss.

*Source:*
*The American Journal of Clinical Nutrition* (61,5:1140)

## Exercise puts the brakes on fractures

Bodybuilders lift weights to bulk up, but exercise bulks up more than just strong muscles. Exercise also helps build strong bones. That's good news for women who must try to hold off the effects of bone loss as they age. Women begin losing about 1 percent of their bone mass per year after age 35, and two to four times that amount after menopause.

Osteoporosis accounts for one and a half million fractures a year, mostly in elderly women. Besides the financial cost, these fractures carry serious consequences. Hip fractures, for example, not only cause great pain, but they increase your risk of dying within a year after the fracture.

Low muscle mass, low muscle strength, and poor balance all increase the risk of bone-breaking falls in the elderly. An exercise program that includes strength training, like weight-lifting, not only helps build strong bones but also increases your balance and coordination. One study of postmenopausal women in Boston found that after a year of exercising at least twice a week, the women had 35 to 70 percent stronger muscles, gained bone density in the neck and spine, and improved their balance. Though other treatments for osteoporosis may increase bone density, they do nothing to counteract the other risk factors for fractures from falls.

If you already have osteoporosis, talk to your doctor before beginning an exercise program. Start slowly, and remember, it's never too late. One study found that even people in their 80s and 90s increased bone mass by marching in place while holding onto a support. Just move it, lift it, or stretch it, and stop fractures from breaking into your life.

*Sources:*
*Medical Tribune for the Internist and Cardiologist* (36,2:17)
*Public Citizen's Health Research Group Health Letter* (11,4:9)
*The Atlanta Journal/Constitution* (July 15, 1993, G4)

# New bone-building treatments

The brittle bones of a person with osteoporosis may become so thin that they snap at any sign of stress. The simple act of standing up can result in a broken bone. Preventing this bone loss from ever happening is your best option. However, for those who already suffer from osteoporosis, new treatments provide bone-building power for those fragile bones.

A three-year study of a new drug, alendronate, found that it increased bone density and cut fracture rates almost in half. Alendronate, sold under the name Fosamax, prevents bones from breaking down while depositing calcium at the same time.

Another treatment for osteoporosis, calcitonin, recently became available in a nasal spray. It previously had to be injected. The commercial name of this spray is Miacalcin. It also increases bone density, and helps ease the pain of fractures. Some people experience nasal irritation or other side effects of the nasal spray, but it is safe for most people.

Many doctors still prefer estrogen replacement therapy instead of the new treatments for osteoporosis because it also helps prevent heart disease and

stroke. However, for women who cannot take estrogen, the new treatments pro-
'ide promising alternatives.

**Source:**
*The Atlanta Journal/Constitution* (Feb. 28, 1996, E3)

# Faster, easier fracture fix

If you or someone you know is fighting the battle of osteoporosis, you know
how you dread falls and accidents that can result in broken bones. As you age,
the healing process gets slower and recovery takes a heavy toll on your body.
But there's great news from the research labs — a new treatment may soon take
away your worries about recovering from broken bones.

Doctors have begun testing a sticky paste that hardens in minutes to form a
natural, bone-like material that quickly heals broken bones. This breakthrough
material may soon replace the painful and expensive pins and screws that are
normally used to help set broken bones. And while it may sound bizarre, it actually works just like your body's bone repair system.

Far from being just a support, such as the wooden beams in a house, normal
bones are alive, very active, and constantly changing. The phrase "dry as a bone"
couldn't be further from the truth. Living bone isn't dry at all but is richly sup-
plied with blood vessels and nerve endings. Not only do bones support our
weight and provide attachment sites for muscles to push and pull against, they
are the primary sites for the production of new blood cells. The inner portion of
bone that manufactures new blood cells is called marrow, while the outer white
portion plays the major role in supporting body weight.

Inside the bone, cells known as *osteoclasts* and *osteoblasts* never rest in their
mission to shape and reshape your bones throughout life. The process is called
'remodeling." The osteoclasts burrow through old, existing areas of bone and
break it down. They are followed soon afterwards by the osteoblasts which lay
down new bone. These remodeling cells are also called into action when you
break a bone, whether from a skiing accident or osteoporosis.

The new bone paste doctors are experimenting with is a mixture of calcium
phosphate and sodium phosphate, both components of natural bone. In the operating room, the paste is mixed and then injected into the fracture site. It hardens
within 10 minutes and actually becomes stronger than natural bone within 12
hours.

Once the paste hardens, the osteoclasts and osteoblasts gradually replace the
material with living bone over the next several months. The bone paste is able
to hold the broken bones together and provide the necessary support to speed up
the healing process.

Be looking for the new bone paste to move out of the research labs and into your doctor's office in the near future.

*Sources:*
*Journal of the American Dietetic Association* (93,9:1000)
*Medical Tribune for the Family Physician* (36,8:14)
*Science* (1995,267:1796)
*The American Medical Association Encyclopedia of Medicine,* Random House, New York, 1989

# Hormone replacement therapy: weighing the risks

When a man has a midlife crisis, he might buy a flashy, hot, new sports car. When a woman hits midlife, she usually just has hot flashes. Doctors often treat the side effects of menopause with hormone replacement therapy (HRT). Should all women automatically take HRT when they reach that "certain age"? Exactly what are the benefits and drawbacks to taking hormones in midlife?

During menopause, which occurs around age 50 for most women, levels of the female hormones estrogen and progesterone gradually decrease. You stop ovulating, and your menstrual period ends. The decline in estrogen causes the unpleasant side effects of menopause such as hot flashes, sleep problems, and vaginal dryness. Estrogen and progesterone also play a part in other aspects of a woman's health, like blood cholesterol levels, building bones, and the condition of your skin and hair.

HRT helps prevent symptoms of menopause like hot flashes and vaginal dryness which can make sexual intercourse painful. It also provides other benefits as well as some drawbacks. You have to weigh the pros and cons and talk to your doctor to decide if hormone replacement therapy can help you.

**Heart protection.** Because HRT reduces the level of LDL ("bad") cholesterol in your blood, which tends to rise sharply after menopause, it provides protection against heart disease. It also reduces the level of fibrinogen, a blood-clotting compound in your blood. This could help prevent blood clots that may cause a heart attack or stroke.

**Building bones.** After menopause, your bones become less dense, making fractures more likely. HRT can help you maintain strong bones, but you also need to exercise, eat right, and make sure you get enough calcium and vitamin D.

**Breast cancer.** Long-term (over five years) HRT use increases your risk of breast cancer. Most doctors believe that women should take HRT because the protection it provides against heart disease outweighs the danger of breast cancer. However, if you are already at risk for breast cancer, HRT may not be for you.

**Asthma.** Research indicates that taking HRT may increase your risk of developing asthma by almost 50 percent.

**Side effects.** Some women experience side effects from HRT. These include breast soreness, bloating, fatigue, and depression. Sometimes these symptoms are only temporary, or they can be relieved by changes in dosage or type of therapy.

Though there are drawbacks to using HRT, doctors continue to recommend it, mostly because of its protective qualities for your heart and bones. Work with your doctor to determine whether HRT provides the best help for your midlife crisis.

*Sources:*
*The Atlanta Journal/Constitution (Nov. 6, 1995, C8)*
*The Journal of the American Medical Association (273,3:240)*
*University of California at Berkeley Wellness Letter (12,1:4)*

# Memory help from hormones

If you've ever spent 20 minutes looking for a pair of glasses that were perched on top of your head the entire time, you might be concerned about your memory. This type of forgetfulness affects most of us from time to time. However, you may be happy to know that a study from Stanford University found that postmenopausal women who took estrogen had better memories than those who did not. The ability to recall names was over one-third better in women who were taking estrogen. So, if you are on estrogen therapy, you may be able to remember the name of your eighth-grade science teacher ... if you remember to take your medicine.

*Source:*
*Geriatrics (50,2:59)*

# Hormones give women another reason to smile

You dazzle people with your beautiful smile, and you'd like to keep it that way. Hormone replacement therapy may help. A recent study found that women on HRT were 19 percent less likely to wear dentures, and over a third less likely to have no teeth, than women who had never taken hormones. Hormone therapy helps prevent osteoporosis, which makes women three times more likely to lose their teeth. Though more research needs to be done on the effects of HRT on tooth loss, if you're already taking hormones for your menopause symptoms, you have even more reason to smile.

*Source:*
*Medical Tribune for the Internist and Cardiologist (37,2:17)*

# Medicine-free menopause

You may be able to put your hot flashes on ice with a little soy. Estrogen replacement therapy may soon be replaced by *phytoestrogens*.

Phytoestrogens are plant hormones similar to human estrogen. These natural compounds may provide relief from menopause symptoms like hot flashes, night sweats, and vaginal thinning, without the increased risk of breast cancer that estrogen replacement therapy (ERT) can cause. Phytoestrogens can be found in about 300 different kinds of plants, including carrots, corn, apples, and barley. Soybean products, however, provide the most phytoestrogen power. In Asian countries, where people eat a lot of soy, the incidence of breast cancer is much lower, and women rarely suffer from menopause symptoms like hot flashes.

Phytoestrogens may provide an alternative for women who want relief from the symptoms of menopause, but don't want to take estrogen. They may also be found to offer protection from heart disease and osteoporosis. Researchers are continuing to study these dietary estrogens.

*Source:*
*Tufts University Diet and Nutrition Newsletter* (12,12:3)

# Heart-smart advice

Even though women tend to develop heart disease at a later age than men, women are just as likely as men to suffer a fatal heart attack, and they are more likely than men to die within a year of having a heart attack.

With your life on the line, learn what you can do to prevent heart disease. Most of the preventative measures recommended for men work well for women, too.

◆ Kick the cigarette habit.
◆ Control your cholesterol.
◆ Keep your blood pressure under control.
◆ Watch your weight.
◆ Exercise regularly.
◆ Eat a low-fat diet.

*Sources:*
*Hope Healthletter* (XVI,2:3)
*The New England Journal of Medicine* (332,26:1758)

# Heart health: Sex makes a difference

Most tactics for combating heart disease benefit both men and women. However, women encounter some factors that men do not. For example:

**Menopause.** Your risk of heart disease increases greatly after menopause. Women who experience a sudden menopause caused by removal of the uterus and ovaries (complete hysterectomy) also experience a sudden, dramatic rise in their risks of heart disease. Women who go through menopause naturally experience a more gradual increase in their risks of heart disease.

**Oral contraceptives.** The older, high-dose oral contraceptives increased the risk of heart disease by raising LDL ("bad") cholesterol levels, reducing HDL ("good") cholesterol levels, raising blood pressure, and increasing the risk of blood clots. This risk increased greatly when combined with cigarette smoking. Whether the new low-dose oral contraceptives carry the same risk remains to be seen.

**Hormone-replacement therapy.** Debate continues over the effect of post-menopausal hormone treatment on women's overall health, but it provides definite benefits in preventing heart disease. Studies show that postmenopausal women taking estrogen reduce their risk of heart disease by almost half.

**Diabetes.** Though men also suffer from diabetes, women with diabetes increase their risk of heart disease even more than men. Women with diabetes are three to seven times more likely to die from heart disease than women without diabetes. Diabetic men are only two to four times more likely to die from heart disease than nondiabetic men.

Heart disease is not a disease for men only. Women should protect their hearts every bit as vigorously as men for a long, healthy life.

*Sources:*
*Hope Healthletter* (XVI,2:3)
*The New England Journal of Medicine* (332,26:1758)

# Vanquish vaginal itch

Have you ever had that embarrassing itch you just can't scratch in public? You will probably experience at least one vaginal yeast infection sometime during your life. These common infections cause itching or burning in the genital area, as well as a discharge with an unusual color, odor, or consistency.

Yeast thrive in a warm, moist environment that is high in glucose. Women with diabetes have yeast infections frequently because of the high level of sugar in their bodies. Yeast infections often develop following antibiotic treatment. Antibiotics kill some of the bacteria which normally live in the vagina, allowing yeast to grow rapidly. Here are some tips for avoiding irritating yeast infections:

- ◆ Don't douche. Douching is not needed for good hygiene, but if you think you must douche, do it only occasionally and use a vinegar and water solution.
- ◆ Wear cotton panties. Underwear and pantyhose made from synthetic fabrics like nylon trap heat and moisture, increasing your risk of developing an infection.
- ◆ Use sanitary pads instead of tampons.
- ◆ Go easy on the sugar. A diet high in simple carbohydrates like sugar, syrup, honey, and molasses provides yeast with lots of glucose to grow on.
- ◆ Don't use vaginal deodorants, powders, or perfumed soaps.
- ◆ Take showers instead of baths. If you do take baths, don't use bubble bath.
- ◆ Avoid tight clothing.
- ◆ Clean spermicide applicators and diaphragms thoroughly.

*Sources:*
*Pharmacy Times* (61,9:20)
*Postgraduate Medicine* (98,4:238)

## An embarrassing female problem few women talk about

If you're embarrassed to say that you suffer from *vaginal prolapse*, you're not alone. As many as one in five postmenopausal women suffer from vaginal prolapse, but rarely do they report it to their doctors. Ignoring the problem may make your condition worsen until it becomes much harder to treat, sometimes even requiring surgery.

A prolapse occurs when pelvic organs, such as the bladder and uterus, move downward, sometimes protruding out of the vagina. This can cause vaginal irritation or bleeding, low back pain, and difficulty urinating or defecating.

Early vaginal prolapse may be treated with Kegel exercises, which involve tightening and releasing the muscles that control urination. Kegel exercises may also help relieve the lower back discomfort which often accompanies vaginal prolapse. However, if the prolapse has extended beyond the mouth of the vagina, Kegel exercises can no longer help.

An ancient treatment which has come back into use is the vaginal pessary. Pessaries are devices which you insert into the vagina to hold the organs in place. Early Greeks and Romans used natural objects like pomegranates as pessaries. Today, many types of pessaries perform different functions. Your doctor can recommend the best type for you, but the daily care of your pessary falls on your shoulders. Many women discontinue using their pessaries because it is too much trouble to clean and care for them. However, considering the options, a little effort now may prevent a lot of pain later on.

If you suspect you suffer from vaginal prolapse, be sure to talk to your doctor. More options than ever are available to help you handle this common problem.

**Source:**
*Postgraduate Medicine* (99,4:171)

## High cholesterol raises risk of this deadly cancer

Women with high cholesterol levels may be hurting more than their hearts. A recent study indicated a link between high levels of cholesterol and ovarian cancer. In this study, the women with the highest levels of cholesterol were three times as likely to develop ovarian cancer as those with the lowest cholesterol levels.

The antioxidant *selenium* (but no other antioxidant) was found to have a protective effect against ovarian cancer. Selenium may be found in small amounts in seafood, grains, muscle meats, garlic, and Brazil nuts.

Cutting the fat also helps ward off ovarian cancer. Eating a low-fat diet that is high in fiber and vegetables provides lots of other health benefits besides.

**Source:**
*Medical Tribune for the Internist and Cardiologist* (37,2:17)

## Caffeine hinders conception

Cut the coffee consumption and increase your chance of getting pregnant. A study of 2,500 pregnancies found that nonsmoking women who drank more than three cups of coffee a day (300 mg of caffeine) usually needed more than a year to become pregnant. Women who consumed less caffeine were more likely to get pregnant within a year. Smoking also decreases your chance of getting pregnant. So, if you cut down on the coffee and stop smoking, you may soon be dealing with bottles and diapers instead.

*Source:*
*Medical Abstracts Newsletter* (16,2:6)

## Infertility breakthrough

When the first "test tube baby" was born, thanks to in vitro fertilization (IVF), thousands of childless couples rejoiced in new hope for the future. However, for many, this was only a dream. Though IVF has helped bring many children into the world, it is an expensive process with a low success rate. Medical bills for IVF run about $9,000 per attempt, and the success rate is only about 18 percent. Nevertheless, many couples continue to attempt IVF.

A new technique may make IVF easier and more affordable. IVF now involves giving women daily hormone injections for a month or more. The hormones cause the women to produce as many as two dozen mature eggs, rather than the one egg she would normally produce. The eggs are then extracted, fertilized in a dish with her husband's sperm, and then implanted in the woman's womb to grow.

The new procedure removes immature eggs from the mother and then bathes them with hormones in a dish, causing them to mature. This would eliminate the need for expensive ($3,000) hormone shots that can cause severe PMS-type symptoms like mood swings, nausea, headaches, and bloating. These hormone shots also raise the risk of ovarian cancer slightly.

Though this technique is still in the preliminary stages, it opens up the possibility of IVF to more couples by making it less expensive and painful. Soon, there may be more bundles of joy to fill the arms of currently childless couples.

*Source:*
*Science News* (149,19:295)

## Pregnant women need 'moo juice'

You're drinking for two, so get as much milk as you can. Calcium, particularly calcium obtained from drinking milk, has been shown to reduce the high blood pressure that sometimes occurs during pregnancy.

High blood pressure during pregnancy may be an indication of *preeclampsia*, which, if untreated, could develop into *eclampsia*. Eclampsia causes seizures and coma and usually results in death. Preventing this from happening to you may be as simple as pouring low-fat milk into a glass and drinking it several times a day.

In a study on the effects of drinking milk on preeclampsia, women who drank less than one glass of milk a day had over a 50 percent greater chance of developing preeclampsia than women who drank two glasses a day. Risk decreased by almost 75 percent in women who drank three glasses of milk a day, but risk more than doubled in women who drank four or more glasses a day. Researchers speculated that this increased risk may be because the women drank mostly whole milk, which is high in fat. The protective benefits of the calcium from milk might be overshadowed by the high fat at higher levels of intake. The best strategy for pregnant women may be to drink skim milk, or keep your milk intake at a moderate level.

***Sources:***
*Medical Tribune for the Internist and Cardiologist* (36,9:10)
*The Journal of the American Medical Association* (275,14:1113)

# Index